Diagnosis of Cutaneous Lymphoid Infiltrates

Antonio Subtil

Diagnosis of Cutaneous Lymphoid Infiltrates

A Visual Approach to Differential Diagnosis and Knowledge Gaps

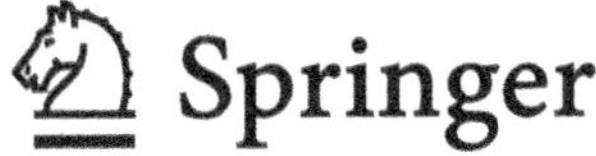

Antonio Subtil
Dermatology and Pathology
Yale University
New Haven, CT
USA

ISBN 978-3-030-11652-1   ISBN 978-3-030-11654-5   (eBook)
https://doi.org/10.1007/978-3-030-11654-5

This Springer imprint is published by the registered company Springer Nature Switzerland AG
The registered company address is: Gewerbestrasse 11, 6330 Cham, Switzerland

Preface

The diagnosis of cutaneous lymphoid infiltrates is one of the most challenging topics of pathology, in part because this area is at the interface of several medical disciplines (dermatopathology, hematopathology, dermatology, and hematology/oncology). As a pathologist trained in both dermatopathology and hematopathology, I have noticed several knowledge gaps by dermatopathologists as well as hematopathologists. In addition, after more than a decade practicing in a referral center for skin lymphomas and participating in a busy consult service, I have witnessed recurring mistakes in the classification of cutaneous lymphoproliferative disorders and pseudolymphomas, some of which with significant clinical impact.

Both dermatology and pathology rely heavily on a visual approach to learning, developing differential diagnoses, and making final diagnoses. Pattern recognition and image decoding skills are essential elements in this process. However, most textbooks do not emphasize images nor adequately use illustrations to demystify important concepts. This disconnect is particularly critical in complicated topics, such as the correct classification of cutaneous lymphomas and pseudolymphomas. The goal of this book is to fill in important knowledge gaps utilizing a visual approach to learning. Both common and rare lymphomas are reviewed. Diagnostic pearls and pitfalls as well as differential diagnoses are covered in detail. In addition to multiple images, several tables, illustrations, and visual clues to the diagnosis are included. In order to highlight what is actually useful to make a diagnosis in real practice, genetic data that is currently only relevant at a research level is included separately in an appendix.

Beyond its usefulness to general pathologists, dermatopathologists, and hematopathologists, this book is also intended to be helpful for dermatologists, hematologists/oncologists, dermatopathology fellows, hematopathology fellows, pathology residents, and dermatology residents.

I would like to acknowledge and thank my mother, Cezina; my late father, Antonio; and my sisters, Adriane and Cristiane, for their lifelong support. Thank you to Larry Gibson, Ifty Ahmed, Jeannine Holden, Peter Heald, Jennifer McNiff, Rick Edelson, Mark Pittelkow, Jean Bolognia, Earl Glusac, Christine Ko, Anjela Galan, Francine Foss, Mike Girardi, Peggy Myung, Shawn Cowper, Irwin Braverman, Kal Watsky, Alistair Robson, Joan Guitart, Christiane Querfeld, Jaqueline Junkins-Hopkins, Catherine Stefanato, Russell Fiorella, Kamani Lankachandra, Edward Gutmann, Carole McArthur, Roberto Miranda, Jamie Skrade, Peter Kragel, Karen Mann, David Jaye,

Shiyong Li, Rich Antaya, Jae Choi, Jennifer Choi, Bob Tigelaar, Mary Tomayko, Kacie Carlson, Ann Putio, Jean Saley, Sasha Finn, Carey Storan, Sikina Rossi, Jinah Kim, Uma Sundram, Youn Kim, Eleanor Knopp, Phil Shapiro, Rossitza Lazova, Steven Billings, Alina Bridges, Margot Peters, Diane Pierson, Adriane Brito, Lola Pettinicchio, Ricardo Macarenco, Jane Grant-Kels, Sharon Weiss, Tony Neto, Stephen Joyner, John Napoli, Gauri Panse, Brian Poligone, Phil LeBoit, Marcus Bosenberg, MaryAnn Ackerman, Debbie Williams, Terri Borrowman, Andrea Harris, Cristina Ishihama, Anini Group (Kelia, Adriane, Thays, Ricardo, Claudiney, Lusmaia, Greice, Maria Cristina, Patrycia, Claudio, Renato), Thanila Macedo, Marilia Ribeiro, Lara Quirino, Lucelia Badan, Celia Revilandia, Scott Freese, Jon Talbert, Marie Valdez, Nancy Talbert, Jack Gryder, Alice Gryder, Leigh Ann Homb, and Norman Homb. Thank you also to Lorraine Coffey, Rebekah Amos, and Samantha Lonuzzi at Springer for their support and outstanding skills. Lastly, thank you to my husband, Nathan, for turning the television volume down so I could write.

New Haven, CT, USA   Antonio Subtil, MD, MBA

Contents

Part I

The Basics

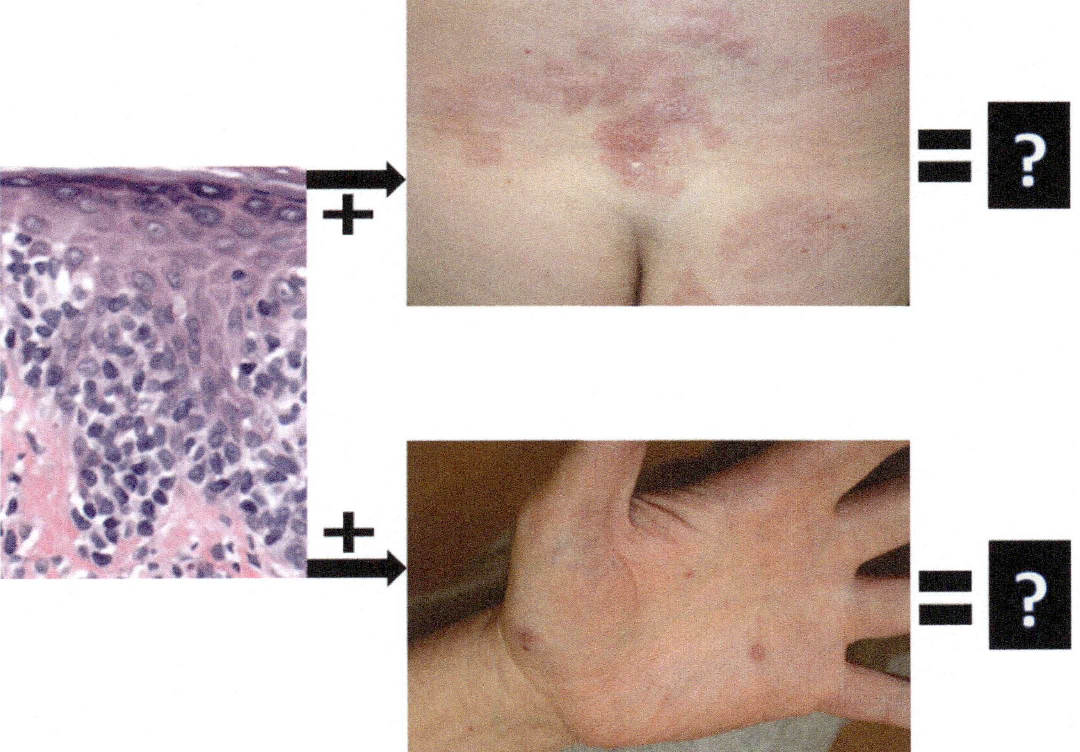

Fig. 1.1 What is the best diagnosis for each clinicopathologic combination?

© Springer Nature Switzerland AG 2019
A. Subtil, *Diagnosis of Cutaneous Lymphoid Infiltrates*,
https://doi.org/10.1007/978-3-030-11654-5_1

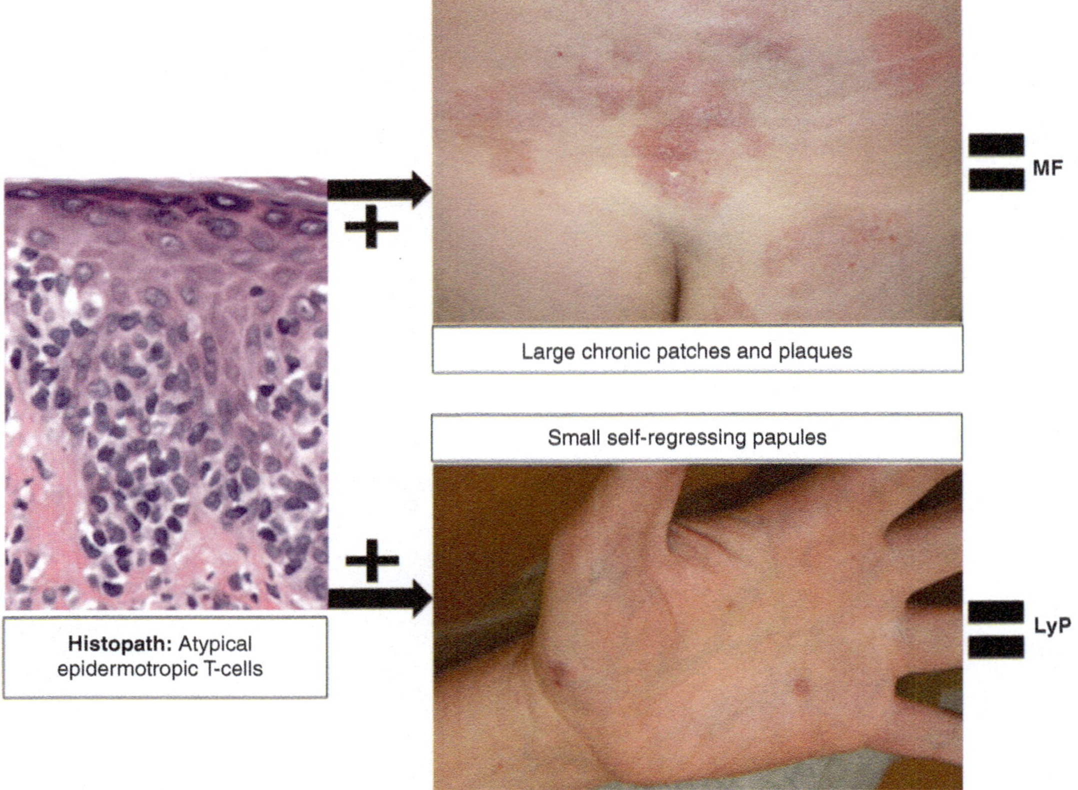

Fig. 1.2 Clinical pathologic correlation is essential to correctly classify cutaneous lymphoid infiltrates. The same histopathologic pattern of epidermotropism would result in different diagnoses depending on the clinical picture: classic mycosis fungoides (large, chronic patches and/or plaques on sun-protected skin) vs. lymphomatoid papulosis (small, self-regressing papules)

Careful correlation of clinical and histopathologic findings is essential to correctly classify cutaneous lymphoid infiltrates. Skin lymphomas would be more appropriately viewed as syndromes, in which a constellation of clinical as well as pathologic changes is needed for each diagnosis. Any given finding cannot be used in a vacuum to make a diagnosis. Ignoring either side of this clinicopathologic equation will often result in misclassification.

A similar histomorphologic pattern is often seen in different cutaneous lymphomas, often with markedly different clinical behaviors. Therefore, depending on the clinical presentation, different diagnoses will be made for similar histopathologic findings (Fig. 1.1). For example, both classic mycosis fungoides (MF) and some variants of lymphomatoid papulosis (LyP) exhibit a histopathologic pattern of epidermotropic atypical T cells (Fig. 1.2). However, MF would present with large, chronic patches and/or plaques on sun-protected skin, while the clinical picture of LyP is of small, self-regressing papules. Epidermotropism may also be seen in aggressive cytotoxic lymphomas, such as primary cutaneous CD8+ aggressive epidermotropic cytotoxic T-cell lymphoma and cutaneous gamma-delta T-cell lymphoma.

Ideally, adequate clinical information should be available to the pathologist evaluating the skin biopsy. Depending on the provided clinical history, different differential diagnoses would be considered (Table 1.1). For example, grouped lesions on the scalp would be a classic presentation for primary cutaneous follicle center lymphoma. Similarly, other differential diagnoses may be discarded depending on the clinical picture. For example, in the absence of erythroderma, Sézary syndrome would not be a diagnostic consideration.

The presence or absence of ulceration can be an important diagnostic feature. Classic mycosis fungoides (the most common type of skin lymphoma) generally is not associated with ulceration, except for late-/tumor-stage disease. Consequently, the presence of ulcerated lesions at the onset would raise a different differential diagnosis. Many aggressive cytotoxic skin lymphomas present with ulcerated lesions in early disease. These include cutaneous gamma-delta T-cell lymphoma, primary cutaneous CD8+ aggressive epidermotropic cytotoxic T-cell lymphoma, and extranodal NK/T-cell lymphoma, nasal type. However, indolent processes such as lymphomatoid papulosis may also ulcerate. It is critical to consider the overall clinical behavior (indolent/self-regressing vs. aggressive/progressive) when evaluating skin biopsies with atypical lymphoid infiltrates (Table 1.1).

In addition, different skin lymphomas tend to preferentially involve certain body regions, and the site of the biopsy can provide important diagnostic clues in the absence of comprehensive clinical information. Table 1.2 lists the classic differential diagnoses for each body site. However, it is important to be aware that exceptions may occur.

Table 1.1 Basic clinical differential diagnoses for atypical cutaneous lymphoid infiltrates

Clinical behavior	Clinical pattern	Main differential diagnosis to consider
Indolent	Chronic large patches and/or plaques on sun-protected skin (back, buttocks, breasts)	Classic mycosis fungoides (MF)
	Small (<2 cm) papular lesions +/− ulceration, self-regressing within 12 weeks	Lymphomatoid papulosis (LyP)
	Solitary or grouped papulonodules, plaques, and/or tumors on scalp or upper/mid back	Primary cutaneous follicle center lymphoma
	Solitary or multifocal papules, plaques, or nodules on trunk and/or arms	Primary cutaneous marginal zone lymphoma
Progressive, intermediate, and aggressive	Alopecia and other follicular-based lesions (comedones, cysts)	Folliculotropic mycosis fungoides (FMF)
	Rapid onset and fast progression of tumors on one or both legs of elderly patients	Primary cutaneous diffuse large B-cell lymphoma
	Erythroderma (>80% of total body surface erythema)	Sézary syndrome (SS)
	Rapid onset and fast progression of multiple, non-regressing skin lesions with frequent ulceration	Aggressive cytotoxic lymphomas (cutaneous gamma-delta T-cell lymphoma, primary cutaneous CD8+ aggressive epidermotropic cytotoxic T-cell lymphoma, extranodal NK/T-cell lymphoma, nasal type)

Table 1.2 Differential diagnosis based on body region

Body region	Differential diagnoses
Face and/or scalp	Folliculotropic mycosis fungoides (FMF)
	Primary cutaneous follicle center lymphoma
	CD4+ small-/medium-sized pleomorphic T-cell lymphoproliferative disorder
Trunk and/or proximal extremities	Classic mycosis fungoides (MF)
	Primary cutaneous follicle center lymphoma
	Primary cutaneous marginal zone lymphoma
Lower extremities	Primary cutaneous diffuse large B-cell lymphoma
	Subcutaneous panniculitis-like T-cell lymphoma (SPTCL)
Acral	Pagetoid reticulosis (Woringer-Kolopp)
>80% body surface erythroderma	Sézary syndrome

Suggested Reading

Subtil A. A general approach to the diagnosis of cutaneous lymphomas and pseudolymphomas. Cutaneous lymphomas (Subtil, ed.). Surg Pathol Clin. 2014;7(2):135–42. Elsevier: Philadelphia.

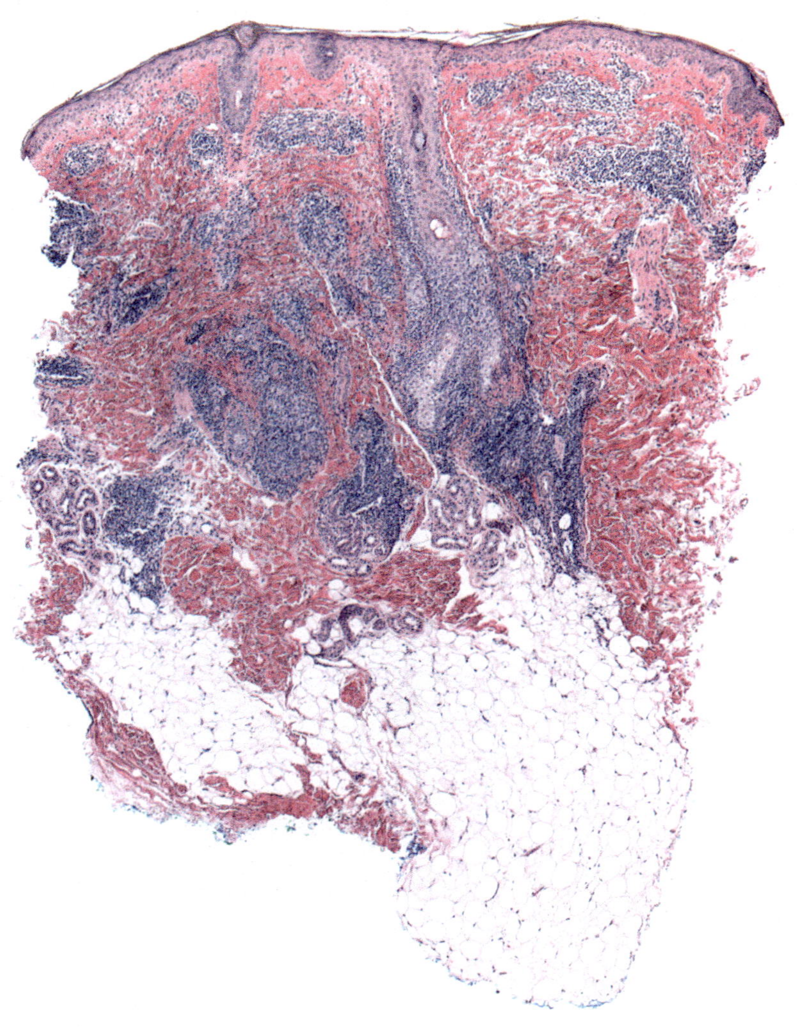

Fig. 2.1 Initial skin biopsy evaluation. How would you approach a skin biopsy with a lymphoid infiltrate? What are important positive and negative findings?

© Springer Nature Switzerland AG 2019
A. Subtil, *Diagnosis of Cutaneous Lymphoid Infiltrates*,
https://doi.org/10.1007/978-3-030-11654-5_2

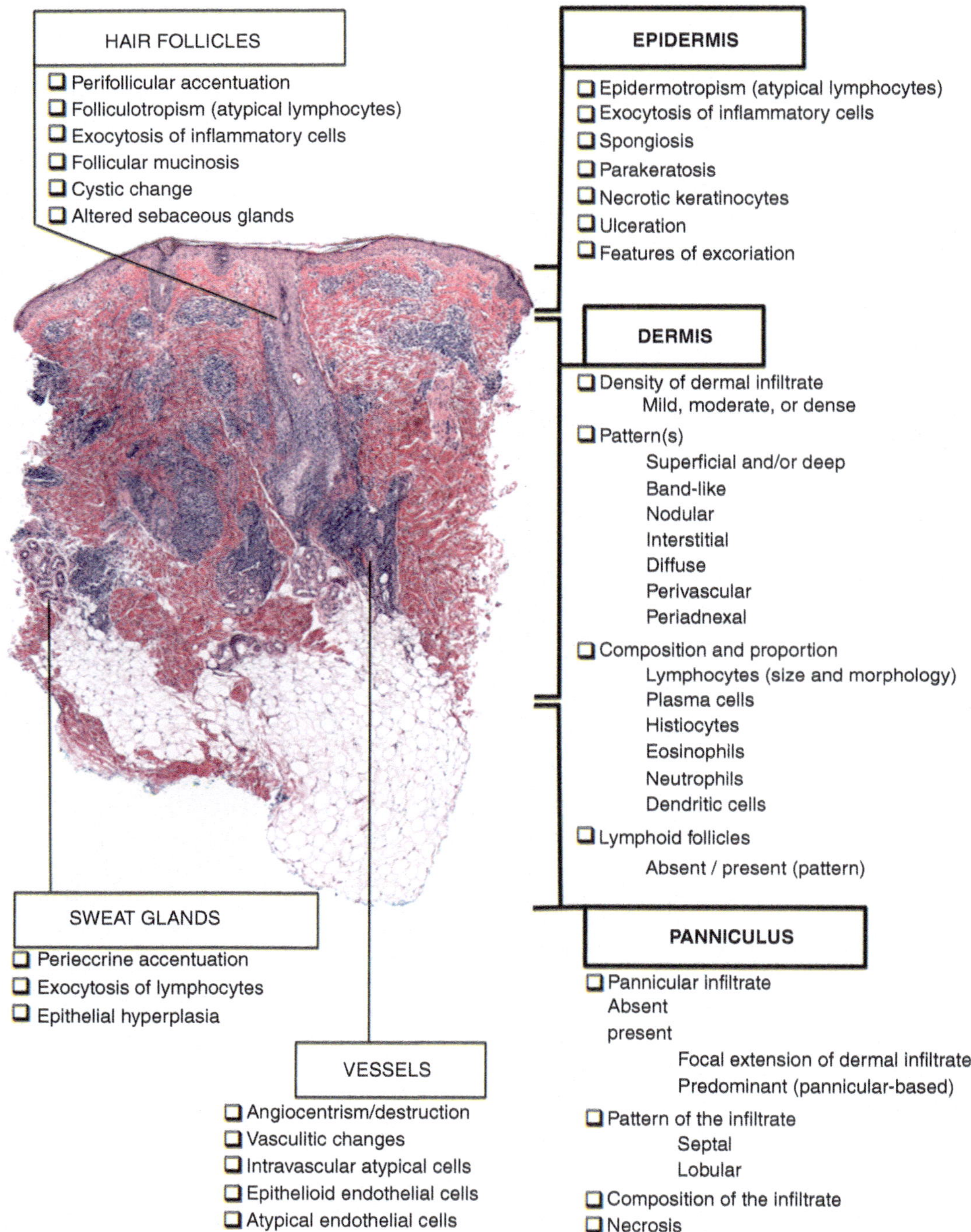

Fig. 2.2 Checklist of possible histomorphologic findings in the initial evaluation of cutaneous lymphoid infiltrates

A large variety of lymphomas and pseudolymphomas may occur in the skin and produce multiple histopathologic patterns. In order to adequately construe differential diagnoses and subsequently decide which immunohistochemical stains to order, it is important to develop a comprehensive approach to analyze positive and negative findings in a skin biopsy (see Fig. 2.1). Failure to identify certain histomorphologic clues may lead to misdiagnosing a cutaneous lymphoid infiltrate.

This introductory chapter provides a checklist of things to look for in a skin biopsy showing a lymphoid infiltrate (see Fig. 2.2 and Table 2.1). This initial approach will allow for accurate microscopic description and will provide the basis for additional workup. In subsequent chapters, the significance and differential diagnosis of key histomorphologic findings will be addressed in further detail.

At low-power magnification, the density of the lymphoid infiltrate can be ascertained (e.g., mild, moderate, or dense). It is important to determine which layer(s) of the skin are involved by the infiltrate: epidermis, dermis (superficial and/or deep), and/or panniculus. Within each of these layers, different features may or may not be present. For example, the epidermis may show exocytosis of lymphocytes or other cell types (eosinophils, neutrophils, etc.) with or without spongiosis, ulceration, and/or features suggestive of excoriation.

The infiltrate generally shows a predominant pattern (or a combination of patterns), such as band-like, nodular, interstitial, diffuse, perivascular, periadnexal (perifollicular and/or perieccrine), perineural, angiocentric, and/or intravascular. If present, lymphoid follicles should be evaluated regarding size and shape (variable vs. homogeneous), well-spaced vs. crowded distribution, presence of mantle zones, presence of tingible body macrophages, and mitotic activity in germinal centers. Additional information on lymphoid follicles can be found in Chaps. 4, 5, 6, 11, and 20.

At high-power magnification, the composition of the infiltrate can be evaluated. It is important to remember that even in the setting of lymphoma, reactive inflammatory cells are also present. Both the size and the morphologic features of lymphocytes must be determined. Lymphocyte morphology is covered in further detail in Chap. 3. In addition to lymphocytes, other cell types may be present, including histiocytes, plasma cells, plasmacytoid cells, eosinophils, neutrophils, and dendritic cells. Their presence and proportion should be noted.

Adnexal structures are frequently overlooked in the evaluation of cutaneous lymphoid infiltrates but may show critical diagnostic features. Eccrine sweat glands may show evidence of syringotropism (exocytosis of lymphocytes and epithelial hyperplasia). Multiple abnormalities may also be found in hair follicles (e.g., folliculotropism of atypical lymphocytes, exocytosis of neutrophils or eosinophils, follicular mucinosis, disrupted architecture, cystic change, and/or altered sebaceous glands).

In addition, blood vessels are often forgotten in the evaluation of lymphoid infiltrates. Features such as angiocentrism, angiodestruction, or intravascular atypical cells are uncommon but have critical diagnostic value. It is also important to evaluate the endothelial cells and determine whether epithelioid or atypical morphology may be present. Vasculitic changes may also occur in some cases. The presence of infarct-like necrosis would suggest the presence of vascular involvement by the lymphoid infiltrate.

Any other histomorphologic findings can be diagnostically useful, particularly in the setting of pseudolymphomas. For example, sebaceous gland necrosis is an important clue for herpes folliculitis. Identification of viral cytopathic effect is of great diagnostic value, since florid inflammation due to viral infection may mimic lymphoma. Finally, artifactual changes (e.g., crushing artifact, electrodessication, fragmentation) or suboptimal sampling (e.g., superficial or small specimen) may prevent adequate evaluation of a lymphoid infiltrate and should be noted in the report.

Table 2.1 Histomorphologic evaluation of cutaneous lymphoid infiltrates

Density of the infiltrate	Mild
	Moderate
	Dense
Location (involved layers of the skin)	Epidermal, dermal (superficial and/or deep), and/or pannicular
Pattern(s) (often several)	Nodular
	Interstitial
	Diffuse
	Band-like
	Perifollicular
	Perieccrine
	Perineural
	Perivascular
	Angiocentric
	Intravascular
Epitheliotropism? (absent/present)	If present, which type?
	Epidermis (epidermotropism)
	Hair follicles (folliculotropism)
	Sweat glands (syringotropism)
Composition of the infiltrate	Lymphocytes (evaluate size, morphology, and proportion)
	Plasma cells/plasmacytoid cells
	Histiocytes/macrophages
	Eosinophils
	Neutrophils
	Dendritic cells
Lymphoid follicles? (absent/present)	If present, evaluate:
	Size and shape: variable or not
	Well-spaced vs. crowded
	Presence of mantle zone
	Presence of polarization in germinal centers
	Mitotic activity in germinal centers
	Presence of tingible body macrophages

Table 2.1 (continued)

Other findings	Ulceration
	Necrosis
	Vasculitis
	Follicular mucinosis
	Increased dermal mucin
	Fibrosis
	Viral cytopathic effect
	Epithelioid or atypical endothelial cells
	Artifactual changes
	Suboptimal sampling
	Other

Suggested Reading

Subtil A. A general approach to the diagnosis of cutaneous lymphomas and pseudolymphomas. Cutaneous lymphomas (Subtil, ed.). Surg Pathol Clin. 2014;7(2):135–42. Elsevier: Philadelphia.

Fig. 3.1 How would you describe these lymphoid cells?

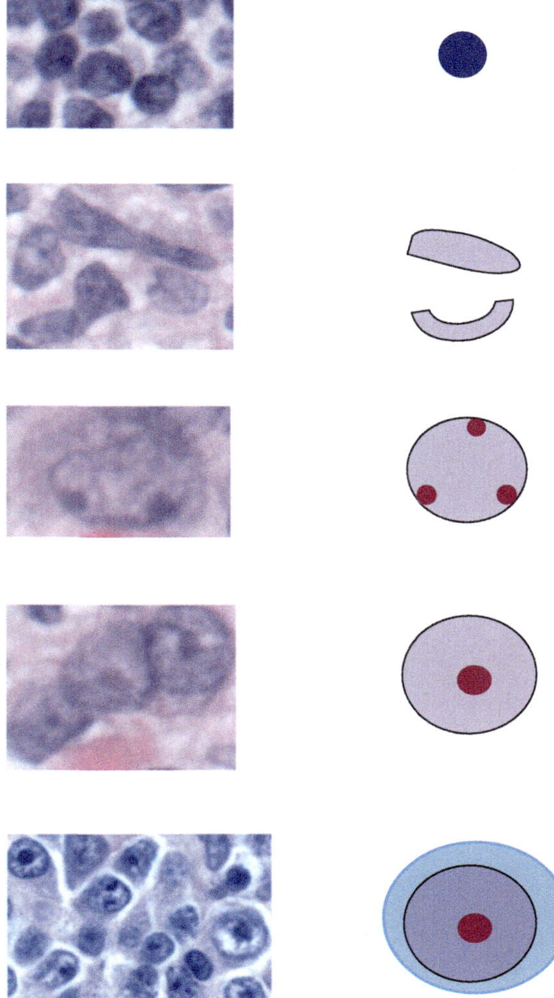

Fig. 3.2 Main types of
lymphoid morphology

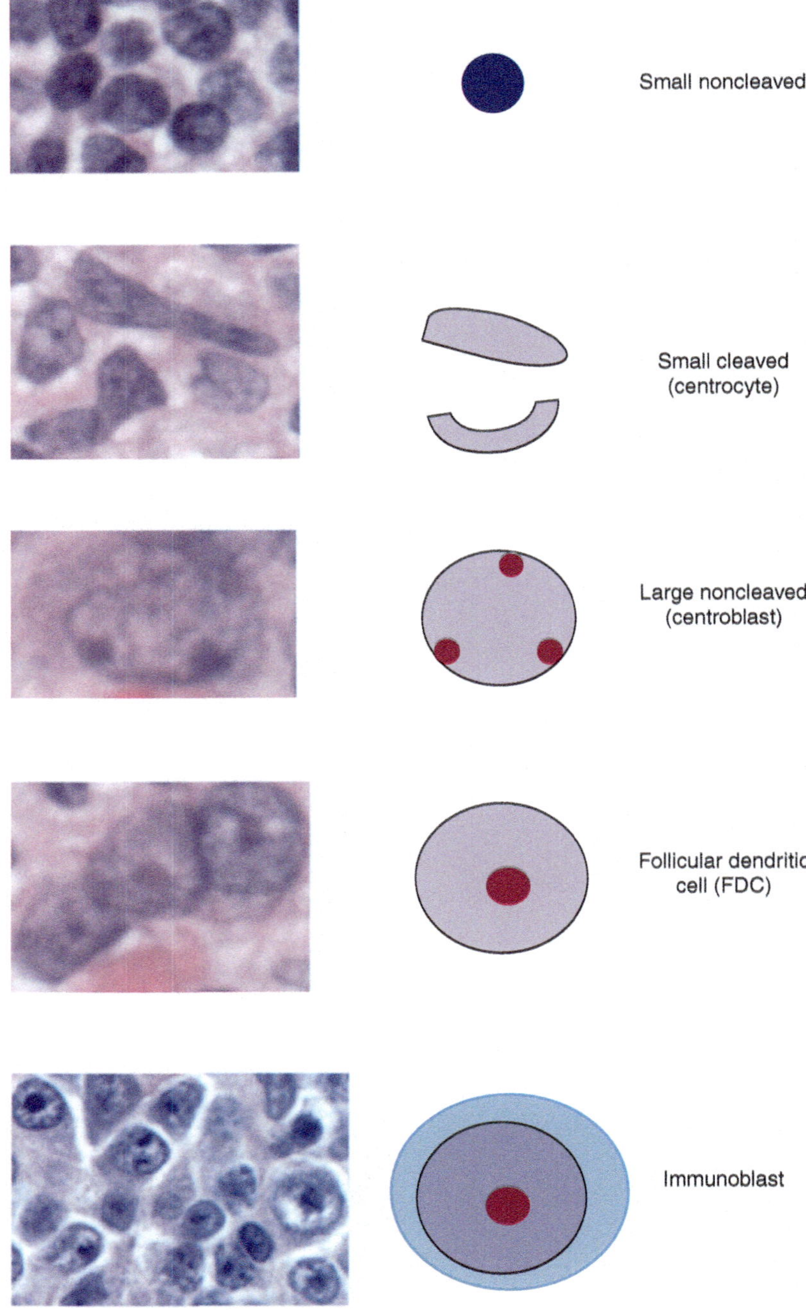

Table 3.1 Basic lymphoid cell morphologies

Lymphoid cell morphology	Dense chromatin	Nuclear shape	Prominent nucleolus	Cytoplasm
Small noncleaved	Yes (dark blue)	Round	No	Scant
Centrocyte (small cleaved)	No	Elongated, spindle-like (cleaved)	No	Scant
Centroblast (large noncleaved)	No	Round	Yes (multiple and peripheral)	Scant
Immunoblast	No	Round	Yes (single and central)	Moderate
Follicular dendritic cell	No	Round	Yes (single and central)	Scant

The cytomorphology of lymphocytes is part of the definition of several lymphomas. For example, the definition of follicular lymphomas includes centrocytes and centroblasts, while diffuse large B-cell lymphomas are composed of immunoblasts and centroblasts. Therefore, being able to properly recognize different types of lymphocytes in a lymphoid infiltrate is critical for the correct diagnosis and classification of lymphomas (Fig. 3.1). In addition, reactive lymphocytes may also show different morphologies, and it is equally important not to confuse them with neoplastic cells.

The majority of lymphoid cells in the skin are of small noncleaved type, which resembles small dark blue dots (see Fig. 3.2). These cells demonstrate a small round nucleus with dense chromatin and scant cytoplasm. Prominent nucleoli are not seen. This histomorphologic type may be seen in memory lymphocytes, NK cells, mantle zone B cells, and follicular helper T cells.

Centrocytes and centroblasts are germinal center B cells. Centrocytes are cleaved cells and usually small to intermediate in size. Their cytoplasm is scant, and nucleoli are inconspicuous. The nucleus is spindle-like and often shows variable, elongated shapes. In contrast, centroblasts are large cells with a noncleaved (round) nucleus. While the cytoplasm is scant, nucleoli are conspicuous, multiple, and peripherally located (see Fig. 3.2).

Immunoblasts are also large cells with a noncleaved (round) nucleus. However, the cytoplasm is not scant. The cells exhibit prominent nucleolus, which is generally single and centrally located (see Fig. 3.2).

Follicular dendritic cells are not lymphocytes but are mentioned here because they are often confused as large lymphocytes in biopsies. They may resemble immunoblasts due to the presence of a single central nucleolus within a large round nucleus. However, the cytoplasm is scant, and the cells are often arranged in small overlapping clusters (see Fig. 3.2). The dendritic processes are not visualized with the standard hematoxylin and eosin stain but can be seen with immunohistochemical stains, such as CD21 (see Chap. 6).

While there are other variations in lymphocyte morphology, these are the basic types to be recognized in the initial evaluation of cutaneous lymphoid infiltrates (see Table 3.1). Other morphologies will be mentioned in the chapters covering specific diagnostic entities (Chaps. 21, 22, 23, 24, 25, 26, 27, 28, 29, 30, 31, 32, 33, 34, 35, 36, 37, 38, 39, 40, 41, 42, and 43).

Suggested Reading

Swerdlow SH, et al., editors. WHO classification of tumors of hematopoietic and lymphoid tissues. Lyon: IARC; 2008.

Willemze R, et al. WHO-EORTC classification for cutaneous lymphomas. Blood. 2005;105:3768–85.

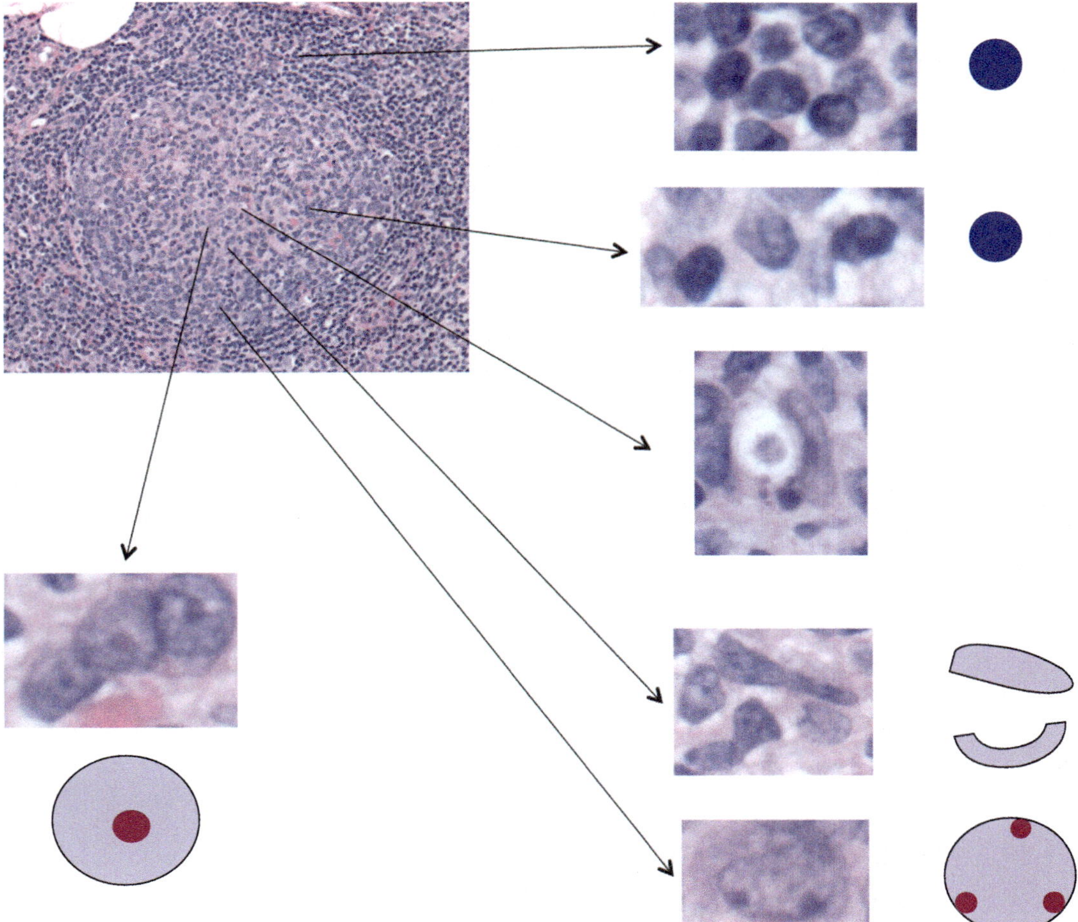

Fig. 4.1 What are the main compartments and cellular components of the lymphoid follicle?

© Springer Nature Switzerland AG 2019

A. Subtil, *Diagnosis of Cutaneous Lymphoid Infiltrates*,

https://doi.org/10.1007/978-3-030-11654-5_4

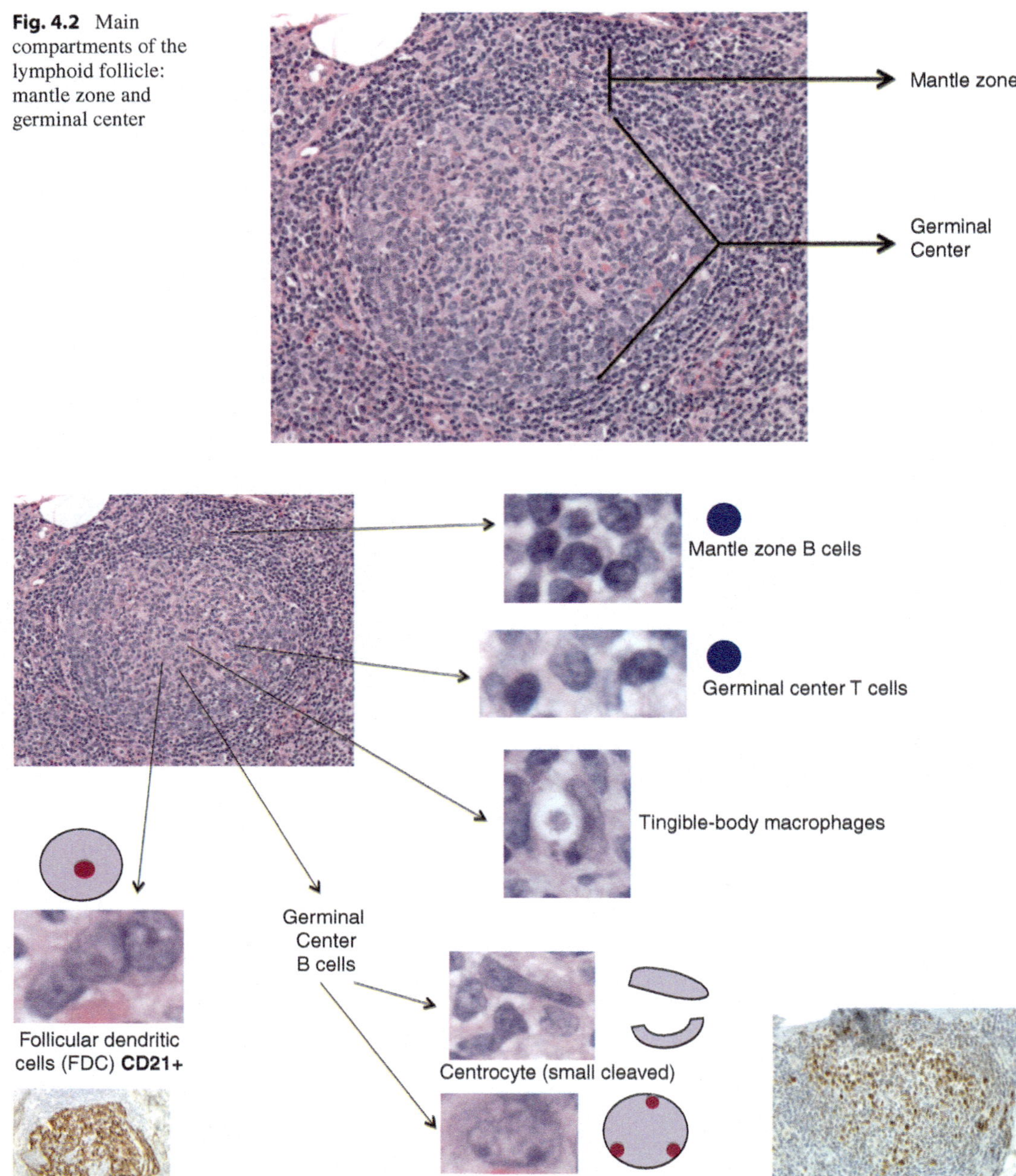

Fig. 4.2 Main compartments of the lymphoid follicle: mantle zone and germinal center

Fig. 4.3 Cellular components of the lymphoid follicle

Table 4.1 Cellular components of reactive lymphoid follicles

Cell type	Location in lymphoid follicle	Cytomorphologic features	Immunophenotype
Follicular dendritic cell (FDC)	Germinal center	Large round noncleaved nucleus with single central nucleolus	CD21+ (immunohistochemical stain highlights the dendritic processes)
Germinal center B cells (centrocytes and centroblasts)	Germinal center	Small cleaved and large noncleaved cells with scant cytoplasm	CD20+, BCL6+, BCL2-
(Tingible body) macrophages	Germinal center	Reniform, elongated nucleus and abundant cytoplasm with apoptotic debris	CD68+
Follicular helper T cells	Germinal center	Small noncleaved	CD3+, BCL2+
Mantle zone B cells	Mantle zone	Small noncleaved	CD20+, BCL6-, BCL2+

Lymphoid follicles are complex structures and consist of several cellular components (see Fig. 4.1). Different cell types show distinct morphologic features and preferential location within separate compartments of the lymphoid follicle. Unlike tonsils and lymph nodes, they are not native to the skin and are often smaller in size. The development of lymphoid follicles in skin is a pathologic finding. Several skin conditions may demonstrate lymphoid follicles, including reactive lymphoid hyperplasia, cutaneous Rosai-Dorfman disease, and lupus panniculitis. In addition, lymphoid follicles are identified in low-grade cutaneous B-cell lymphomas (marginal zone lymphoma and follicle center lymphoma).

It is important to emphasize the fact that lymphoid follicles can be reactive (benign) or neoplastic (malignant). In order to identify what is abnormal, one must be able to recognize what is normal. Since many students of cutaneous pathology may not be very familiar with lymphoid follicles, this introductory chapter offers a basic review of their composition (see Table 4.1 and Figs. 4.2 and 4.3). In subsequent Chaps. 5, 6, 20, and 40, the distinguishing features of benign and malignant follicles will be reviewed.

Reactive secondary lymphoid follicles show two main compartments: the mantle zone and the germinal center (Fig. 4.2). The *mantle zone* is located at the periphery of the follicle and consists predominantly of mantle zone B cells (small noncleaved lymphocytes with dense chromatin, inconspicuous nucleoli, and scant cytoplasm). The other cell types are located in the *germinal center* and include (a) *follicular dendritic cells* (single or clustered large cells with round, noncleaved nuclei and single central nucleolus), (b) *centrocytes* (small germinal center B cells with cleaved nuclei and inconspicuous nucleoli), (c) *centroblasts* (large germinal center B cells with round, noncleaved nuclei and multiple conspicuous peripheral nucleoli), (d) *follicular helper T cells* (small noncleaved lymphocytes with dense chromatin, inconspicuous nucleoli, and scant cytoplasm), and (e) *tingible body macrophages* (histiocytes with reniform, elongated nucleus and abundant cytoplasm with apoptotic fragments) (see Fig. 4.3). The immunophenotype of these cell types is listed in Table 4.1.

Suggested Readings

Ioachim HL, Medeiros LJ. Ioachim's lymph node pathology. 4th ed. Philadelphia: Lippincott Williams & Wilkins; 2009.

Orazi A, Weiss LM, Foucar K, Knowles DM. Knowles' neoplastic hematopathology. 3rd ed. Philadelphia: Lippincott Williams & Wilkins; 2014.

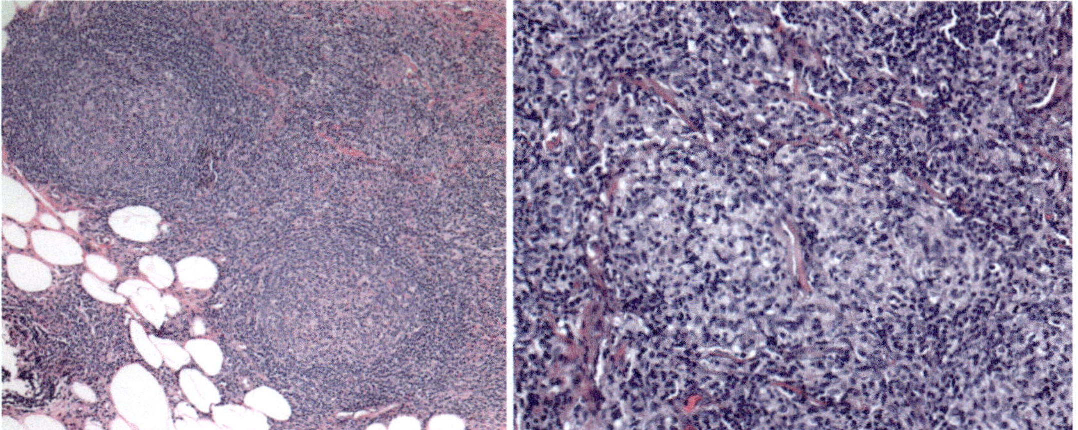

Fig. 5.1 Which of these lymphoid follicles are reactive, and which are neoplastic? What are the distinguishing histo-morphologic features?

© Springer Nature Switzerland AG 2019

A. Subtil, *Diagnosis of Cutaneous Lymphoid Infiltrates*,

https://doi.org/10.1007/978-3-030-11654-5_5

- Well spaced lymphoid follicles
- Mantle zones generally well preserved
- Frequent mitoses
- Tingible-body macrophages
- Germinal centers often polarized

- Back to back follicles (crowding)
- Mantle zones diminished to absent
- Less frequent mitoses (exception: high grade)
- Less frequent tingible-body macrophages

Reactive   VS.   Neoplastic

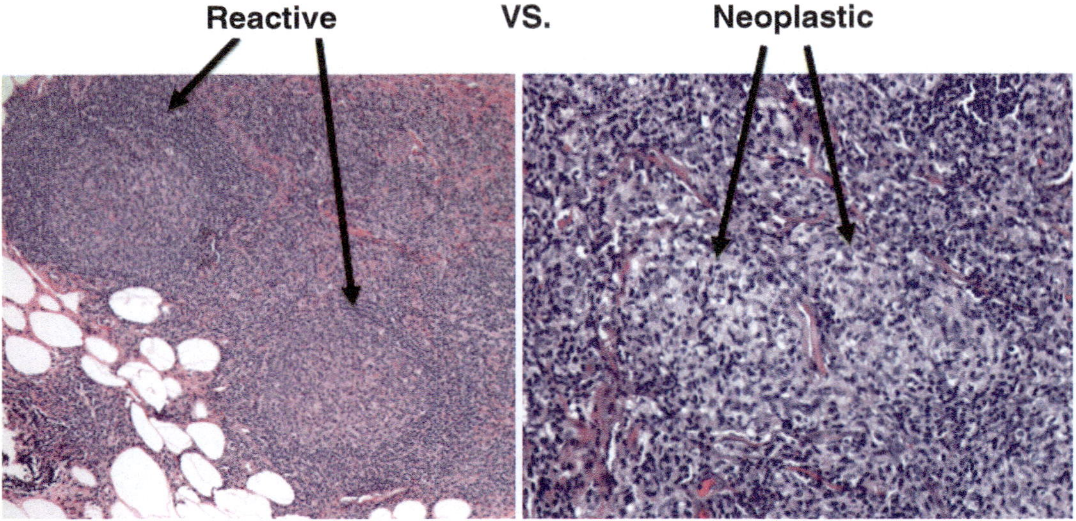

Fig. 5.2 Histomorphologic features of reactive and neoplastic lymphoid follicles

Ki-67 (MIB-1)

• **Reactive:**

High and polarized

• **Neoplastic:**

Decreased and non-polarized

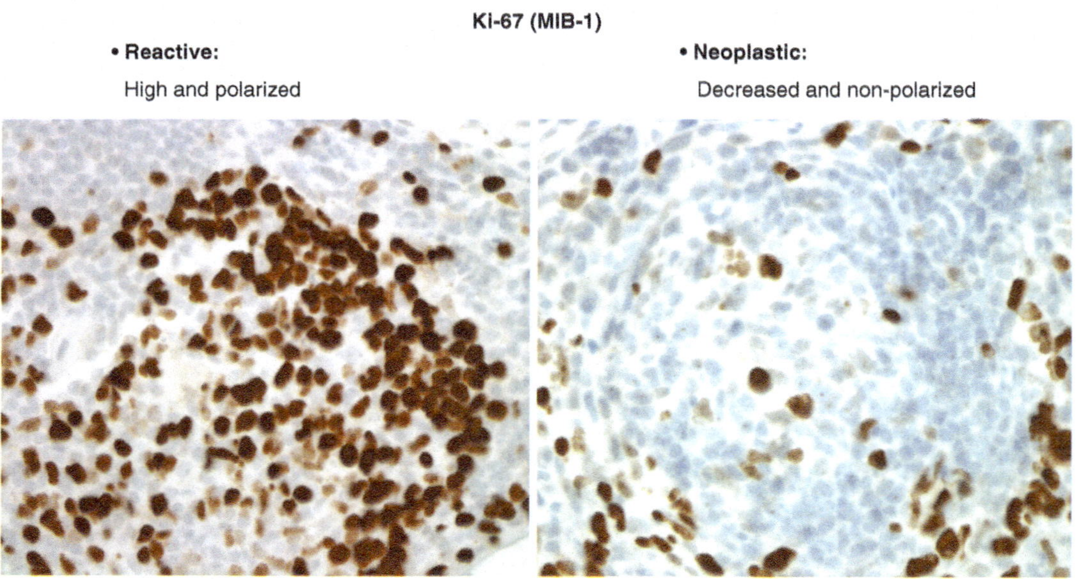

Fig. 5.3 Comparison of Ki-67 staining in reactive and neoplastic lymphoid follicles

As reviewed in Chap. 4, lymphoid follicles are complex structures and consist of several cellular components, which are distributed in two main compartments: the mantle zone (at the periphery) and the germinal center. They are not native to the skin, and their presence in the dermis represents a pathologic finding. Several reactive cutaneous diseases may exhibit lymphoid follicles, including reactive lymphoid hyperplasia, Rosai-Dorfman disease, and lupus profundus. In addition, lymphoid follicles are identified in low-grade cutaneous B-cell lymphomas. In pseudolymphomas (Fig. 5.1, left) and in marginal zone lymphoma, lymphoid follicles are reactive (benign), while in follicle center (follicular) lymphoma, lymphoid follicles are neoplastic (malignant) (Fig. 5.1, right).

Several histomorphologic features can be used to differentiate reactive from neoplastic lymphoid follicles (Fig. 5.2 and Table 5.1). At lower magnification, reactive follicles are generally well spaced from each other and show rounded outlines. In contrast, neoplastic follicles tend to be crowded (back to back) and irregular. The mantle zones are usually well preserved in reactive follicles, while their absence is common in neoplastic follicles. However, since lymphoid follicles are not native to the skin, it is not unusual to see partially diminished mantle zones in reactive follicles. Tingible body macrophages and high mitotic activity are frequent in reactive follicles and tend to be diminished in neoplastic follicles. However, in high-grade follicular lymphoma, mitoses can be frequent. Depending on sectioning, reactive germinal centers may show a polarized pattern with a lighter-staining zone (rich in centrocytes) and a darker-staining zone (rich in centroblasts). This polarization is generally not seen in neoplastic follicles.

In addition to the histomorphology, immunohistochemistry can be helpful in the differential of reactive versus neoplastic follicles. The proliferation rate can be assessed with Ki-67 staining (Fig. 5.3). In reactive follicles, there is high and often polarized staining of the germinal center with Ki-67. In contrast, neoplastic follicles generally show diminished staining with Ki-67, often in scattered distribution. The use and interpretation of other immunohistochemical stains for the evaluation of lymphoid follicles will be covered in Chaps. 6 (BCL6 and CD21) and 20 (BCL2).

Table 5.1 Histomorphologic features of reactive and neoplastic lymphoid follicles

	Reactive follicles	Neoplastic follicles
Distribution	Well-spaced follicles	Back-to-back follicles (crowding)
Mantle zones	Generally well preserved	Diminished to absent
Mitoses	Frequent	Diminished (exception: high grade)
Tingible body macrophages	Frequent	Diminished
Polarization of germinal centers	Common	Rare

Suggested Readings

Leinweber B, Colli C, Chott A, Kerl H, Cerroni L. Differential diagnosis of cutaneous infiltrates of B lymphocytes with follicular growth pattern. Am J Dermatopathol. 2004;26(1):4–13.

Subtil A. A general approach to the diagnosis of cutaneous lymphomas and pseudolymphomas. Cutaneous lymphomas (Subtil, ed.). Surg Pathol Clin. 2014;7(2):135–42. Elsevier: Philadelphia.

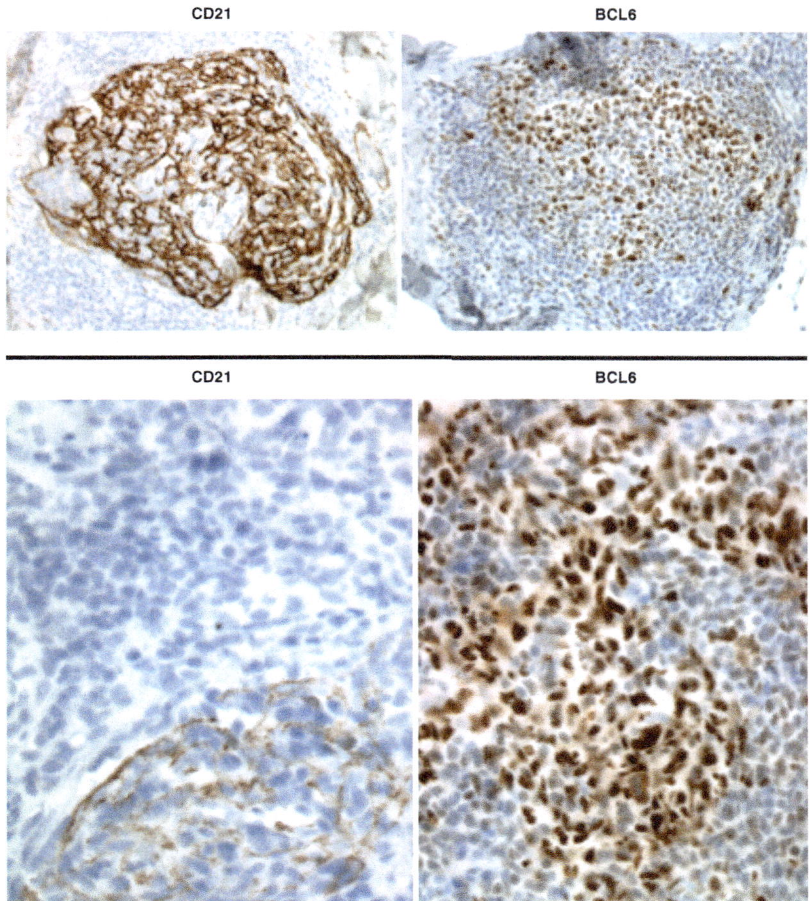

Fig. 6.1 Lymphoid follicles from two different biopsies (one from follicle center lymphoma and another from cutaneous reactive lymphoid hyperplasia) are compared with immunohistochemical stains. Which cells are highlighted by BCL6? What is the structure demonstrated by CD21? Which of these follicles is neoplastic?

© Springer Nature Switzerland AG 2019
A. Subtil, *Diagnosis of Cutaneous Lymphoid Infiltrates*,
https://doi.org/10.1007/978-3-030-11654-5_6

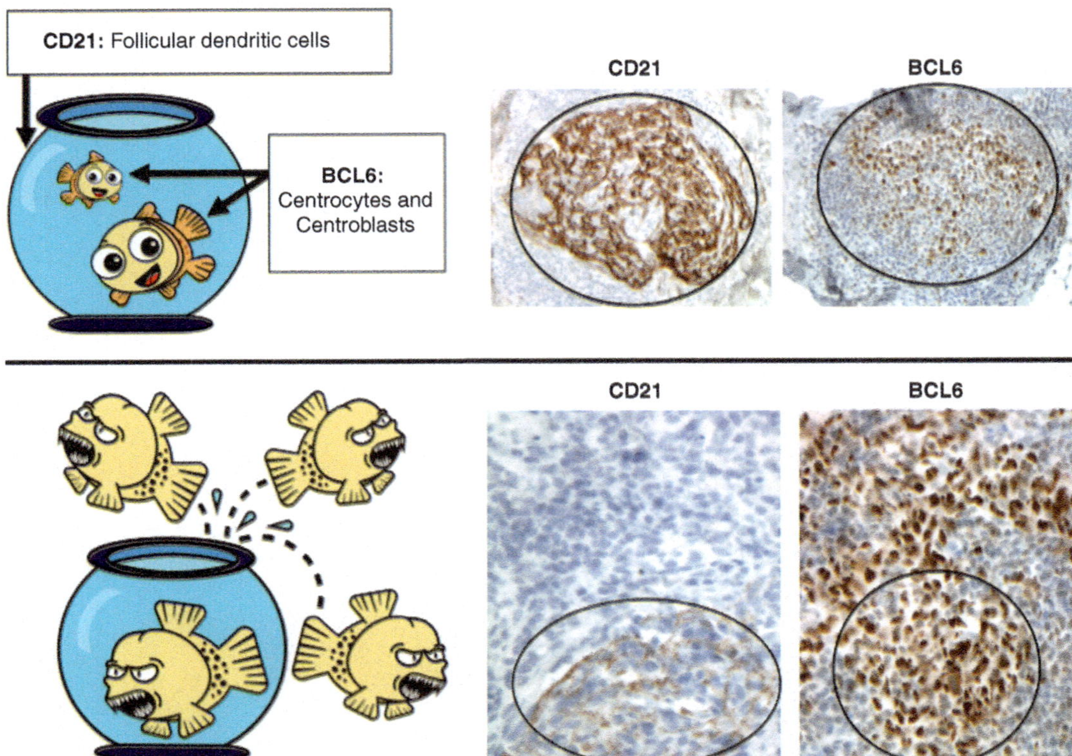

Fig. 6.2 BCL6 marks germinal center B cells (centrocytes and centroblasts), while CD21 highlights the lymphoid follicle by staining follicular dendritic cell meshworks. As an analogy, if centrocytes and centroblasts were fish, the follicular dendritic cell meshwork of the lymphoid follicle would be a fishbowl. In a benign process (reactive lymphoid hyperplasia, top panel), benign fish (goldfish) would stay inside the fishbowl (lymphoid follicle), and the foci of staining with both CD21 and BCL6 would match. In a malignant process (follicular lymphoma, bottom panel), it would be common for malignant fish (piranhas) to jump out of the fishbowl (lymphoid follicle). This extrafollicular spread of germinal center B cells is highlighted by a mismatch between the staining pattern of BCL6 and CD21 (clusters of BCL6-positive cells are identified both within and outside the CD21-positive lymphoid follicle)

Recognizing neoplastic versus reactive lymphoid follicles is a critical step in the differential diagnosis of cutaneous follicle center lymphoma versus reactive lymphoid hyperplasia. The composition and architecture of lymphoid follicles were reviewed in Chaps. 4 and 5. Another useful parameter in this differential is related to the growth pattern of germinal center B cells beyond the confines of the lymphoid follicle. Extrafollicular spread of centrocytes and centroblasts is diagnostic of follicular lymphoma and can be demonstrated with immunohistochemical stains (Fig. 6.1).

BCL6 marks germinal center B cells (centrocytes and centroblasts), while CD21 highlights the lymphoid follicle by staining follicular dendritic cell meshworks. In reactive secondary lymphoid follicles, centrocytes and centroblasts are present only within the germinal center. Therefore, the foci of staining with both CD21 and BCL6 match (Fig. 6.1, top panel). In follicular lymphoma, it is frequent to identify a proliferation of centrocytes and centroblasts beyond the lymphoid follicle into interfollicular tissues. This extrafollicular spread of germinal center B cells is highlighted by a mismatch between the staining pattern of BCL6 and CD21 (i.e., clusters of BCL6-positive cells are identified both within and outside the CD21-positive lymphoid follicle) (Fig. 6.1, bottom panel).

As an analogy (Fig. 6.2), if centrocytes and centroblasts were to represent fish, the follicular dendritic cell meshwork of the lymphoid follicle would be a fishbowl. In a benign process (reactive lymphoid hyperplasia), benign fish (goldfish) would stay inside the fishbowl (lymphoid follicle), and the foci of staining with both CD21 and BCL6 would always match (Fig. 6.2, top panel). In a malignant process (follicular lymphoma), it would be common for malignant fish (piranhas) to jump out of the fishbowl (lymphoid follicle), and there would be a mismatch between the staining pattern of BCL6 and CD21 (Fig. 6.2, bottom panel).

Pearls and Pitfalls

1. Extrafollicular spread of germinal center B cells is a useful feature in the diagnosis of follicle center lymphoma; however, it is not always present. Cases of follicular lymphoma without a diffuse/interstitial component would lack this finding.
2. It is important to remember that there must be clusters of BCL6-positive cells. Only a few scattered cells staining with BCL6 should be ignored.
3. BCL6 may be a technically difficult special stain, and it would be judicious to be careful with overstained or understained BCL6. Always confirm that the morphology of cells staining with BCL6 is that of centrocytes (cleaved) and centroblasts (large noncleaved cells with multiple peripheral nucleoli).
4. In addition, CD21 stain may be a technically difficult stain. If follicular dendritic cells (large noncleaved nucleus with single central nucleolus and scant cytoplasm, often in small clusters) are identified in a lymphoid infiltrate, there should be some staining with CD21. If follicular dendritic cells are visualized in the infiltrate and CD21 stain looks completely negative, it likely represents a false negative, and the stain should be repeated.

Suggested Reading

Nybakken G, Warnke R, Natkunam Y. Follicular lymphoma. In: Orazi A, Foucar K, editors. Knowles' neoplastic hematopathology. 3rd ed. Philadelphia: Lippincott Williams & Wilkins; 2014.

Part II

Histomorphologic Differential Diagnoses (DDx)

Fig. 7.1 This skin biopsy shows epidermotropism. What is the differential diagnosis for this histopathologic finding?

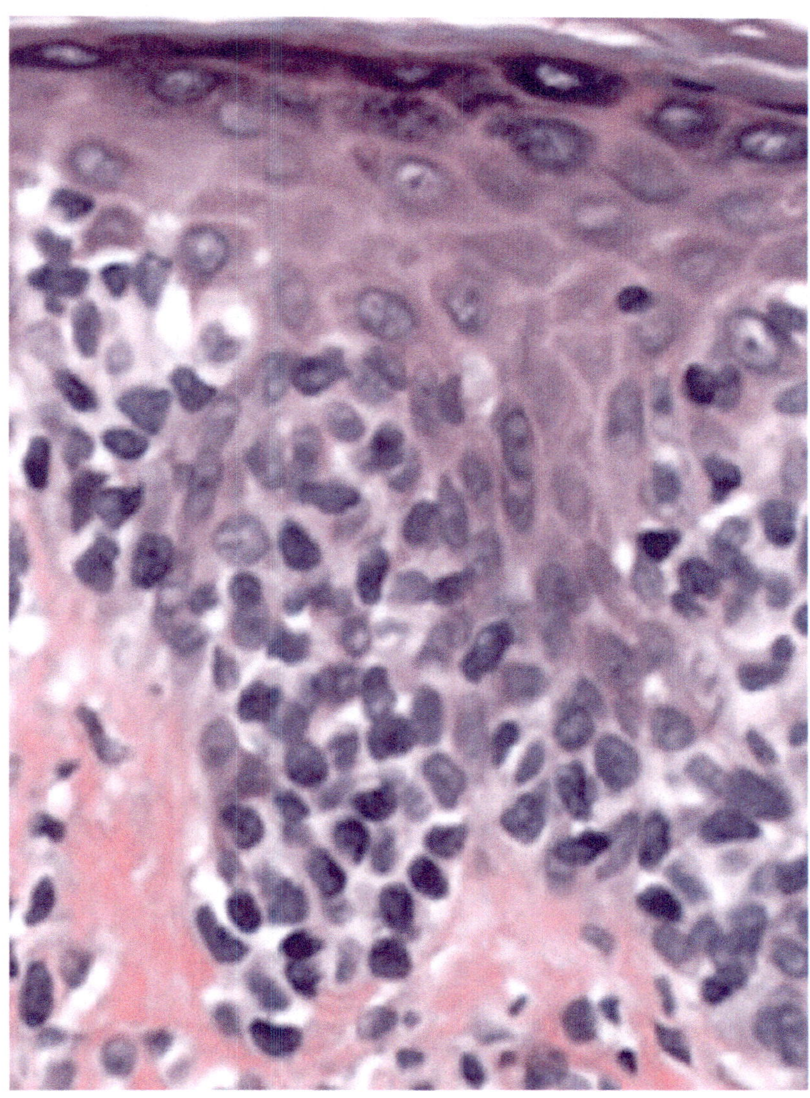

© Springer Nature Switzerland AG 2019
A. Subtil, *Diagnosis of Cutaneous Lymphoid Infiltrates*,
https://doi.org/10.1007/978-3-030-11654-5_7

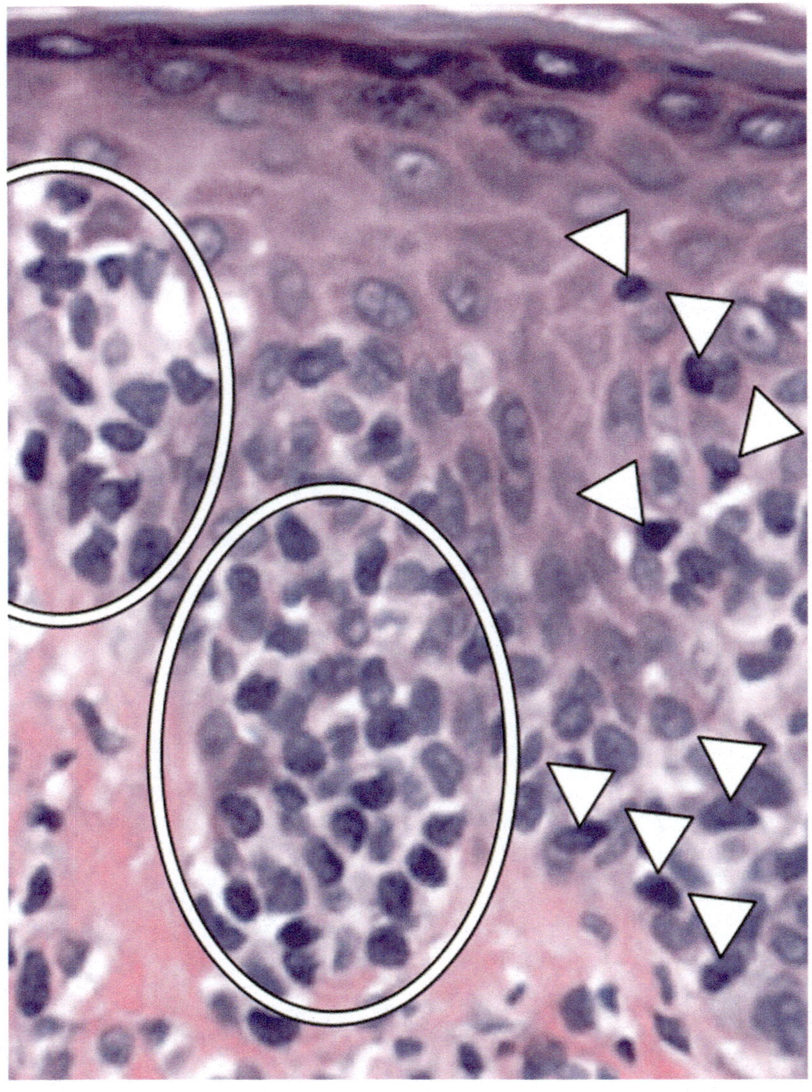

Fig. 7.2 Epidermotropism is present in this skin biopsy of classic mycosis fungoides. Intraepidermal lymphocytes are highlighted by arrowheads (single) and circles (clusters or Pautrier microabscesses). Prominent spongiosis is not seen

Fig. 7.4 Since the same histopathologic pattern may occur in several entities, clinical pathologic correlation and/or immunophenotyping is necessary to correctly classify cutaneous lymphoid infiltrates. An epidermotropic histopathologic pattern will result in different diagnoses depending on the clinical picture: large, chronic patches and/or plaques on sun-protected skin for classic mycosis fungoides vs. small, self-regressing papules for lymphomatoid papulosis

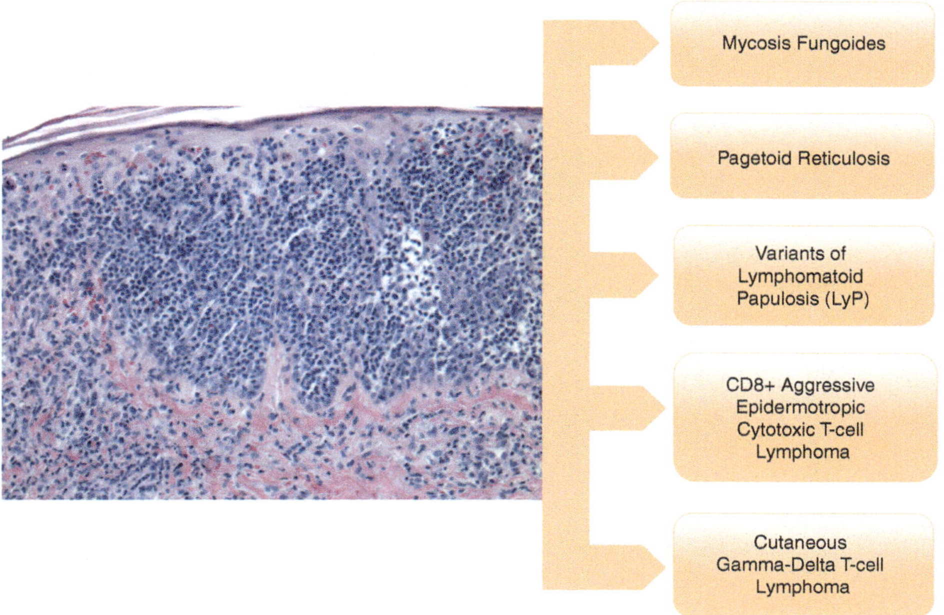

Fig. 7.3 Differential diagnosis of epidermotropism. Several entities besides mycosis fungoides may exhibit prominent intraepidermal lymphocytes. For example, marked epidermotropism is present in this biopsy of type D lymphomatoid papulosis (LyP)

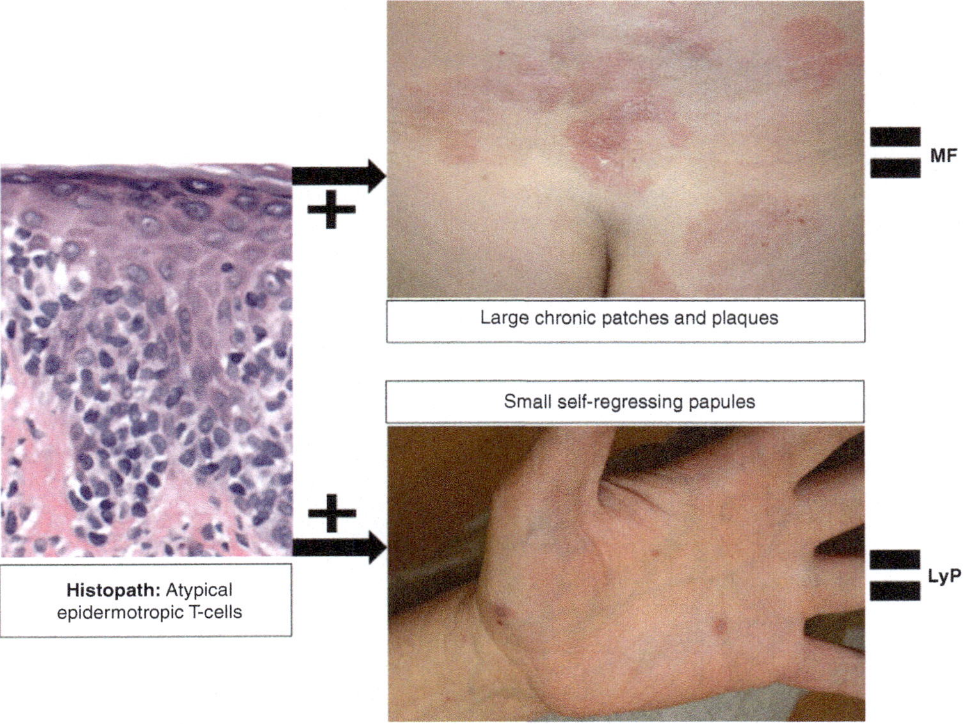

Normal human skin lacks inflammatory cells within the epidermis, except for Langerhans cells in the stratum spinosum. Exocytosis is the process of migration of inflammatory cells into the epidermis and occurs in a variety of benign dermatoses. In spongiotic/eczematous dermatitis, exocytosis of a relatively small number of lymphocytes is associated with prominent intercellular edema (spongiosis). The presence of atypical lymphocytes within the epidermis is described as epidermotropism (Fig. 7.1) and is usually associated with scant spongiosis.

Mycosis fungoides (MF) is the most common type of skin lymphoma and is the prototype of epidermotropic disorders. The neoplastic lymphocytes of classic MF demonstrate tropism for the epidermis and characteristically exhibit atypical cytologic features with hyperchromatic, cerebriform nuclei (Fig. 7.2). The intraepidermal lymphocytes are arranged as single cells and/or in aggregates (Pautrier microabscesses). Epidermotropism is present in both patch and plaque stages but may be absent in tumor-stage MF. Epidermotropism may also be absent in biopsies of treated lesions of MF, which could lead to misdiagnosis particularly in early-stage disease. Folliculotropic mycosis fungoides is a variant of MF with tropism for hair follicles and often lacks epidermotropism.

The presence of epidermotropic T cells is not specific for mycosis fungoides and may occur in other lymphoproliferative disorders and lymphomas (Fig. 7.3). There are variants of lymphomatoid papulosis (LyP) with epidermotropic T cells. Type B LyP shows a predominantly intraepidermal lymphocytic infiltrate mimicking MF. Type

D LyP is a CD8-positive cytotoxic T-cell variant with prominent epidermotropism. LyP with 6p25.3 rearrangement shows a biphasic growth pattern, with small cerebriform lymphocytes in the epidermis and large lymphocytes in the dermis. Careful clinical pathologic correlation is essential to correctly classify epidermotropic lymphoid infiltrates (Fig. 7.4).

Both indolent and aggressive non-MF cutaneous lymphomas may exhibit prominent epidermotropism. Pagetoid reticulosis (localized type, Woringer-Kolopp) is a variant of mycosis fungoides with excellent prognosis and generally presents with localized patches or plaques on distal extremities. Aggressive epidermotropic CD8-positive cytotoxic T-cell lymphoma is a rare cytotoxic cutaneous lymphoma with poor prognosis and is associated with marked epitheliotropism. Gamma-delta T-cell lymphoma is an aggressive cutaneous lymphoma and may variably involve one or several layers of the skin (epidermis, dermis, and/or panniculus).

Prominent exocytosis of lymphocytes in the epidermis is not definitively diagnostic of lymphoma and may be observed in several benign dermatoses, such as inflammatory stage of vitiligo, pityriasis lichenoides, lymphomatoid lichenoid keratosis, early lichen sclerosus, pigmented purpuric dermatoses, lymphomatoid drug reaction, pseudolymphomatous tattoo reaction, and CD8-positive cutaneous infiltrates in the setting of acquired immunodeficiency syndrome (AIDS) (Table 7.1). Identification of other diagnostic histopathologic findings as well as clinical correlation will prove helpful to prevent misdiagnosis.

Table 7.1 Differential diagnosis of frequent intraepidermal lymphocytes

Lymphomas/lymphoproliferative disorders	Benign dermatoses
Mycosis fungoides	Inflammatory stage of vitiligo
Pagetoid reticulosis	Pityriasis lichenoides
Lymphomatoid papulosis (LyP types B and D and with 6p25.3 rearrangement)	Lymphomatoid lichenoid keratosis
Primary cutaneous aggressive epidermotropic CD8-positive cytotoxic T-cell lymphoma	Early lichen sclerosus
Cutaneous gamma-delta T-cell lymphoma	Pigmented purpuric dermatoses
	Lymphomatoid drug reaction
	Pseudolymphomatous tattoo reaction
	CD8-positive cutaneous infiltrates in the setting of acquired immunodeficiency syndrome

Pearls and Pitfalls

1. Too much epidermotropism would be unusual for classic mycosis fungoides and would raise the possibility of another epidermotropic process, including type D lymphomatoid papulosis (LyP), pagetoid reticulosis, and aggressive epidermotropic CD8-positive cytotoxic T-cell lymphoma.
2. Epidermotropism is often absent in tumor-stage mycosis fungoides, in partially treated lesions of early mycosis fungoides, and in folliculotropic mycosis fungoides.

Suggested Reading

Karai LJ, Kadin ME, Hsi ED, et al. Chromosomal rearrangements of 6p25.3 define a new subtype of lymphomatoid papulosis. Am J Surg Pathol. 2013;37(8):1173–81.

Pimpinelli N, Olsen EA, Santucci M, et al. Defining early mycosis fungoides. J Am Acad Dermatol. 2005;53(6):1053–63.

Saggini A, Gulia A, Argenyi Z, et al. A variant of lymphomatoid papulosis simulating primary cutaneous aggressive epidermotropic CD8+ cytotoxic T-cell lymphoma. Description of 9 cases. Am J Surg Pathol. 2010;34(8):1168–75.

Suchak R, Verdolini R, Robson A, Stefanato CM. Extragenital lichen sclerosus et atrophicus mimicking cutaneous T-cell lymphoma: report of a case. J Cutan Pathol. 2010;37(9):982–6.

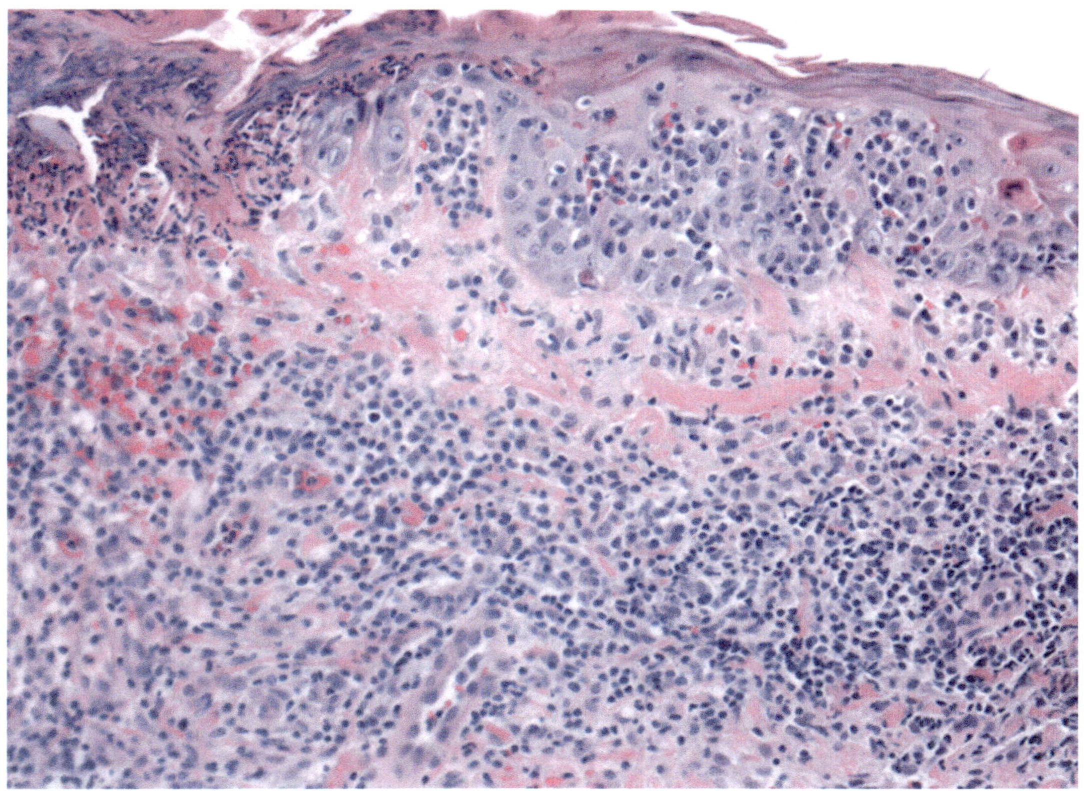

Fig. 8.1 While epidermotropism is present in this skin biopsy, this patient does not have mycosis fungoides. What is the clue seen here for a different diagnosis?

A. Subtil, *Diagnosis of Cutaneous Lymphoid Infiltrates*,
https://doi.org/10.1007/978-3-030-11654-5_8

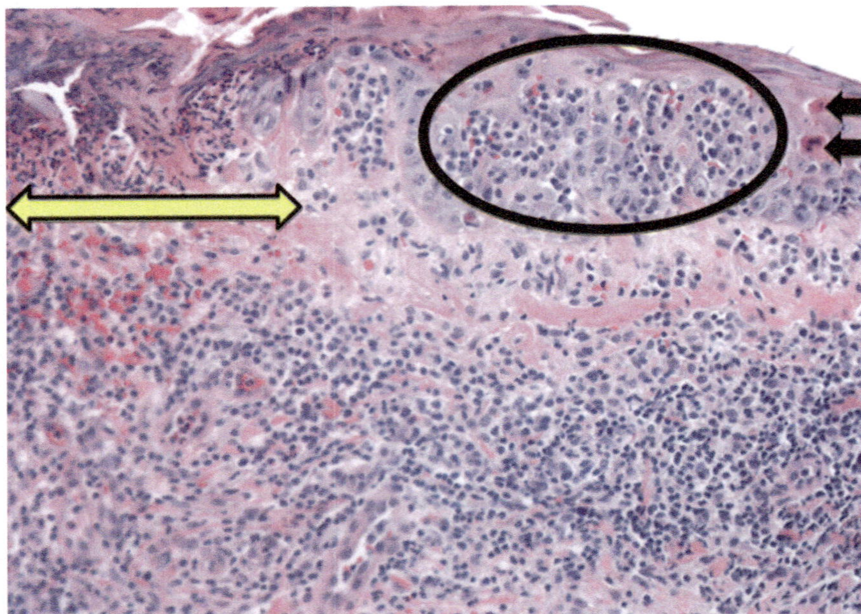

Fig. 8.2 Ulceration is generally absent in mycosis fungoides (MF), except for advanced tumor-stage disease, which only occurs in a small subset of patients after several years. While this biopsy shows epidermotropism (circle), the presence of ulceration (yellow arrow) would suggest a non-MF process (in this case, lymphomatoid papulosis type D). Apoptotic keratinocytes (black arrows) are also seen

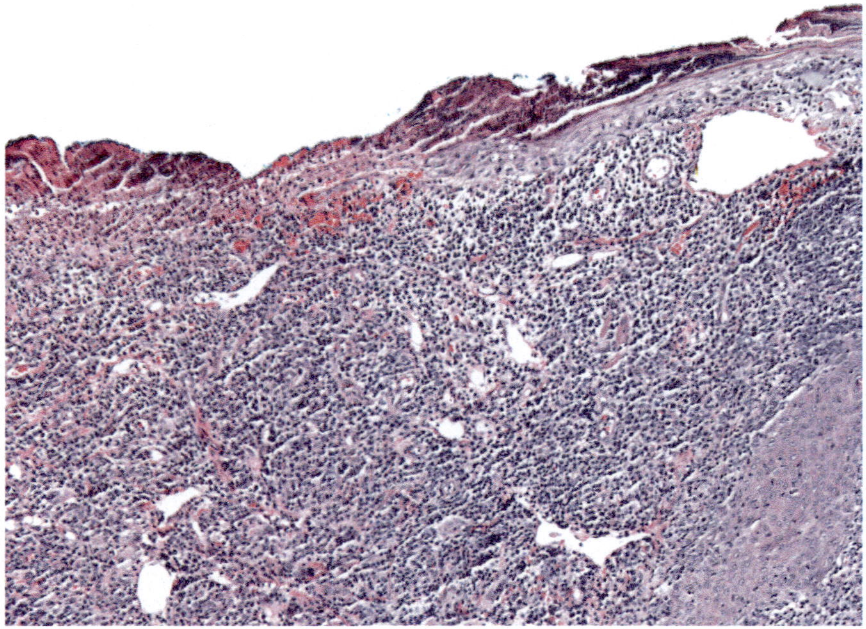

Fig. 8.3 Primary cutaneous aggressive epidermotropic CD8-positive cytotoxic T-cell lymphoma. Ulceration was present in this first skin biopsy of an enlarging nodule of 3-month duration. While the histopathology resembles tumor-stage mycosis fungoides, the patient had no patches or plaques. The presence of tumor-induced ulceration at an early onset is a clue that this cutaneous lymphoma is not mycosis fungoides

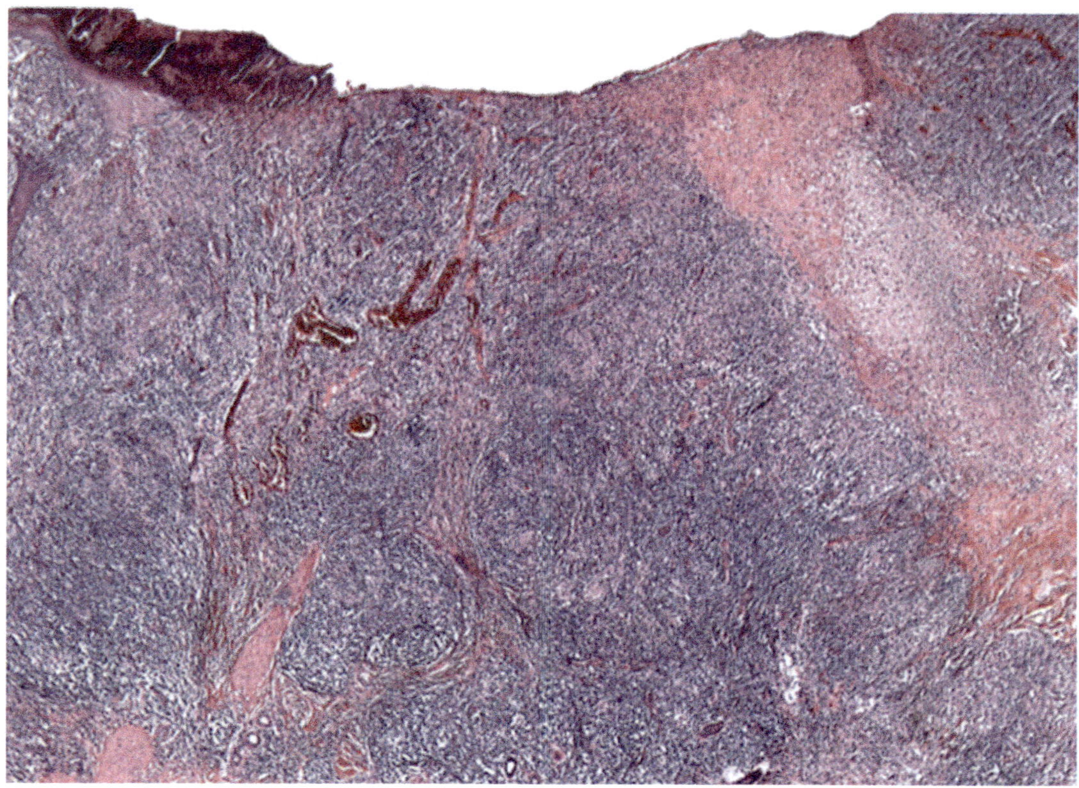

Fig. 8.4 Cutaneous leishmaniasis with ulceration. Some infectious processes may be associated with dense lympho-histiocytic infiltrates resembling lymphoma

The presence of ulceration is an important histopathologic finding in the evaluation of skin biopsies with lymphoid infiltrates. Full-thickness epidermal loss is generally associated with necrotic keratinocytes, mixed inflammation with prominent neutrophils, fibrin deposition, and reactive changes in the adjacent epidermis. Mycosis fungoides (MF) is the most common type of cutaneous lymphoma. However, ulceration is generally absent in MF, except in some cases of advanced tumor-stage disease, which only occurs in a small subset of patients after several years. Therefore, the presence of ulceration at an early onset would raise the possibility of a non-MF cutaneous lymphoproliferative process.

Both indolent and aggressive cutaneous lymphoproliferative conditions may be associated with ulceration. Therefore, careful correlation of clinical and histopathologic findings is essential.

Primary cutaneous CD30-positive lymphoproliferative disorders include lymphomatoid papulosis (LyP) (Figs. 8.1 and 8.2) and cutaneous anaplastic large cell lymphoma (C-ALCL). Both LyP and C-ALCL are indolent and often develop ulceration. A variety of histopathologic types have been described for LyP and will be covered in detail in Chap. 28.

Several aggressive cutaneous lymphomas often develop ulceration. These generally exhibit a cytotoxic immunophenotype. Primary cutaneous aggressive epidermotropic CD8-positive cytotoxic T-cell lymphoma is frequently associated with eroded and ulcerated skin lesions (Fig. 8.3). Angioinvasion and angiodestruction may also occur and result in extensive infarct-type necrosis, particularly in extranodal NK/T-cell lymphoma, nasal type, and some cases of cutaneous gamma-delta T-cell lymphoma.

Table 8.1 Differential diagnosis of ulceration

Lymphomas/lymphoproliferative disorders	Benign dermatoses/pseudolymphomas
Tumor-stage mycosis fungoides	Pityriasis lichenoides et varioliformis acuta (PLEVA)
CD30-positive lymphoproliferative disorders: lymphomatoid papulosis, cutaneous anaplastic large cell lymphoma	Inflamed molluscum contagiosum
Primary cutaneous aggressive epidermotropic CD8-positive cytotoxic T-cell lymphoma	Herpesvirus infection
Cutaneous gamma-delta T-cell lymphoma	Primary syphilis
Extranodal NK/T-cell lymphoma, nasal type	Leishmania infection

Some benign dermatoses may also demonstrate ulceration, such as pityriasis lichenoides et varioliformis acuta (PLEVA). Infectious processes may be associated with dense lymphohistiocytic infiltrates resembling lymphoma (Table 8.1). Entities that may also demonstrate ulceration include primary syphilis, inflamed molluscum contagiosum, herpesvirus infection, and leishmaniasis (Fig. 8.4).

Pearls and Pitfalls

1. Ulceration is seen in some cases of advanced, tumor-stage mycosis fungoides (MF). The presence of ulceration at initial presentation would suggest a non-MF process.
2. Some pseudolymphomas may also demonstrate ulceration. These include pityriasis lichenoides and infectious processes, such as leishmaniasis and inflamed molluscum contagiosum.
3. If ulceration is not seen in the skin biopsy, it does not necessarily mean that the patient does not have ulcerated lesions elsewhere, since dermatologists often avoid biopsying lesions with secondary changes. Careful correlation of clinical and histopathologic findings is essential.
4. Ulceration or angioinvasion may not be present in the early stage of aggressive cytotoxic skin lymphomas. While immunophenotyping may provide clues to the diagnosis, close follow-up and rebiopsy of changed lesions may prove helpful.

Suggested Reading

Guitart J, Weisenburger DD, Subtil A, et al. Cutaneous gamma-delta T-cell lymphomas: a spectrum of presentations with overlap with other cytotoxic lymphomas. Am J Surg Pathol. 2012;36(11):1656–65.

Handler MZ, Patel PA, Kapila R, et al. Cutaneous and mucocutaneous leishmaniasis: clinical perspectives. J Am Acad Dermatol. 2015;73(6):897–908.

Kempf W. Cutaneous CD30-positive lymphoproliferative disorders. Surg Pathol Clin. 2014;7(2):203–28.

Willemze R, Jaffe ES, Burg G, et al. WHO-EORTC classification for cutaneous lymphomas. Blood. 2005;105(10):3768–85.

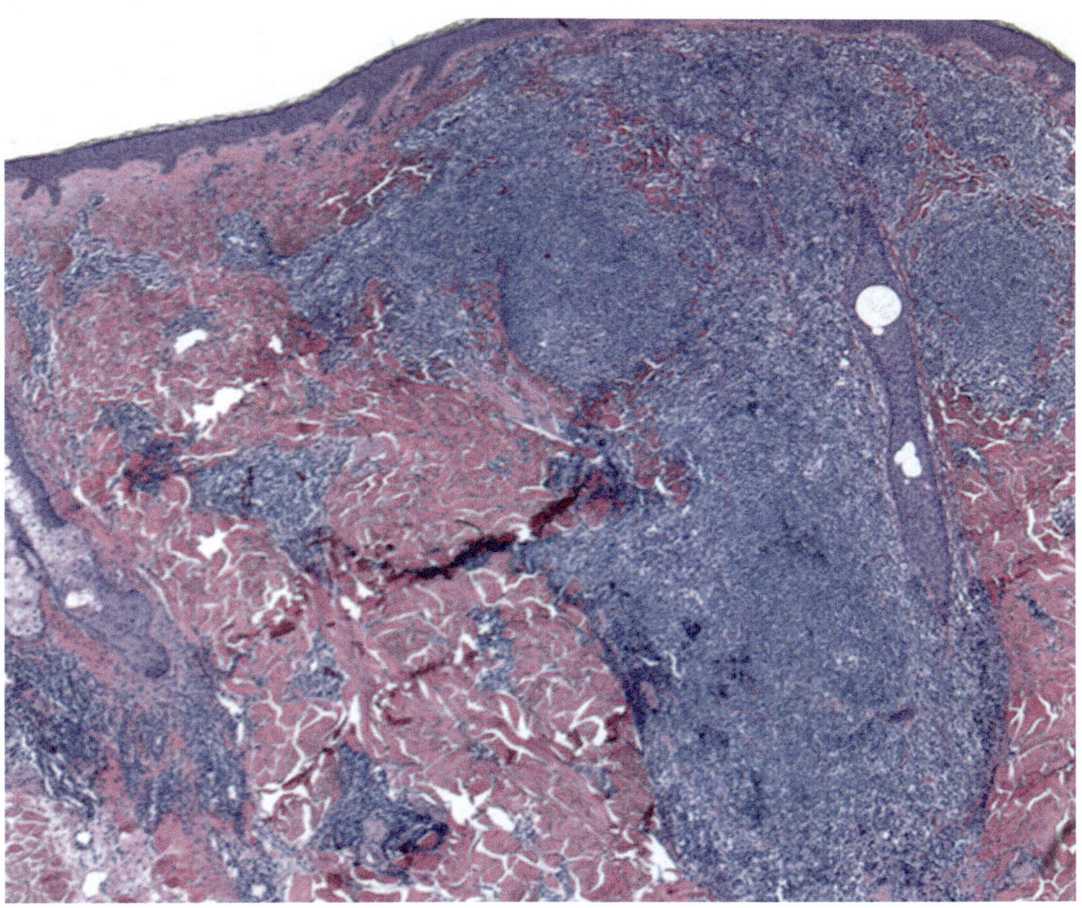

Fig. 9.1 Some cutaneous lymphoid infiltrates may exhibit perifollicular accentuation. What is the differential diagnosis for this pattern?

© Springer Nature Switzerland AG 2019

A. Subtil, *Diagnosis of Cutaneous Lymphoid Infiltrates*,

https://doi.org/10.1007/978-3-030-11654-5_9

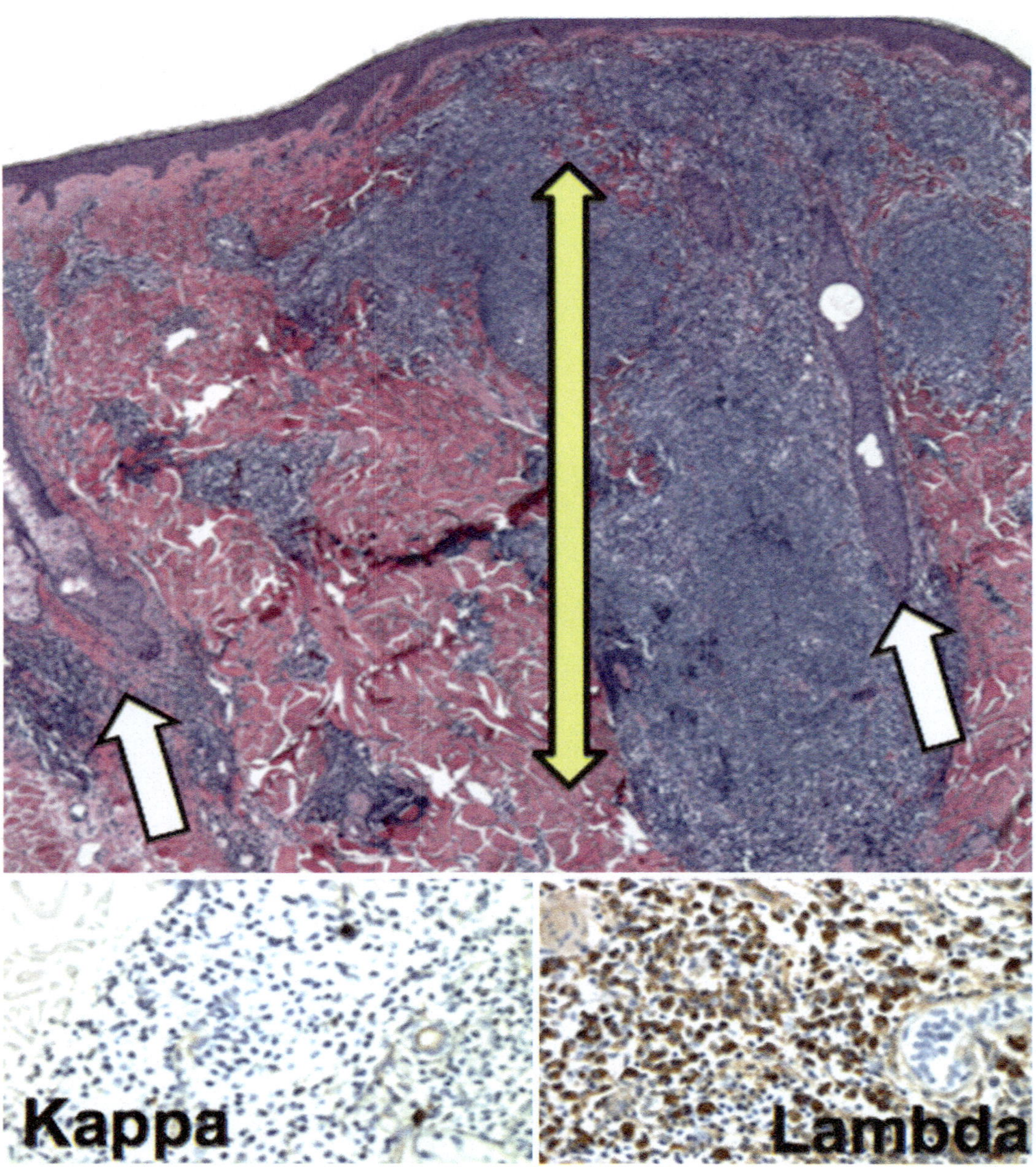

Fig. 9.2 Cutaneous marginal zone B-cell lymphoma showing perifollicular accentuation. A vertical orientation (yellow arrow) of the infiltrate resembling a column adjacent to a hair follicle (white arrow) is a common pattern. Immunoglobulin light chain stains demonstrate a marked predominance of lambda compared to that seen with kappa, consistent with a monotypic pattern

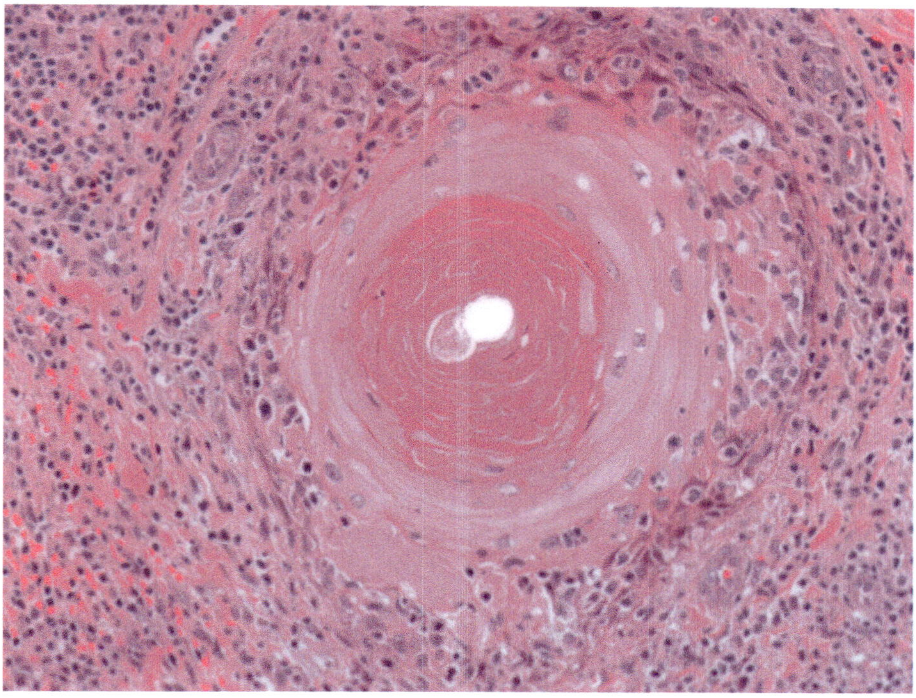

Fig. 9.3 Primary cutaneous aggressive epidermotropic CD8-positive cytotoxic T-cell lymphoma. Involvement of hair follicles is a common finding in this lymphoma

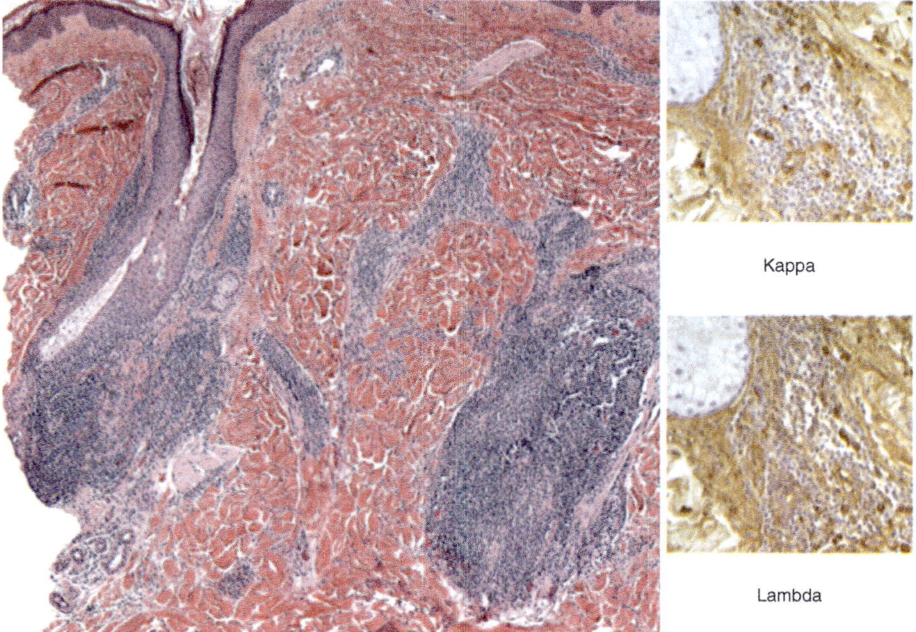

Fig. 9.4 Lymphomatoid drug eruption due to carbamazepine showing vertical orientation of the infiltrate adjacent to a hair follicle. Kappa and lambda immunoglobulin light chain stains demonstrate a polytypic pattern in scattered plasma cells

Some benign and malignant cutaneous lymphoid infiltrates may exhibit accentuation around hair follicles (Fig. 9.1 and Table 9.1). This perifollicular pattern may or may not be associated with disruption of follicular architecture and infiltration of the follicular epithelium by lymphocytes (folliculotropism). Sebaceous glands are often diminished. A perifollicular distribution may be the main pattern or may be associated with other histopathologic patterns.

Cutaneous marginal zone B-cell lymphoma frequently demonstrates vertical orientation of the lymphoplasmacytic infiltrate adjacent to hair follicles. This pattern resembles a blue column in the dermis (Fig. 9.2). Plasma cells are generally present at the periphery of the infiltrate, and monotypic expression of immunoglobulin light chain can be detected via immunohistochemistry or in situ hybridization.

Folliculotropic mycosis fungoides is a variant of mycosis fungoides showing tropism for hair follicles. There is prominent infiltration of the follicular epithelium by atypical lymphocytes. Disruption of follicular architecture is also present and may manifest in several forms: cystic change, follicular destruction with granuloma formation, telogen shift, and basaloid folliculolymphoid hyperplasia. Cases of folliculotropic mycosis fungoides with mucin deposition must be distinguished from primary benign follicular mucinosis.

Folliculotropism may also be identified in primary cutaneous aggressive epidermotropic CD8-positive cytotoxic T-cell lymphoma (Fig. 9.3). Correlation with clinical findings and identification of an immature cytotoxic alpha-beta CD8-positive T-cell phenotype would help distinguish this aggressive lymphoma from mycosis fungoides. Another condition to consider in this differential would be lymphomatoid papulosis (LyP), which may occasionally demonstrate a follicular pattern. A clinical presentation of self-regressing papules and CD30 expression would favor LyP.

Some benign dermatoses may also demonstrate lymphocytic infiltrates with perifollicular accentuation. Some cases of lymphomatoid drug eruption show vertical orientation of the infiltrate adjacent to a hair follicle reminiscent of marginal zone B-cell lymphoma. However, a polytypic pattern is present with kappa and lambda immunoglobulin light chain stains (Fig. 9.4).

Pseudolymphomatous folliculitis (PF) is a clinicopathologic variant of cutaneous pseudolymphoma and generally presents with a solitary lesion showing a dense dermal lymphohistiocytic infiltrate with follicular architecture disruption. PF classically lacks T-cell clonality and does not recur after excision. Herpes folliculitis may also show a dense dermal lymphocytic infiltrate. The presence of sebaceous gland necrosis is a clue to the diagnosis and should elicit searching for herpetic viral cytopathic effect within hair follicles.

Graft-versus-host disease and alopecia areata are also associated with perifollicular lymphocytic inflammation; however, the density of the infiltrate is quite mild. Discoid lupus erythematosus, lichen planopilaris, and lichen striatus exhibit more prominent lymphocytic interface inflammation (often in both epidermal and perifollicular distribution), but the degree is unlikely to raise the possibility of lymphoma. In contrast to folliculotropic mycosis fungoides, these entities lack prominent infiltration of the follicular epithelium by atypical lymphocytes. Arthropod bite reactions are also unlikely to raise the possibility of lymphoma; however, the density of the infiltrate may occasionally be denser than usual. Persistent nodular scabies may occasionally exhibit folliculotropism. Careful clinical correlation will prove helpful to prevent misdiagnosis.

Table 9.1 Differential diagnosis of cutaneous lymphocytic infiltrates with perifollicular accentuation

Lymphomas/lymphoproliferative disorders	Benign dermatoses
Cutaneous marginal zone B-cell lymphoma	Lymphomatoid drug eruption
Folliculotropic mycosis fungoides	Pseudolymphomatous folliculitis
Follicular lymphomatoid papulosis	Primary follicular mucinosis
Primary cutaneous aggressive epidermotropic CD8-positive cytotoxic T-cell lymphoma	Arthropod bite reaction (including persistent nodular scabies)
	Herpes folliculitis
	Lichen striatus
	Lupus erythematosus
	Lichen planopilaris
	Alopecia areata
	Graft-versus-host disease
	Infundibulofolliculitis

Pearls and Pitfalls
1. The involved hair follicle may not be present in a particular histological section. Serial sections are generally necessary in conditions with follicular involvement.
2. A perifollicular pattern may or may not be associated with disruption of follicular architecture and infiltration of the follicular epithelium by atypical lymphocytes (folliculotropism).

Suggested Reading

Arai E, Okubo H, Tsuchida T, et al. Pseudolymphomatous folliculitis: a clinicopathologic study of 15 cases of cutaneous pseudolymphoma with follicular invasion. Am J Surg Pathol. 1999;23(11):1313–9.

Brown HA, Gibson LE, Pujol RM, et al. Primary follicular mucinosis: long-term follow-up of patients younger than 40 years with and without clonal T-cell receptor gene rearrangement. J Am Acad Dermatol. 2002;47(6):856–62.

Gerami P, Guitart J. The spectrum of histopathologic and immunohistochemical findings in folliculotropic mycosis fungoides. Am J Surg Pathol. 2007;31(9):1430–8.

Kempf W, Kazakov DV, Baumgartner HP, et al. Follicular lymphomatoid papulosis revisited: a study of 11 cases, with new histopathological findings. J Am Acad Dermatol. 2013;68(5):809–16.

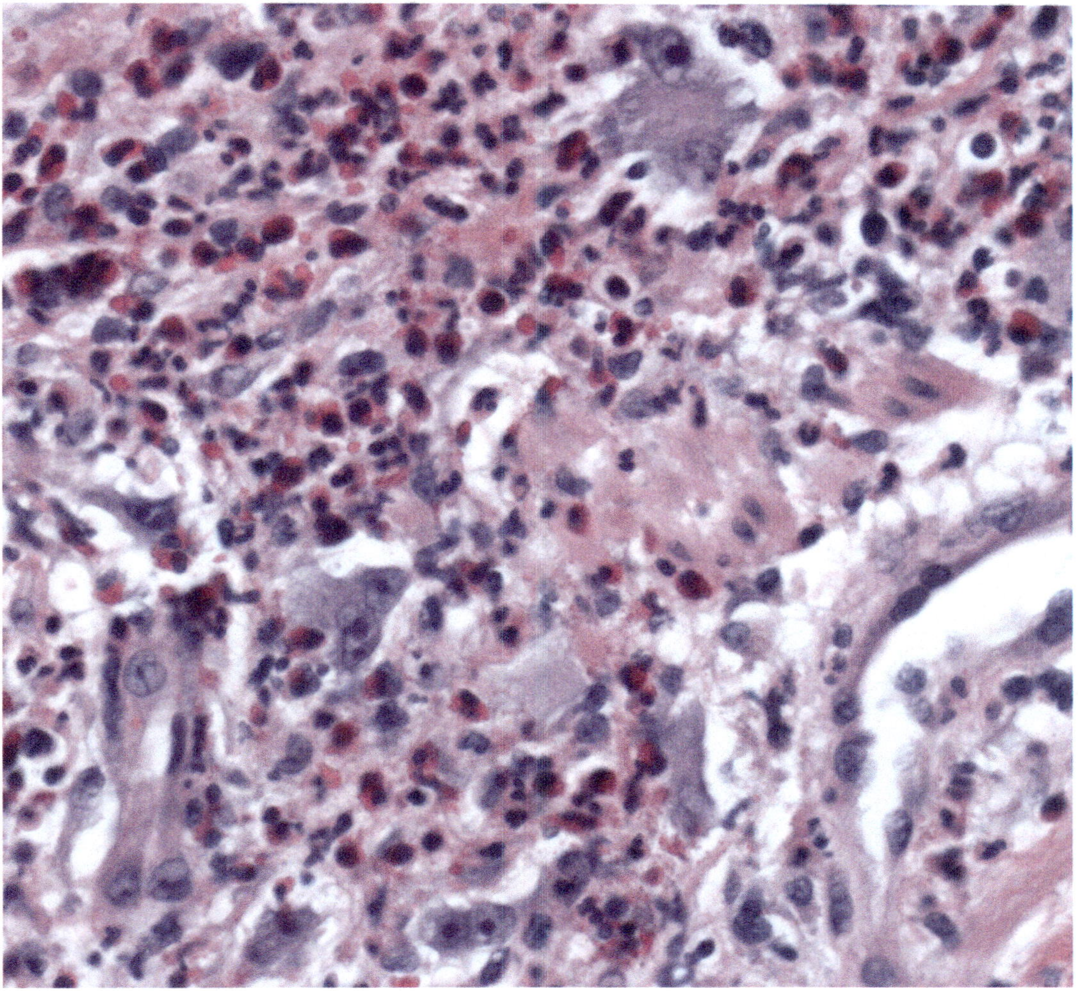

Fig. 10.1 This skin biopsy shows an atypical lymphoid infiltrate with frequent eosinophils. What is the differential diagnosis for this histopathologic pattern?

© Springer Nature Switzerland AG 2019

A. Subtil, *Diagnosis of Cutaneous Lymphoid Infiltrates*,

https://doi.org/10.1007/978-3-030-11654-5_10

Fig. 10.2
Lymphomatoid
papulosis (type A)
showing atypical large
lymphoid cells admixed
with a mixed dermal
inflammatory infiltrate
including prominent
eosinophils and
neutrophils. The large
atypical cells are
immunoreactive with
CD30 stain

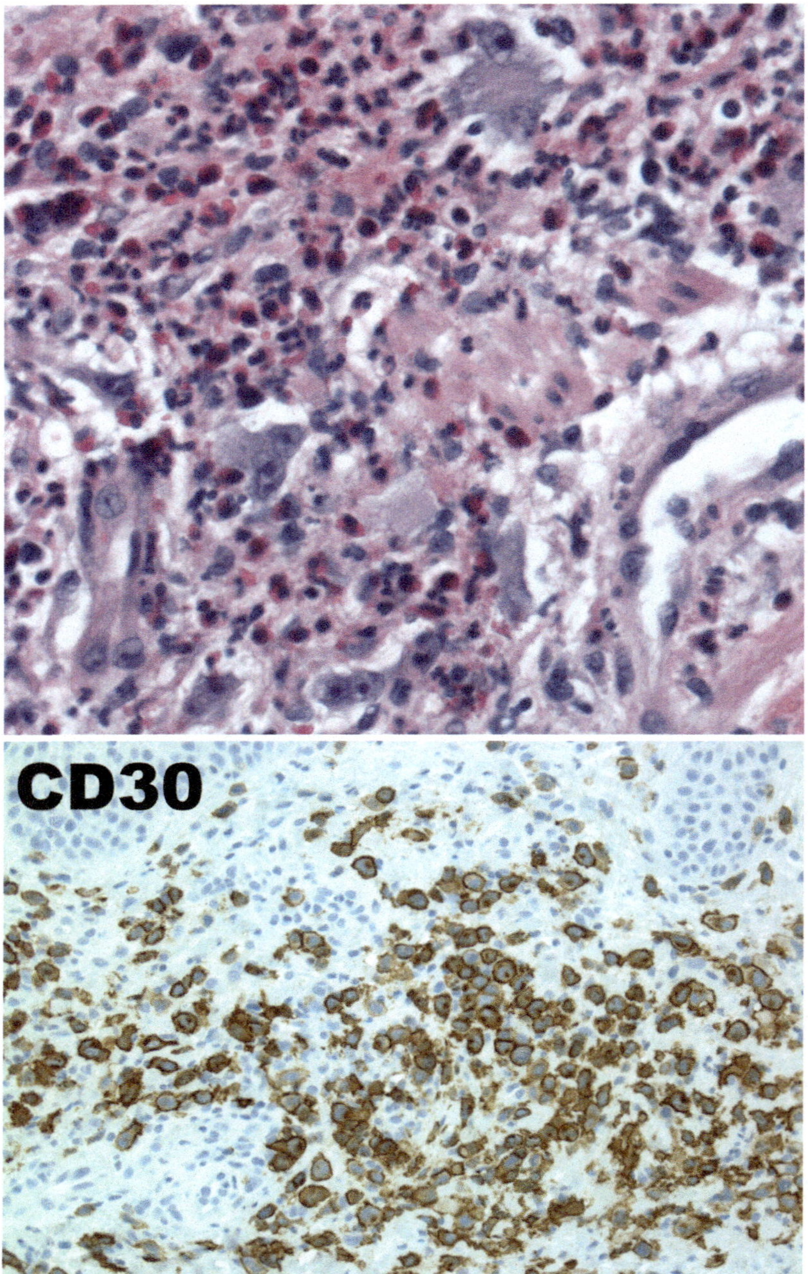

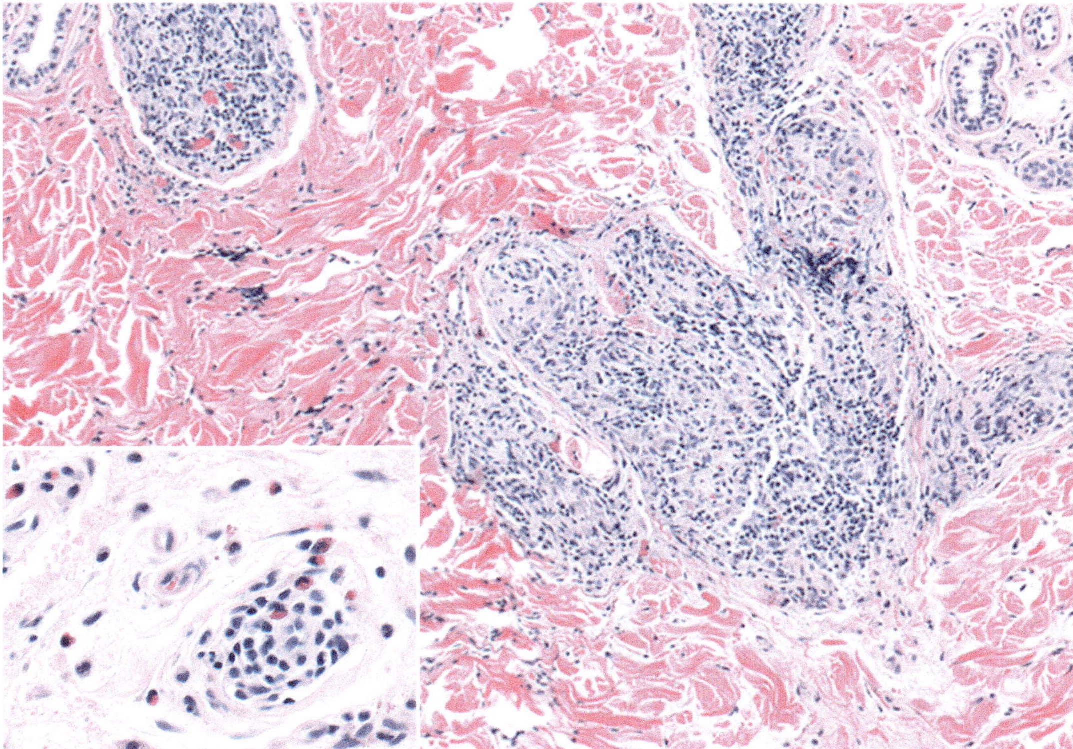

Fig. 10.3 Exaggerated arthropod bite-like reaction in a patient with systemic low-grade B-cell lymphoma. Dermal inflammatory infiltrate with small lymphocytes and prominent eosinophils

Eosinophils are frequently found in a variety of common reactive cutaneous inflammatory infiltrates, such as drug eruptions, arthropod bite reactions, urticaria, and immunobullous disorders. In cutaneous pseudolymphomas, the inflammatory infiltrate is generally denser (thus mimicking lymphoma); however, eosinophils are also frequently present. Examples would include cutaneous reactive lymphoid hyperplasia, lymphomatoid drug eruption, and persistent arthropod bite reaction (including nodular scabies) (Table 10.1).

While eosinophils are generally associated with a reactive process, they may also be present in cutaneous lymphoproliferative disorders and lymphomas, particularly of T-cell origin. Lymphomatoid papulosis (LyP) is part of the spectrum of CD30-positive lymphoproliferative disorders. LyP type A is the most common histopathologic subtype and exhibits a mixed dermal inflammatory infiltrate including prominent eosinophils admixed with atypical large

lymphoid cells that mark with CD30 (Figs. 10.1 and 10.2).

Mycosis fungoides (MF) is the most common type of skin lymphoma and includes a variety of clinicopathologic stages and variants. While a prominent component of eosinophils would be unusual in early patch-stage MF, eosinophils (as well as plasma cells) are frequently found in plaque- and tumor-stage disease. Folliculotropic MF is a variant showing tropism for hair follicles. There is prominent infiltration of the follicular epithelium by atypical lymphocytes and disruption of follicular architecture. In addition, eosinophils are frequently present, sometimes in association with granulomatous inflammation.

Systemic B-cell lymphomas may occasionally be associated with a persistent, pruritic hypersensitivity-like reaction in the skin (exaggerated arthropod bite-like reaction/eosinophilic dermatosis of myeloproliferative disease). While lesions may occur at insect bite sites, a history of

Table 10.1 Differential diagnosis of cutaneous lymphoid infiltrates with frequent eosinophils

Lymphomas/lymphoproliferative disorders	Benign dermatoses/pseudolymphomas
Folliculotropic mycosis fungoides	Cutaneous reactive lymphoid hyperplasia
Plaque- and tumor-stage mycosis fungoides	Lymphomatoid drug eruption
Lymphomatoid papulosis, type A	Arthropod bite reaction (including persistent nodular scabies)
	Exaggerated arthropod bite-like reaction/eosinophilic dermatosis of myeloproliferative disease

bites may not be present. The most common association is chronic lymphocytic leukemia/small lymphocytic lymphoma, but this process can also be seen in patients with mantle cell lymphoma, follicular lymphoma (Fig. 10.3), and myelodysplastic syndromes.

> **Pearls and Pitfalls**
> 1. The presence of eosinophils in a skin biopsy does not exclude the possibility of cutaneous (T-cell) or systemic (B-cell) lymphoma.

Suggested Reading

Byrd JA, Scherschun L, Chaffins ML, et al. Eosinophilic dermatosis of myeloproliferative disease: characterization of a unique eruption in patients with hematologic disorders. Arch Dermatol. 2001;137(10):1378–80.

El Shabrawi-Caelen L, Kerl H, Cerroni L. Lymphomatoid papulosis: reappraisal of clinicopathologic presentation and classification into subtypes A, B, and C. Arch Dermatol. 2004;140:441–7.

Gerami P, Guitart J. The spectrum of histopathologic and immunohistochemical findings in folliculotropic mycosis fungoides. Am J Surg Pathol. 2007;31(9):1430–8.

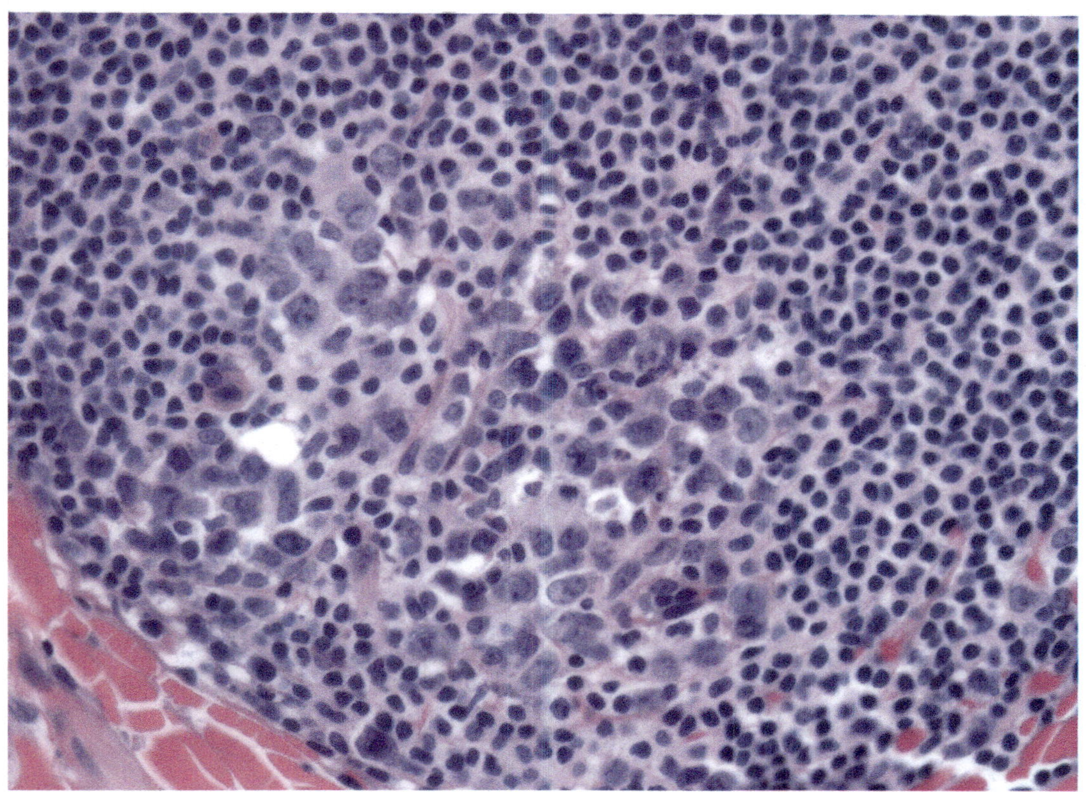

Fig. 11.1 What is the differential diagnosis of a cutaneous lymphoid infiltrate with lymphoid follicles?

© Springer Nature Switzerland AG 2019

A. Subtil, *Diagnosis of Cutaneous Lymphoid Infiltrates*,

https://doi.org/10.1007/978-3-030-11654-5_11

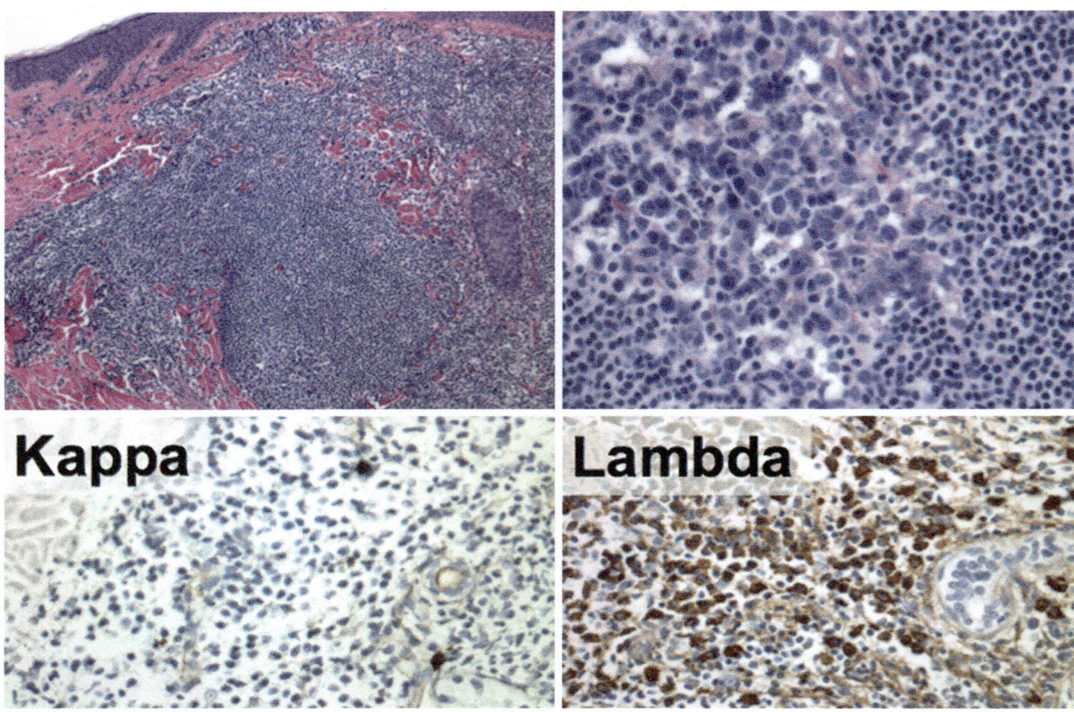

Fig. 11.2 Cutaneous marginal zone B-cell lymphoma. Nodular dermal lymphoid infiltrate with reactive lymphoid follicles and lambda-restricted plasma cells

Fig. 11.3 Cutaneous reactive lymphoid hyperplasia (pseudolymphoma). Reactive lymphoid follicles are well-spaced and show preserved mantle zones

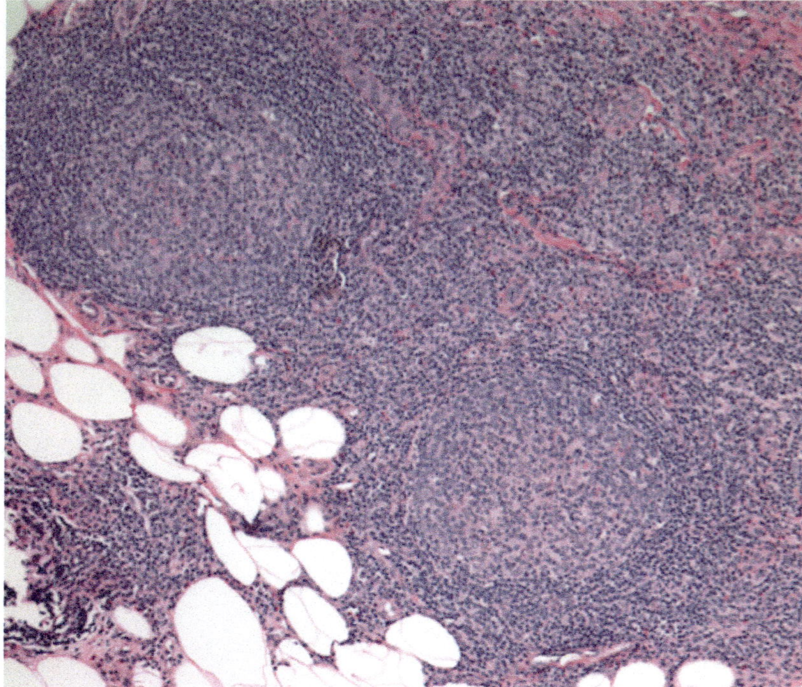

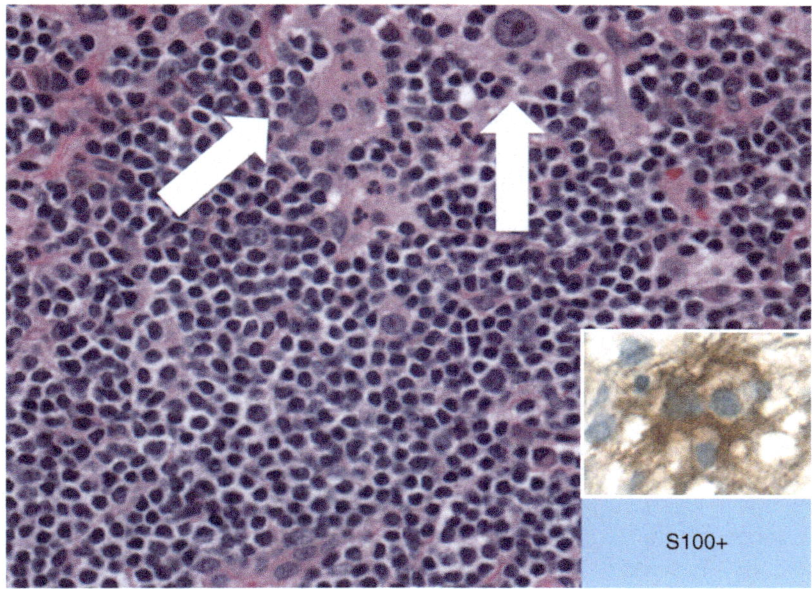

Fig. 11.4 Rosai-Dorfman disease. Dermal lymphoplasmacytic infiltrate with lymphoid follicles. Histiocytes show emperipolesis (arrows) and S100 expression (inset)

Fig. 11.5 Primary cutaneous follicle center lymphoma. Dense nodular lymphoid infiltrate showing crowded lymphoid follicles with diminished mantle zones

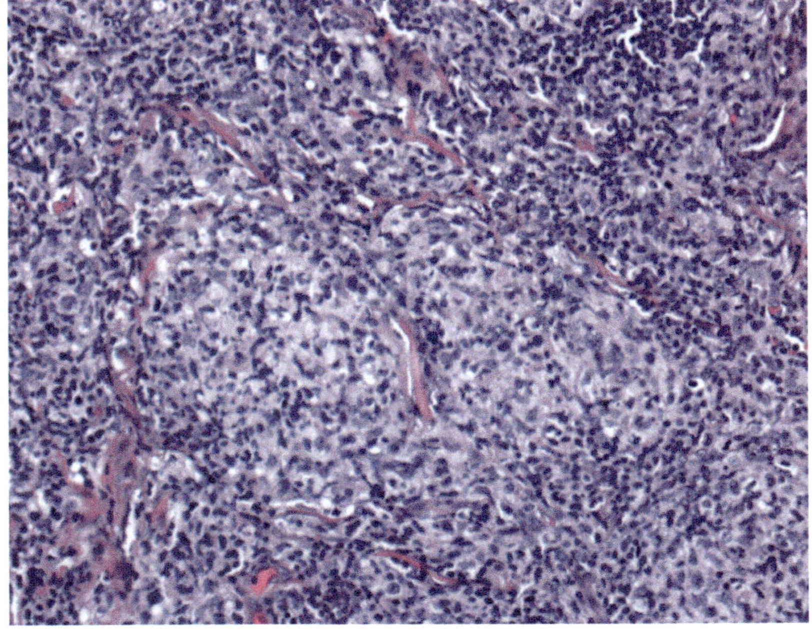

The presence of lymphoid follicles in a skin biopsy is always a pathologic finding (Figs. 11.1 and 11.2). Unlike tonsils, lymph nodes, or portions of the gastrointestinal tract, they are not native to the dermis and are not found in normal skin.

Several skin conditions may demonstrate significant lymphoid follicle formation, including reactive lymphoid hyperplasia (such as may occur due to vaccinations, arthropod bites, medications, and spirochetal infections, Fig. 11.3), cutaneous Rosai-Dorfman disease (Fig. 11.4), lupus panniculitis, and cutaneous IgG4-related disease. In addition, lymphoid follicles are frequently identified in low-grade cutaneous B-cell lymphomas (marginal zone lymphoma and follicle center lymphoma) and occasionally in tumor-stage mycosis fungoides.

As reviewed in Chap. 5, it is important to remember that lymphoid follicles can be reactive (benign) or neoplastic (malignant). In pseudolymphomas and in marginal zone lymphoma (Fig. 11.2), lymphoid follicles are reactive, while in follicle center (follicular) lymphoma (Fig. 11.5), lymphoid follicles are malignant and are composed of an admixture of neoplastic centrocytes and centroblasts (generally with a diminished component of the other cellular elements of the follicle).

Since lymphoid follicles are composed predominantly of B cells, their presence in a cutaneous infiltrate will be associated with prominent staining with CD20 and CD79a. While a prominent component of B cells might raise the possibility of a B-cell lymphoma, evaluation of other histomorphologic parameters is necessary to determine whether the infiltrate represents a specific type of skin lymphoma or a B-cell-predominant pseudolymphoma.

Lymphocytic infiltrates with prominent involvement of the subcutaneous adipose tissue occur in some entities such as lupus erythematosus panniculitis (LEP), subcutaneous panniculitis-like T-cell lymphoma, and some cases of gamma-delta T-cell lymphoma. The presence of lymphoid follicles would favor a diagnosis of LEP but may occasionally be found in some cases of lymphoma (Table 11.1).

Table 11.1 Differential diagnosis of cutaneous lymphoid infiltrates with lymphoid follicle formation

Reactive/lymphoproliferative disorders	Lymphomas
Cutaneous reactive lymphoid hyperplasia (such as may occur due to vaccinations, arthropod bites, medications, and spirochetal infections)	Primary cutaneous follicle center lymphoma
Cutaneous Rosai-Dorfman disease	Secondary cutaneous involvement by systemic/nodal follicular lymphoma
Cutaneous IgG4-related disease	Cutaneous marginal zone lymphoma
Lupus panniculitis	Some cases of tumor-stage mycosis fungoides

Pearls and Pitfalls
1. In pseudolymphomas and in marginal zone lymphoma, lymphoid follicles are reactive, while in follicle center (follicular) lymphoma, lymphoid follicles are neoplastic.
2. Lymphoid follicles in marginal zone lymphoma can be colonized by BCL2-positive neoplastic B cells and mimic BCL2-positive follicular lymphoma (ref. Chap. 20).

Suggested Reading

LeBlanc RE, Tavallaee M, Kim YH, et al. Useful parameters for distinguishing subcutaneous panniculitis-like T-cell lymphoma from lupus erythematosus panniculitis. Am J Surg Pathol. 2016 Jun;40(6):745–54.

Leinweber B, Colli C, Chott A, Kerl H, Cerroni L. Differential diagnosis of cutaneous infiltrates of B lymphocytes with follicular growth pattern. Am J Dermatopathol. 2004 Feb;26(1):4–13.

Subtil A. A general approach to the diagnosis of cutaneous lymphomas and pseudolymphomas. Cutaneous lymphomas (Subtil, ed.). Surg Pathol Clin. 2014;7(2):135–42. Elsevier: Philadelphia.

Fig. 12.1 This atypical cutaneous lymphoid infiltrate shows angiocentrism and necrosis. Two affected vessels are highlighted. What is the differential diagnosis for this pattern?

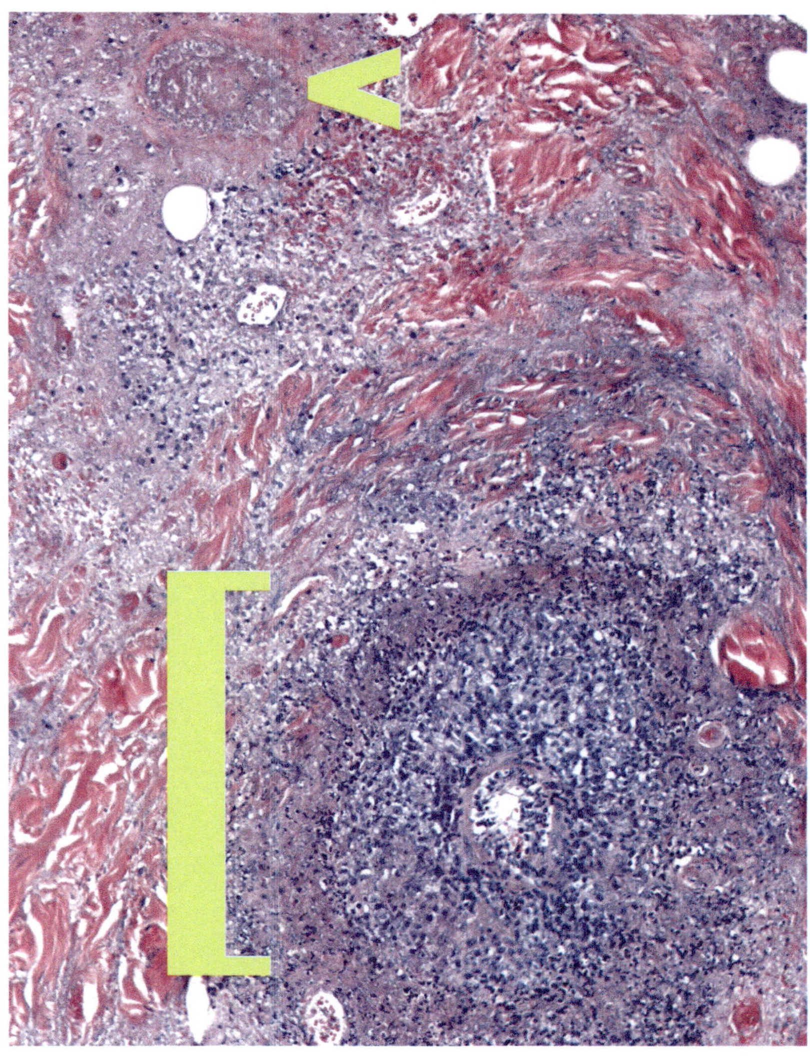

© Springer Nature Switzerland AG 2019
A. Subtil, *Diagnosis of Cutaneous Lymphoid Infiltrates*,
https://doi.org/10.1007/978-3-030-11654-5_12

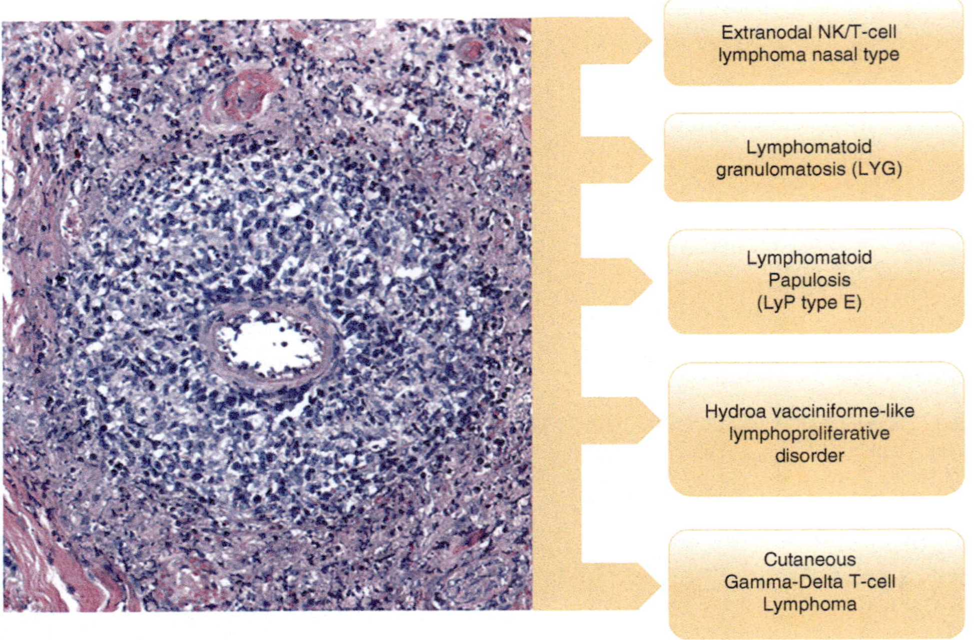

Fig. 12.2 Differential diagnosis of atypical lymphoid infiltrate with angiocentrism

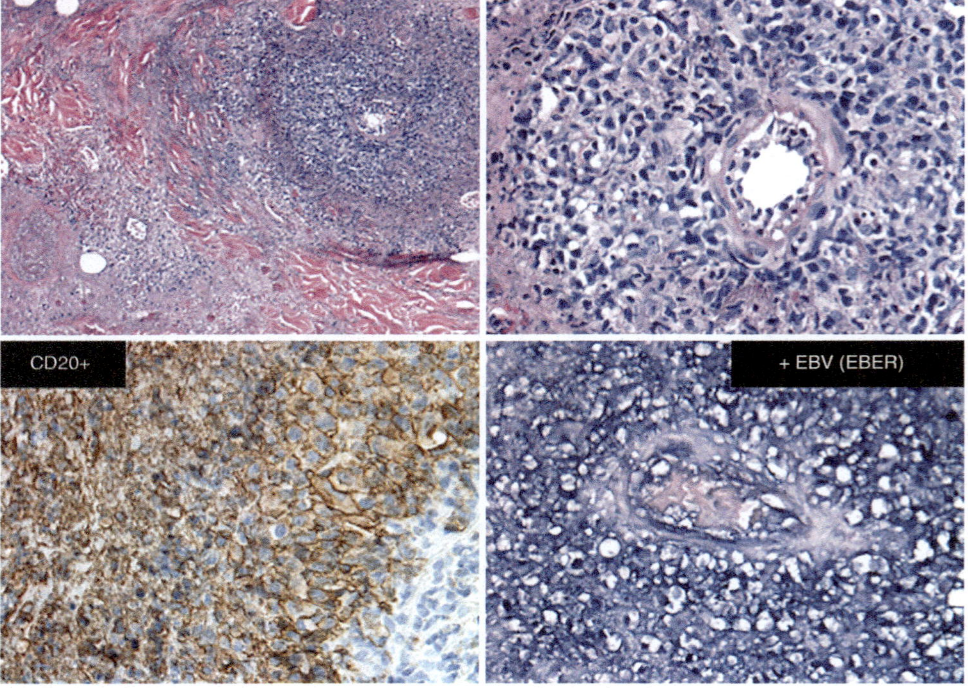

Fig. 12.3 Lymphomatoid granulomatosis. This skin biopsy shows an atypical lymphoid infiltrate with angiocentrism and necrosis. The large atypical lymphocytes infiltrating the blood vessel walls are predominantly CD20-positive B cells. EBV in situ hybridization is positive

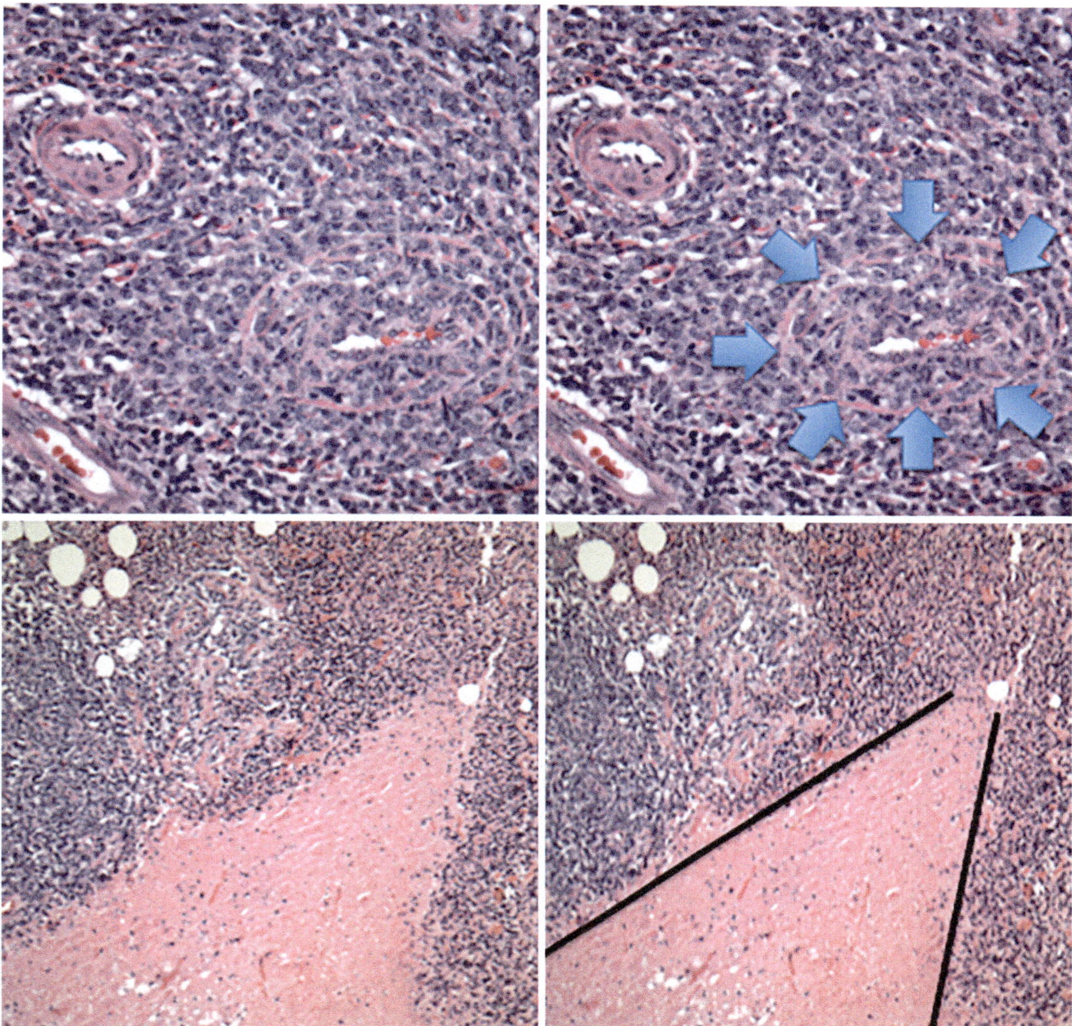

Fig. 12.4 Extranodal NK/T-cell lymphoma, nasal type. Angiocentrism is not always easily recognizable in a biopsy of an angioinvasive lymphoid process. Arrows highlight subtle infiltration of a blood vessel by atypical lymphocytes. An important clue for angiocentrism and angiodestruction is the presence of extensive, infarct-like necrosis (highlighted by lines)

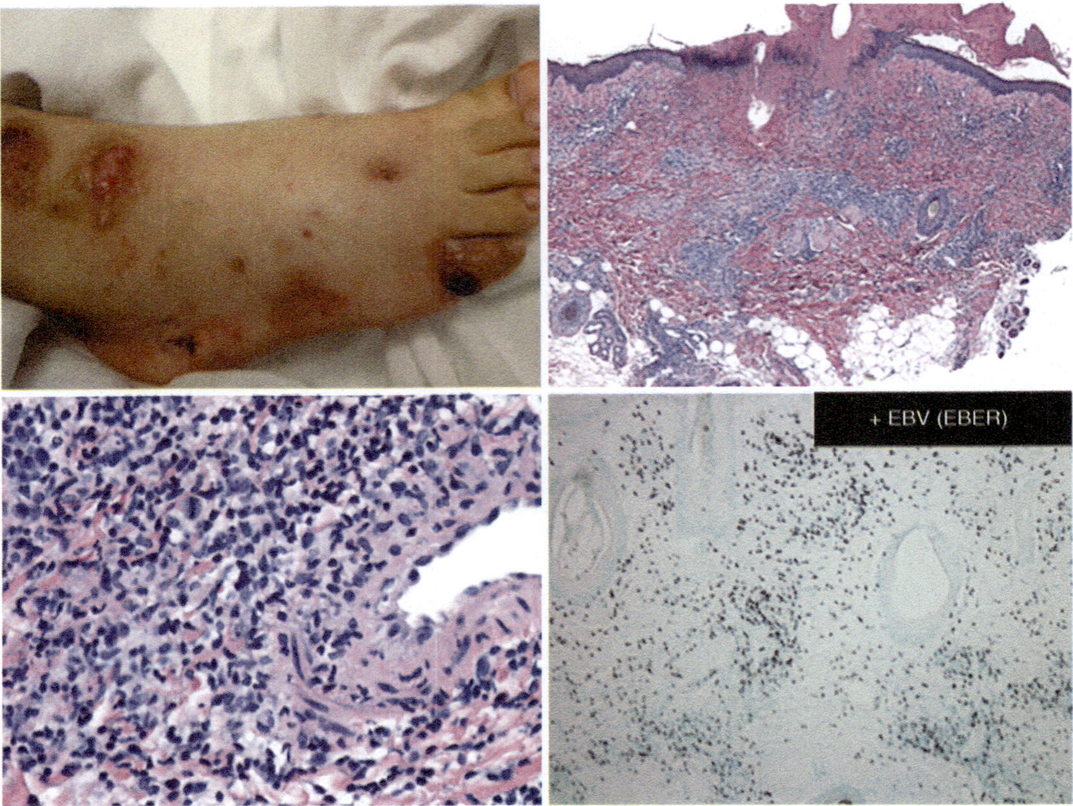

Fig. 12.5 This child with hydroa vacciniforme-like lymphoproliferative disorder initially presented with edema and ulcerated necrotic lesions on sun-exposed skin. Biopsy showed abrupt necrosis of epidermis and dermis in association with an atypical EBV-positive lymphoid infiltrate with angiocentrism

A cutaneous lymphoid infiltrate may occasionally demonstrate infiltration of blood vessel walls by atypical cells (Fig. 12.1). Angiodestruction and prominent necrosis are often present in this setting. Angiocentrism would raise the possibility of several disorders, many of which are associated with Epstein-Barr virus (Fig. 12.2).

Angioinvasion may be a feature of aggressive lymphomas, such as extranodal NK/T-cell lymphoma nasal type and gamma-delta T-cell lymphoma. However, it may also occur in an indolent process, such as angioinvasive lymphomatoid papulosis (LyP type E). Considering the disparate prognoses of the entities with an angiocentric pattern, it is critical to obtain comprehensive immunophenotyping, EBV in situ hybridization, and careful clinical correlation for accurate classification (Table 12.1).

While angiocentrism is generally a feature of entities with a NK- or T-cell immunophenotype, it may occur in a B-cell process, such as lymphomatoid granulomatosis (Fig. 12.3). LYG is an angiocentric lymphoproliferative disease involving extranodal sites (particularly the lung and skin) composed of EBV-positive B cells admixed with reactive T cells. There is a spectrum of histopathologic grade and clinical aggressiveness, which are related to the proportion of large B cells.

Extranodal NK/T-cell lymphoma, nasal type, most commonly involves the upper aerodigestive tract but frequently presents in the skin (Fig. 12.4). This EBV-positive angiodestructive malignant process is designated "NK/T" because the immunophenotype can be NK cell or cytotoxic T cell. Another EBV-positive condition

Table 12.1 Differential diagnosis of an atypical angiocentric lymphoid infiltrate in relation to Epstein-Barr virus (EBV) and immunophenotype

EBV	Angiocentric process	Immunophenotype
Positive (+)	Extranodal NK/T-cell lymphoma nasal type	T cell or NK cell
	Hydroa vacciniforme-like lymphoproliferative disorder	T cell or NK cell
	Lymphomatoid granulomatosis (LYG)	B cell
Negative (−)	Cutaneous gamma-delta T-cell lymphoma	Gamma-delta T cell
	Lymphomatoid papulosis (LyP type E)	CD30-positive T cell

with NK- or T-cell phenotype is hydroa vacciniforme-like lymphoproliferative disorder. This rare entity affects children and usually presents with ulcerated necrotic lesions on sun-exposed skin. Angiocentrism and necrosis are usually present (Fig. 12.5).

> **Pearls and Pitfalls**
> 1. Angiocentrism is not always present in a biopsy of an angioinvasive lymphoid process. Clues for the diagnosis would include infarct-like necrosis and cytotoxic immunophenotype. EBV in situ hybridization and careful clinical pathologic correlation would be essential for proper classification.
> 2. Infiltration and destruction of blood vessel walls is generally not a feature of intravascular lymphomas (atypical lymphocytes within vessel lumens).

Suggested Reading

Kempf W, Kazakov DV, Scharer L, et al. Angioinvasive lymphomatoid papulosis. A new variant simulating aggressive lymphomas. Am J Surg Pathol. 2013;37:1–13.

Song JY, Pittaluga S, Dunleavy K, et al. Lymphomatoid granulomatosis. A single institution experience: pathologic findings and clinical correlations. Am J Surg Pathol. 2015;39(2):141–56.

Swerdlow SH, et al., editors. WHO classification of tumors of hematopoietic and lymphoid tissues. Lyon: IARC; 2008.

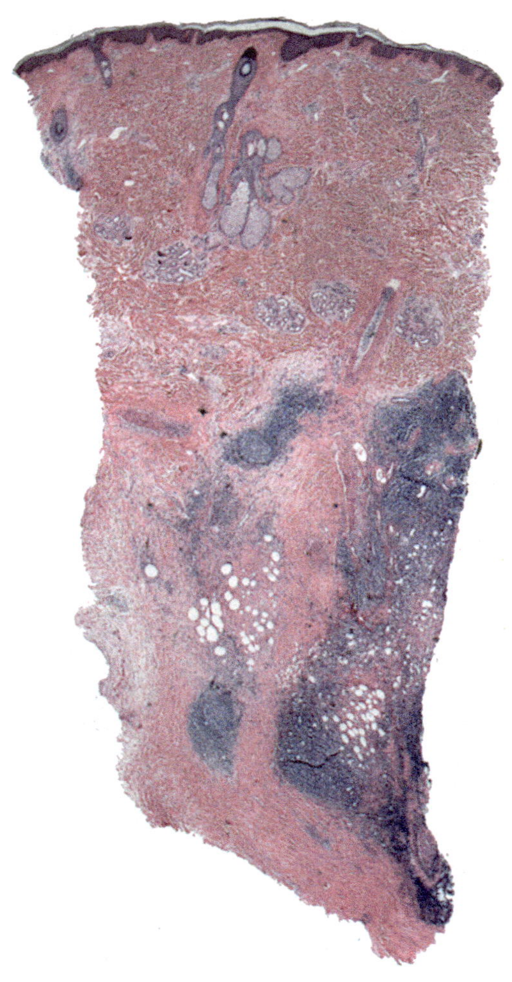

Fig. 13.1 What is the differential diagnosis of a pannicular lymphocytic infiltrate?

© Springer Nature Switzerland AG 2019
A. Subtil, *Diagnosis of Cutaneous Lymphoid Infiltrates*,
https://doi.org/10.1007/978-3-030-11654-5_13

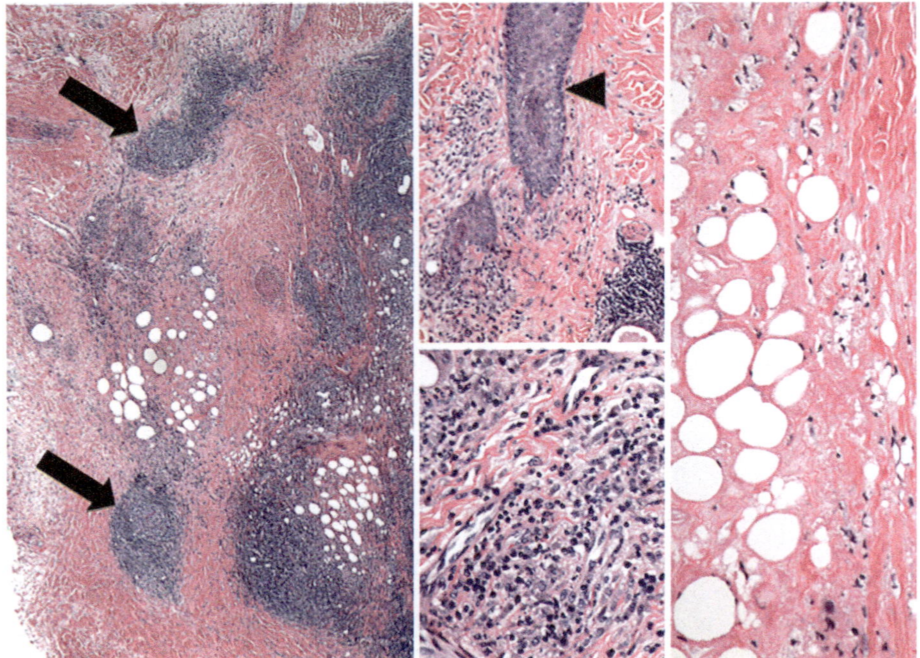

Fig. 13.2 Lupus erythematosus panniculitis. Lobular panniculitis composed predominantly of lymphocytes and plasma cells. Lymphoid follicles (arrows) and hyaline fat necrosis (right panel) are present. The overlying skin shows changes of discoid lupus erythematosus, including perifollicular (arrowhead) and perieccrine inflammation

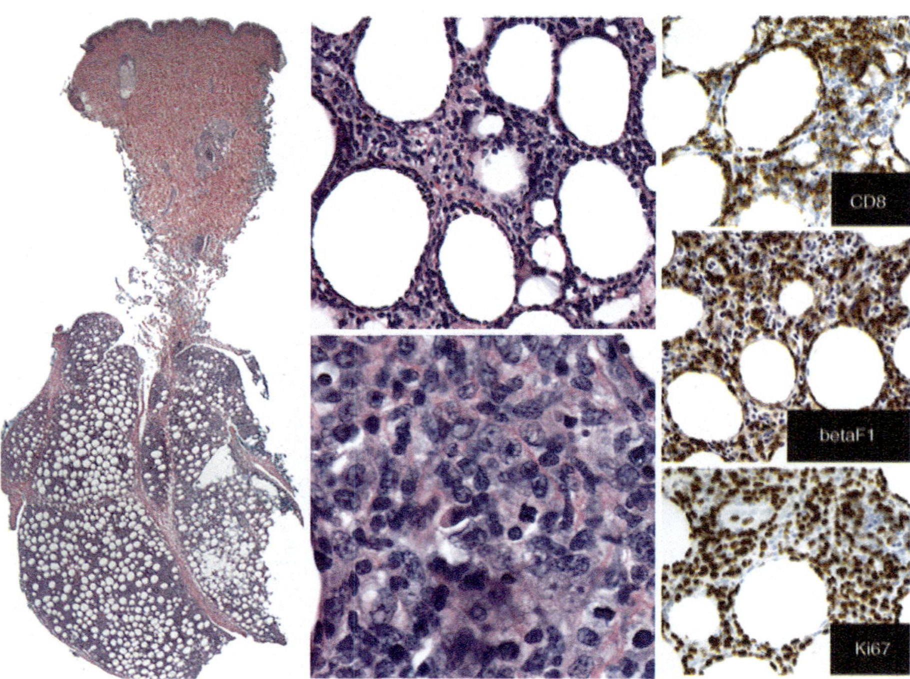

Fig. 13.3 Subcutaneous panniculitis-like T-cell lymphoma. Pannicular-based infiltrate of atypical lymphocytes with rimming of adipocytes. Mitotic figures and apoptosis are common. The infiltrate is composed of cytotoxic alpha-beta T cells (CD8+, TCRbetaF1+). There is a high proliferation rate with Ki-67 stain

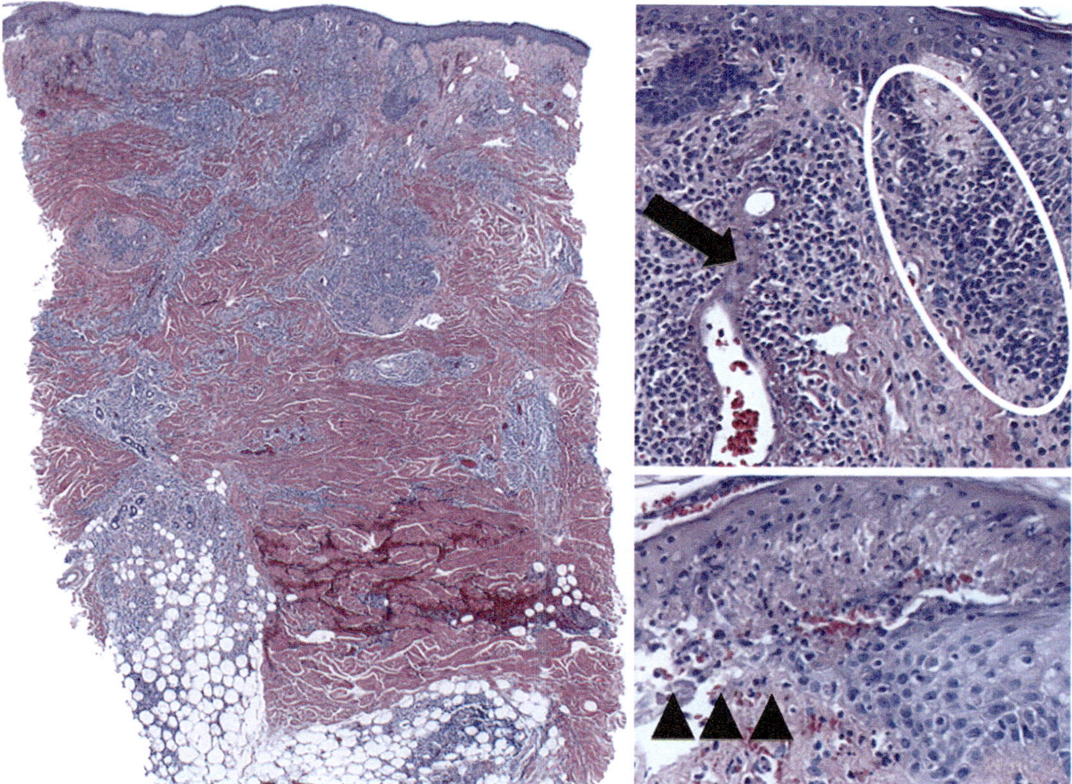

Fig. 13.4 Gamma-delta T-cell lymphoma involving all layers of the skin (epidermis, dermis, and panniculus). The epidermis shows intraepithelial atypical lymphocytes (circle) and ulceration (arrowheads). Vasculitic changes with fibrin deposition are present (arrow)

Some lymphocytic infiltrates show prominent involvement of the subcutaneous adipose tissue (Fig. 13.1). The entities in this differential diagnosis show marked differences in prognosis, and correct classification is essential for proper clinical management. Adequate sampling of the panniculus is important, and small or superficial biopsies are often nondiagnostic. Since the overlying skin may also show diagnostic clues, the biopsy of a pannicular infiltrate should also include epidermis and dermis.

Lupus erythematosus panniculitis (LEP) and subcutaneous panniculitis-like T-cell lymphoma (SPTCL) may demonstrate significant clinical and histopathologic overlap. In addition, a significant subset of patients with SPTCL has a history of autoimmune disease, particularly lupus. While the differential diagnosis for a pannicular lymphocytic infiltrate includes LEP and SPTCL, a few patients may have both entities. A prominent component of CD20-positive B cells (often forming CD21+ lymphoid follicles), plasma cells (CD79a+, CD138+), and plasmacytoid dendritic cells (CD123+) as well as hyaline fat necrosis would favor a diagnosis of LEP (Fig. 13.2). Lymphocytic atypia, adipocyte rimming by cytotoxic alpha-beta T cells (betaF1+, CD3+, CD4-, CD8+, CD56-, TIA1+), and an increased proliferation rate (overall Ki-67 index >20% and/or "hotspots" of lymphocytic aggregates with Ki-67 > 30%) would favor SPTCL (Fig. 13.3).

Gamma-delta T-cell lymphoma (GDTCL) is an important differential diagnosis in this setting. While SPTCL is an indolent lymphoma of alpha-beta T cells involving the panniculus, GDTCL is an aggressive lymphoma of gamma-delta T cells (betaF1−, CD3+, CD5−, CD4−, CD8−/+, CD56+, TIA1+) that may involve any combination of panniculus, dermis, and epidermis (Fig. 13.4). Ulceration and angiocentrism may also occur. Other lymphomas that may show variable involvement of the subcutaneous adipose tissue include tumor-stage mycosis fungoides and diffuse large B-cell lymphoma, leg type.

Besides LEP, other benign conditions and indolent lymphoproliferative disorders may also demonstrate pannicular infiltrates including lymphocytes (Table 13.1). The differential diagnosis would also include necrobiosis lipoidica, morphea, cold panniculitis, and Rosai-Dorfman disease. Careful evaluation of clinical and histopathologic findings is essential for accurate diagnosis.

Table 13.1 Differential diagnosis of lymphocytic infiltrates with pannicular involvement

Lymphomas	Benign conditions/indolent lymphoproliferative disorders
Subcutaneous panniculitis-like T-cell lymphoma	Lupus erythematosus panniculitis
Gamma-delta T-cell lymphoma	Rosai-Dorfman disease
Tumor-stage mycosis fungoides	Cold panniculitis
Diffuse large B-cell lymphoma, leg type	Morphea
	Necrobiosis lipoidica

Pearls and Pitfalls

1. Subcutaneous lymphomas often demonstrate patchy distribution in the panniculus. Therefore, a large and deep specimen is generally necessary for diagnosis.
2. Manuscripts published prior to the 2005 WHO-EORTC classification include gamma-delta T-cell lymphomas in the subcutaneous panniculitis-like T-cell lymphoma category (beware of marked differences in prognosis).

Suggested Reading

LeBlanc RE, Tavallaee M, Kim YH, et al. Useful parameters for distinguishing subcutaneous panniculitis-like T-cell lymphoma from lupus erythematosus panniculitis. Am J Surg Pathol. 2016;40(6):745–54.

Pincus LB, Leboit PE, McCalmont TH, et al. Subcutaneous Panniculitis-like T-cell lymphoma with overlapping clinicopathologic features of lupus erythematosus: coexistence of 2 entities? Am J Dermatopathol. 2009;31:520–6.

Swerdlow SH, et al., editors. WHO classification of tumors of hematopoietic and lymphoid tissues. Lyon: IARC; 2008.

Willemze R, Jaffe ES, Burg G, et al. WHO-EORTC classification for cutaneous lymphomas. Blood. 2005;105:3768–85.

Differential Diagnosis of Large Cell Infiltrate

14

Fig. 14.1 This skin biopsy shows an atypical large cell lymphoid infiltrate. What is the differential diagnosis?

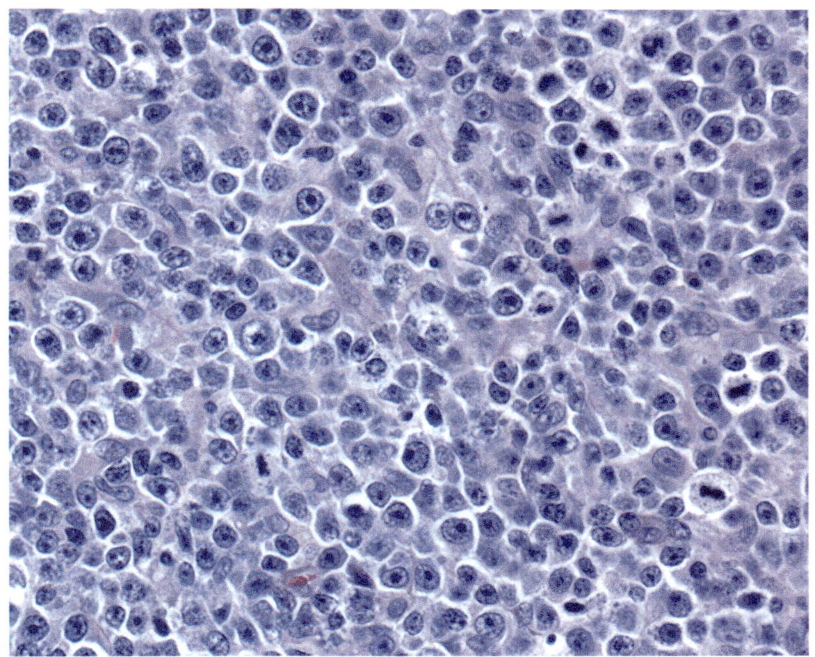

A. Subtil, *Diagnosis of Cutaneous Lymphoid Infiltrates*,
https://doi.org/10.1007/978-3-030-11654-5_14

Fig. 14.2 Differential diagnosis of atypical cutaneous large cell lymphoid infiltrate

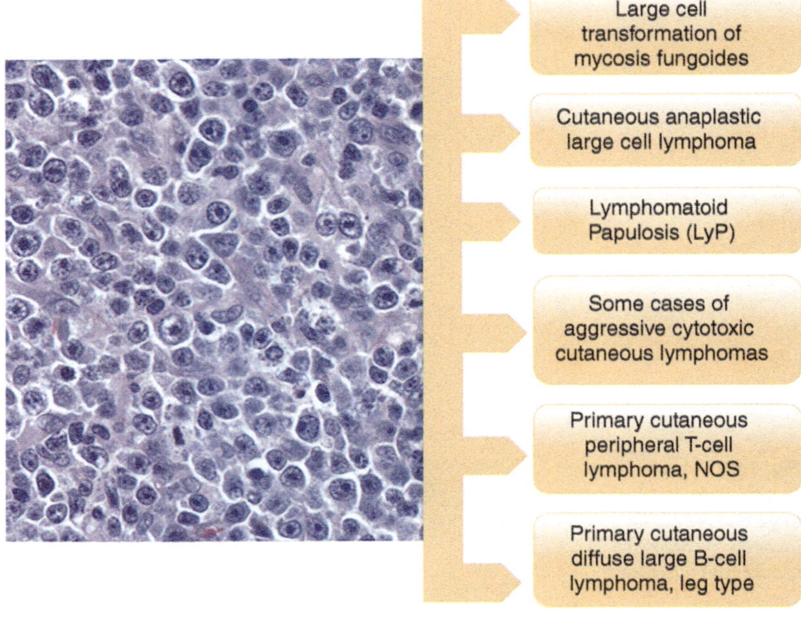

Fig. 14.3 Lymphomatoid papulosis. Large atypical lymphocytes admixed with inflammatory cells, predominantly neutrophils

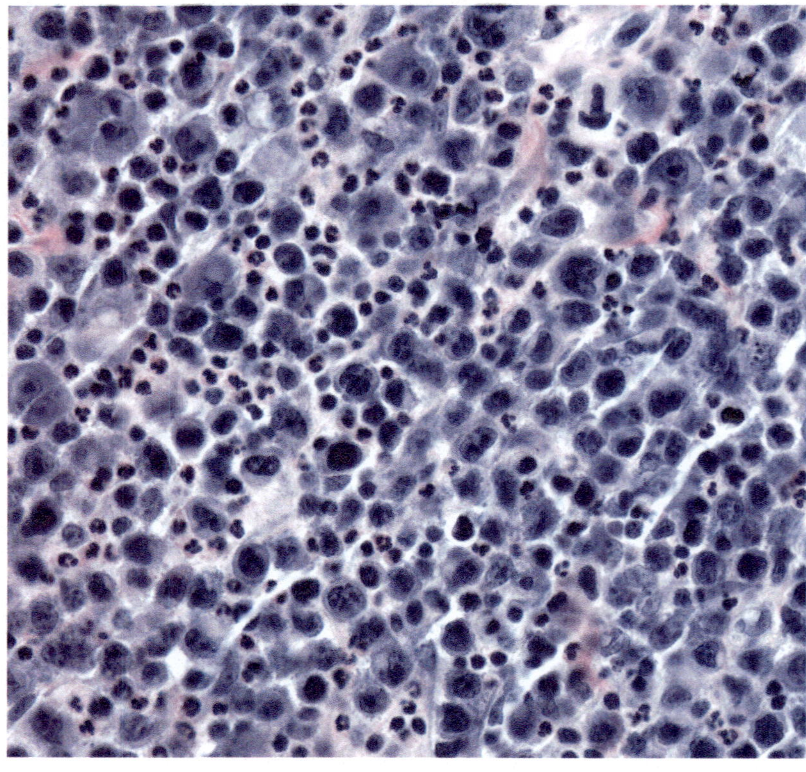

Fig. 14.4 Primary cutaneous diffuse large B-cell lymphoma, leg type. Dense diffuse dermal infiltrate of large lymphocytes. Most atypical cells show immunoblastic cytomorphology with large noncleaved nucleus with prominent central nucleolus. Mitotic figures are frequent

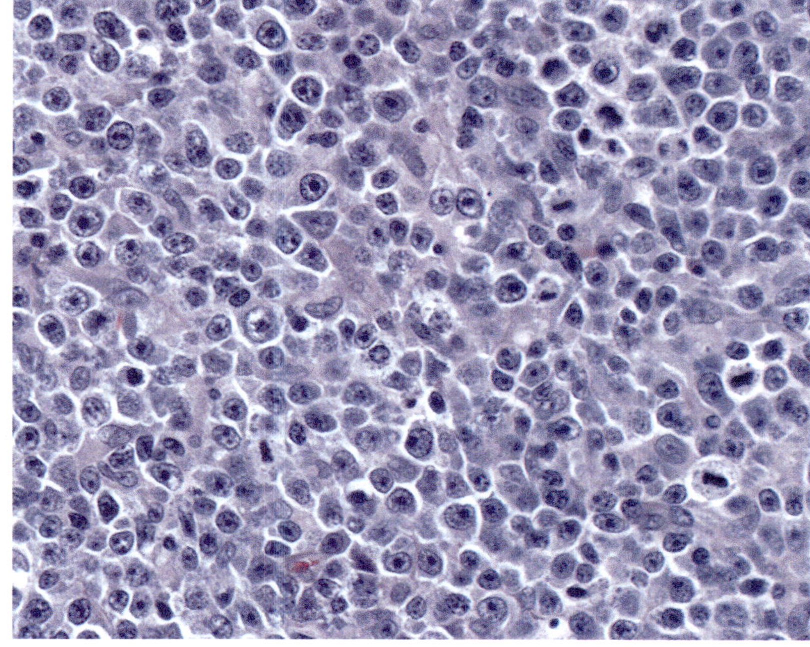

Fig. 14.5 Extranodal NK/T-cell lymphoma, nasal type. Some cases of aggressive cytotoxic cutaneous lymphomas may exhibit large cell infiltrates. Subtle infiltration of blood vessel wall (angiocentrism) is present in the lower half of the figure

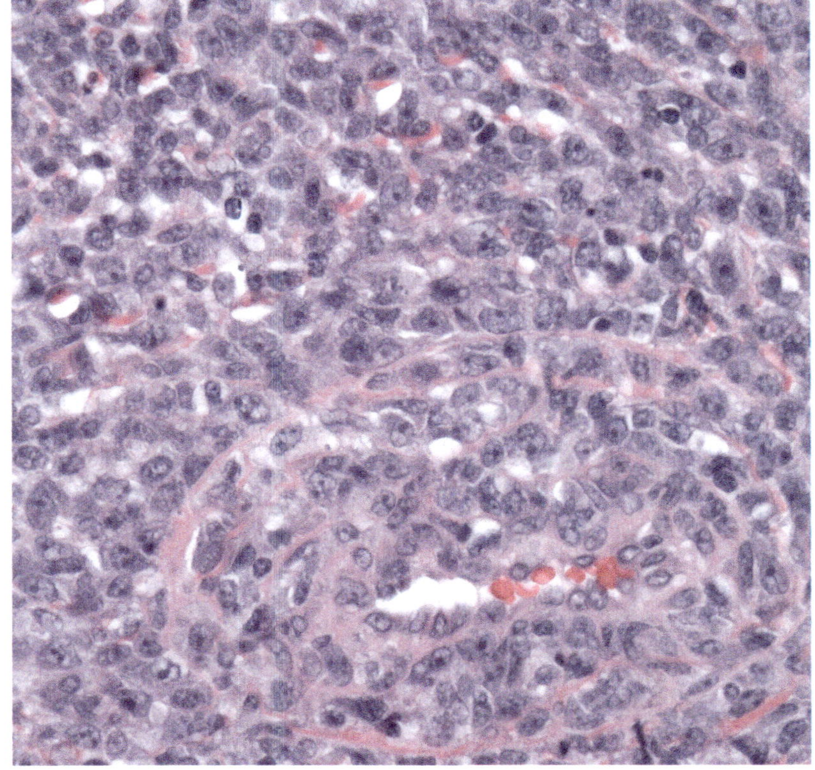

The majority of cutaneous lymphoid infiltrates are composed of small- and/or intermediate-sized lymphocytes. While less common, a large cell-predominant infiltrate (Fig. 14.1) raises an important differential diagnosis, including several aggressive lymphomas. However, indolent conditions such as CD30-positive lymphoproliferative disorders should also be considered (Fig. 14.2 and Table 14.1).

The minimum proportion of large cells in an atypical cutaneous large cell lymphoid infiltrate is rather small (less than one third). Large cell transformation of mycosis fungoides requires at least 25% of large atypical cells or formation of microscopic nodules of large cells. It is important not to overcall medium-sized cells with dense chromatin as large cells, which are defined as at least 4 times the size of a small lymphocyte and generally exhibit vesicular chromatin and conspicuous nucleoli. The category of primary cutaneous peripheral T-cell lymphoma, unspecified is used for rare cases of cutaneous T-cell lymphomas that do not fit into any of the better-defined subtypes of skin lymphomas (including provisional entities). This diagnosis of exclusion requires at least 30% large neoplastic cells of the total tumor cell population.

Cutaneous CD30-positive lymphoproliferative disorders are indolent conditions, in spite of the atypical histomorphology of large lymphoid cells. Some variants of lymphomatoid papulosis (LyP type C; Fig. 14.3) can mimic cutaneous anaplastic large cell lymphoma in the biopsy. Therefore, careful clinicopathologic correlation and/or close follow-up are generally necessary to correctly distinguish between these two ends of the CD30-positive lymphoproliferative spectrum.

Most of the conditions in the differential diagnosis of atypical cutaneous large cell lymphoid infiltrate are of T-cell origin. However, cutaneous B-cell infiltrates may rarely be composed of large cells. Primary cutaneous diffuse large B-cell lymphoma, leg type (Fig. 14.4) is composed of an admixture of immunoblasts (cells with large noncleaved nucleus and prominent central nucleolus) and centroblasts (cells with large noncleaved nucleus and multiple peripheral nucleoli). Unlike primary cutaneous follicle center lymphoma, follicular dendritic cell meshworks and centrocytes (small cleaved germinal center B cells) are absent.

Some cases of aggressive cytotoxic cutaneous lymphomas (such as extranodal NK/T-cell lymphoma, nasal type; Fig. 14.5) may demonstrate large cell infiltrates in the initial biopsy. It is important to include them in the differential diagnosis of large T-cell infiltrates. Since variable CD30 expression may occur in cytotoxic lymphomas, these aggressive cases may be misdiagnosed as anaplastic large cell lymphoma (an indolent process).

Table 14.1 Differential diagnosis of atypical large cell lymphoid infiltrate (>25–30% large cells)

Large cell transformation of mycosis fungoides
Cutaneous anaplastic large cell lymphoma
Lymphomatoid papulosis (LyP), type C
Some cases of aggressive cytotoxic cutaneous lymphomas
Primary cutaneous peripheral T-cell lymphoma, unspecified
Primary cutaneous diffuse large B-cell lymphoma, leg type

Pearls and Pitfalls

1. Immunoblasts (large noncleaved lymphocytes with central nucleolus) are often seen in inflammatory infiltrates due to viral infection, such as herpes folliculitis and inflamed molluscum contagiosum. However, the proportion of large cells in this setting is generally small. Identification of viral cytopathic effect would facilitate the diagnosis.

Suggested Reading

Subtil A. A general approach to the diagnosis of cutaneous lymphomas and pseudolymphomas. Cutaneous lymphomas (Subtil, ed.). Surg Pathol Clin. 2014;7(2):135–42. Elsevier: Philadelphia.

Swerdlow SH, et al., editors. WHO classification of tumors of hematopoietic and lymphoid tissues. Lyon: IARC; 2008.

Willemze R, Jaffe ES, Burg G, et al. WHO-EORTC classification for cutaneous lymphomas. Blood. 2005;105(10):3768–85.

Part III

Special Techniques

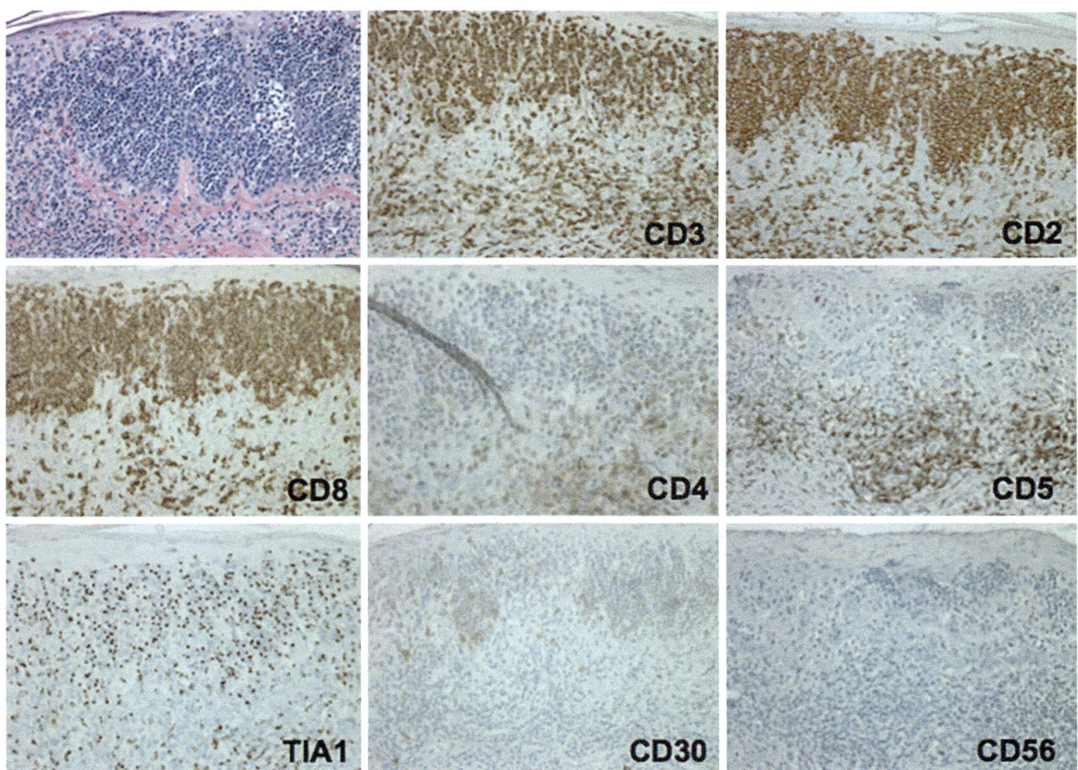

Fig. 15.1 Immunohistochemical stains are generally performed in the evaluation of a cutaneous lymphoid infiltrate. Which markers should be tested? What are the parameters for selecting initial and additional special stains?

© Springer Nature Switzerland AG 2019

A. Subtil, *Diagnosis of Cutaneous Lymphoid Infiltrates*,

https://doi.org/10.1007/978-3-030-11654-5_15

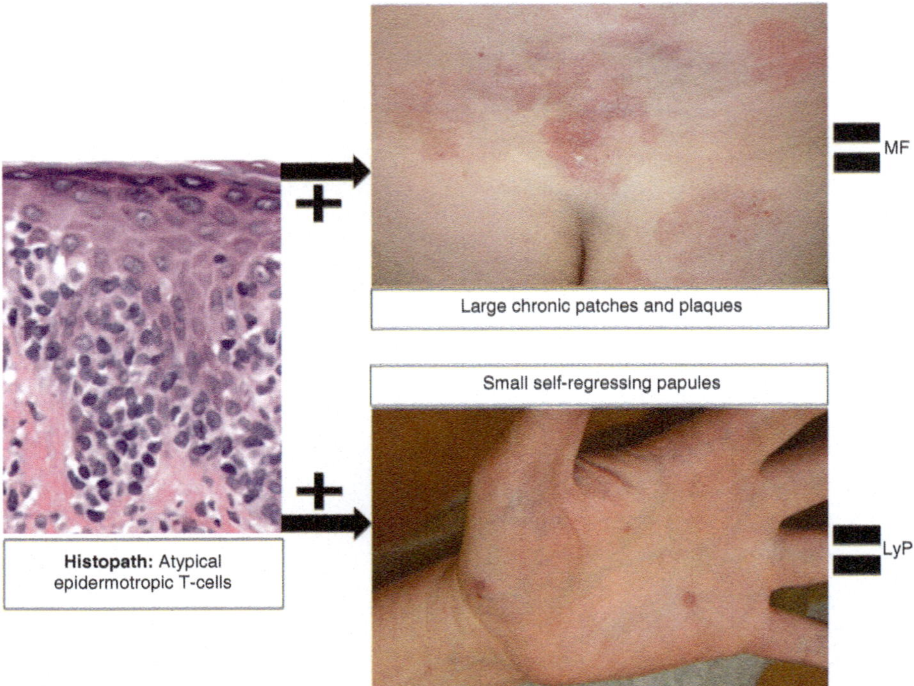

Fig. 15.2 Immunophenotyping (even when extensive) cannot replace the basic equation for the diagnosis of cutaneous lymphoid infiltrates: clinical pathologic correlation

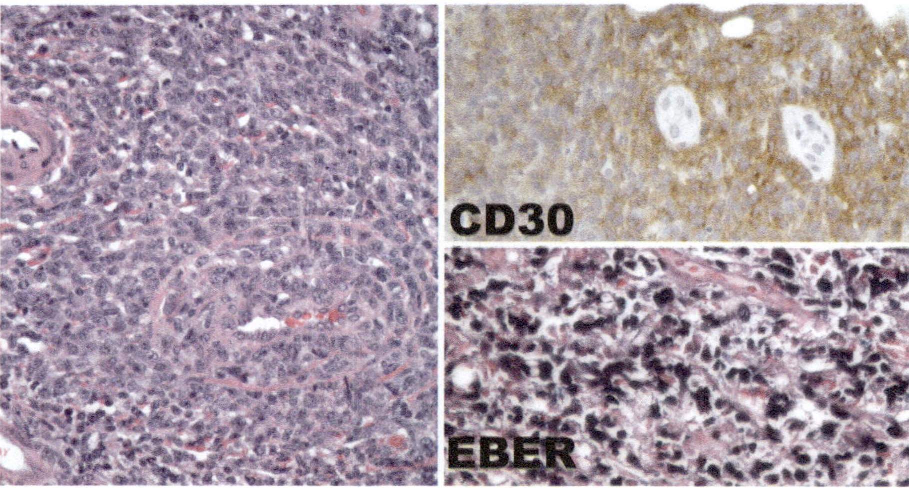

Fig. 15.3 Extranodal NK/T-cell lymphoma, nasal type. Some cases of aggressive cytotoxic lymphomas may exhibit variable CD30 expression (such as this example of extranodal NK/T-cell lymphoma, nasal type). However, the proportion of cells marking with CD30 stain is below the positivity threshold of 75% used for anaplastic large cell lymphoma (one of the cutaneous CD30-positive lym- phoproliferative disorders). Therefore, this infiltrate is classified as a CD30-negative process, despite the signifi- cant level of staining. Subtle infiltration of the walls of a blood vessel (angiocentrism) is present in the lower half of the figure. EBV in situ hybridization (EBER) is positive

Several immunohistochemical stains are generally performed in the evaluation of cutaneous lymphoid infiltrates (Fig. 15.1). However, the selection of stains varies significantly from case to case. Immunophenotyping (even when extensive) cannot replace the basic equation for the diagnosis of cutaneous lymphoid infiltrates: clinical pathologic correlation (Fig. 15.2). Therefore, immunostains should not be the starting point. The first step is to determine the differential diagnosis from the clinical pattern and the histomorphologic findings on hematoxylin and eosin-stained sections (pattern and composition of the infiltrate). The selection of immunostains will be based on that differential. A second (and occasionally a third) round of additional markers may be performed depending on the results of the initial stains (Tables 15.1, 15.2, 15.3, and 15.4).

It is also important to recognize that immunophenotype is not destiny. There are immunophenotypic variants of cutaneous lymphomas without significant prognostic differences (e.g., CD8-positive mycosis fungoides, gamma-delta mycosis fungoides, CD8-positive lymphomatoid papulosis, etc.). Therefore, correlation with clinical findings is invariably necessary for final classification. In addition, the classic staining pattern of different lymphomas is not always identified. Aberrant phenotype or unexpected absence of certain markers occurs frequently (e.g., up to 25% of mantle cell lymphomas lack CD5).

Table 15.1 Basic panel of initial markers in the evaluation of cutaneous lymphoid infiltrates (ordered in almost all cases)

CD3 (T cell)
CD20 (B cell) (add CD79a if history of rituximab treatment or if infiltrate is plasmacytoid or immunoblastic)
CD30
If plasma cells are present in the infiltrate: kappa and lambda

Table 15.2 Markers for the evaluation of cutaneous T-cell infiltrates

Initial panel (Table 15.1)
CD4
CD8
CD2
CD5
CD7
CD56
TIA-1 (cytotoxic marker)
If dense infiltrate: add Ki-67
If CD30+: add ALK and CD15
If CD8+, CD2-, CD7+: add CD45RA and CD45RO
If cytotoxic or angiocentric infiltrate: add EBV(EBER) ISH and betaF1 (+/− TCR gamma stain)

Table 15.3 Markers for the evaluation of cutaneous B-cell infiltrates

Initial panel (Table 15.1)
Kappa and lambda
CD21
Bcl-2
Bcl-6
Ki-67
CD5
CD10
CD23
CD43
Cyclin D1
MUM1
If high-grade/large cell infiltrate: add MYC, ALK, HHV8, TdT

Table 15.4 Initial markers for the evaluation of leukemia cutis

CD3 (T cell)
CD79a (B cell)
CD30
CD43 (T cell and myeloid)
Myeloperoxidase (MPO)
TdT (B and T lymphoblastic)

Pearls and Pitfalls

1. The more stains are performed, the higher the chance that a given stain might not have worked and would need to be repeated. Recognition of technical problems is critically important in the interpretation of special stains. Careful examination of the composition and cytomorphology of the infiltrate may be helpful. For example, if follicular dendritic cells (large noncleaved nucleus with fine vesicular chromatin and conspicuous central nucleolus, often in small clusters) are identified in the infiltrate, CD21 and/or CD23 should show some positivity (otherwise, these stains did not work and should be repeated).

2. The threshold of positivity is variable for different markers. For example, for anaplastic large cell lymphoma (ALCL; one of the cutaneous CD30-positive lymphoproliferative disorders), CD30 must be positive in at least 75% of atypical cells (i.e., even if 60% of an infiltrate marks with CD30, that level of staining is not sufficient for ALCL, and other entities should be considered in the differential diagnosis; Fig. 15.3). A high cutoff is also used for CD56 (i.e., if only a small subset of cells stain with CD56 in a lymphoid infiltrate, that process is considered CD56-negative).

3. Tissue immunohistochemistry results often do not perfectly match flow cytometry results. For example, it is common for an acute myeloid leukemia to be CD34-positive in peripheral blood flow cytometry while not marking with CD34 immunostain in a biopsy of leukemia cutis. This frequent mismatch may be multifactorial (e.g., greater sensitivity of flow cytometry in detecting dim expression, use of different antibodies with different epitope targets, downregulation of certain proteins during the process of tissue infiltration).

4. If plasma cells are present in a cutaneous lymphoid infiltrate, do not forget to check kappa and lambda immunoglobulin light chains (via immunohistochemistry or in situ hybridization; Table 15.1). Cutaneous marginal zone lymphoma often exhibits mixed infiltrates (T-cell-rich or with reactive lymphoid follicles) and may be misdiagnosed as reactive lymphoid hyperplasia if kappa and lambda are not performed.

Suggested Reading

Higgins RA, Blankenship JE, Kinney MC. Application of immunohistochemistry in the diagnosis of non-Hodgkin and Hodgkin lymphoma. Arch Pathol Lab Med. 2008;132:441–61.

Hodak E, David M, Maron L, et al. CD4/CD8 double-negative epidermotropic cutaneous T-cell lymphoma: an immunohistochemical variant of mycosis fungoides. J Am Acad Dermatol. 2006;55:276–84.

Swerdlow SH, Campo E, Harris NL, et al., editors. WHO classification of tumors of hematopoietic and lymphoid tissues. Lyon: IARC; 2008.

Fig. 16.1 This atypical epidermotropic T-cell infiltrate is CD8-positive. Is this an aggressive or indolent process?

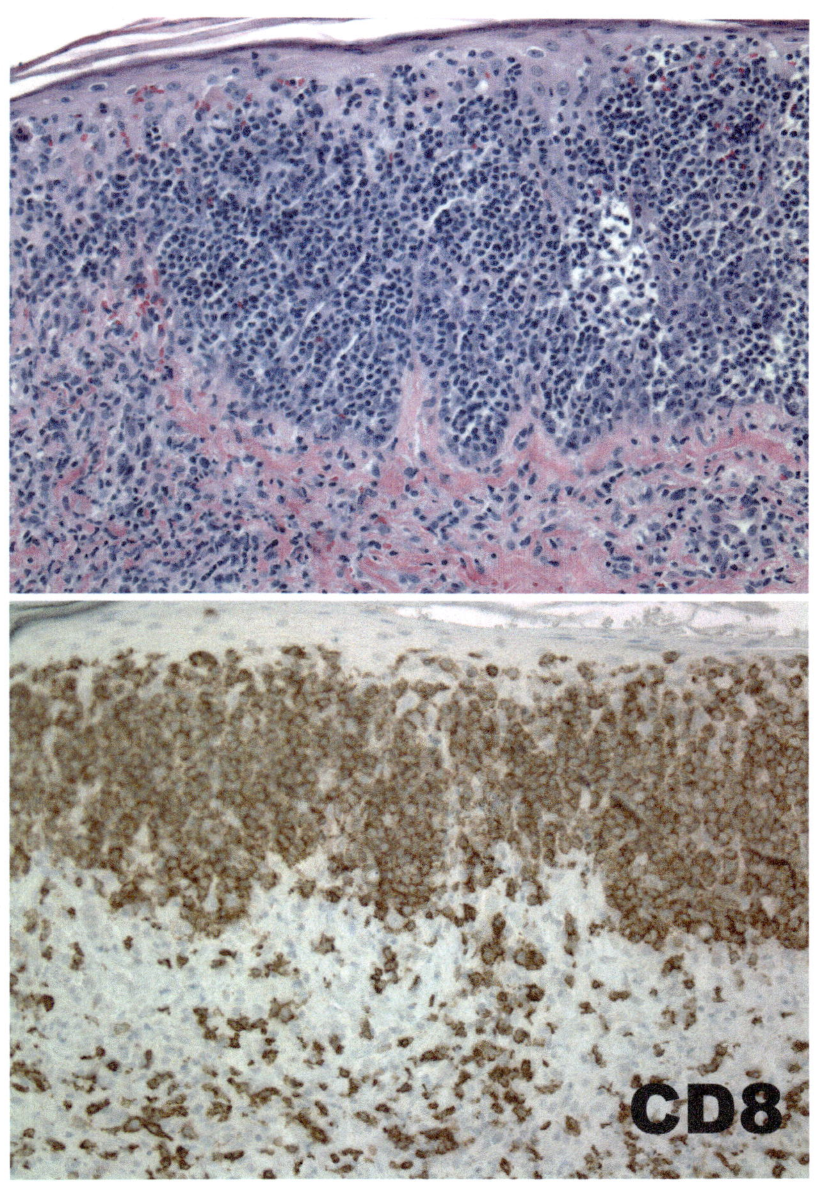

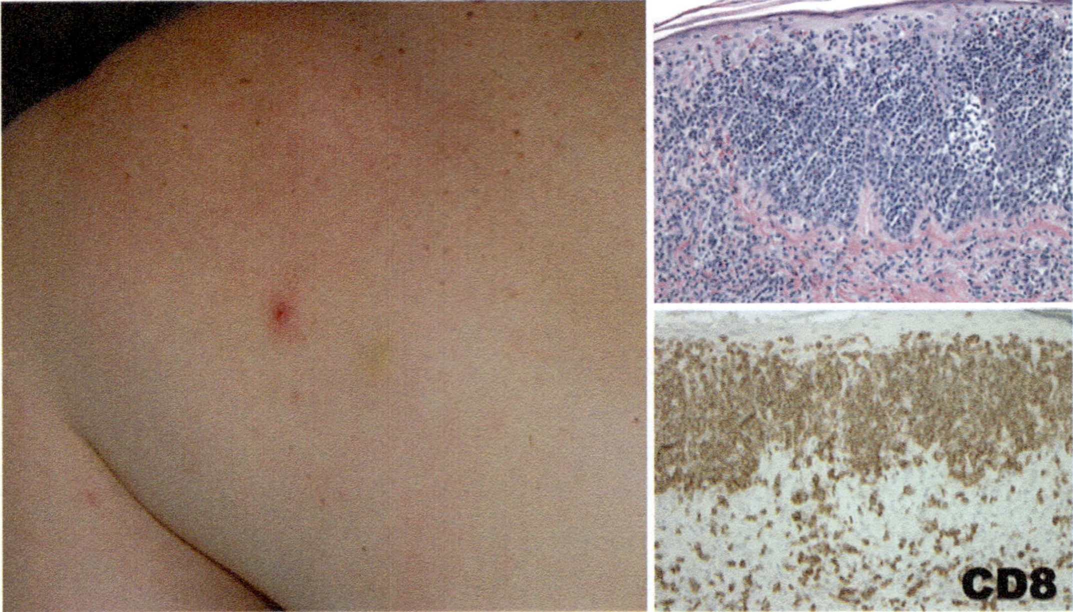

Fig. 16.2 Lymphomatoid papulosis type D (CD8-positive). While the histopathology of an atypical cytotoxic infiltrate with marked epidermotropism appears concerning, the clinical presentation and follow-up are benign (small, self-regressing papules)

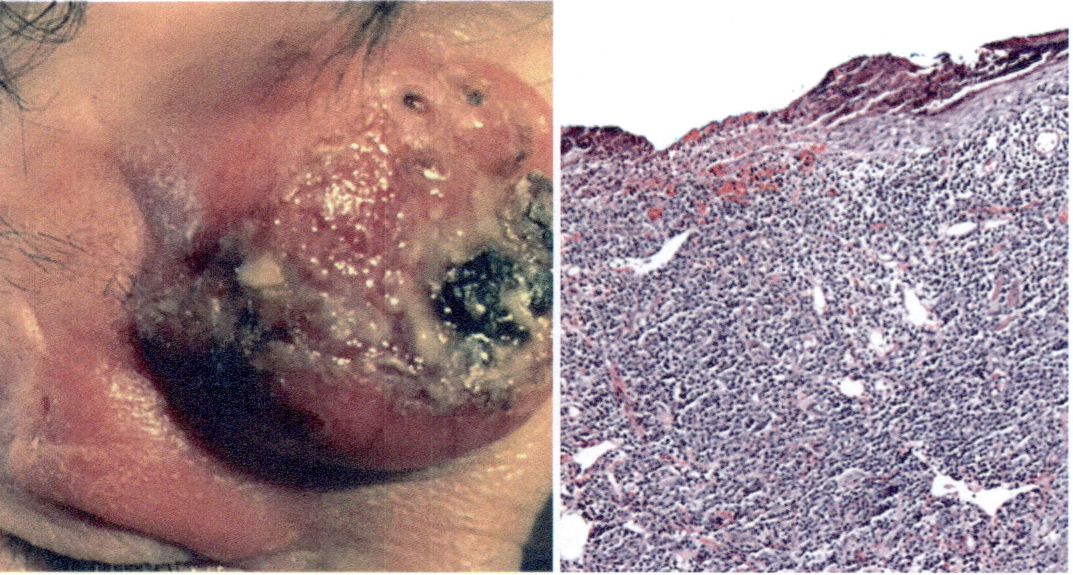

Fig. 16.3 Primary cutaneous CD8-positive aggressive epidermotropic cytotoxic T-cell lymphoma. Initial clinical presentation with large, ulcerated tumor on the forehead with fast progression. The dense atypical lymphoid infiltrate shows epidermotropism and ulceration

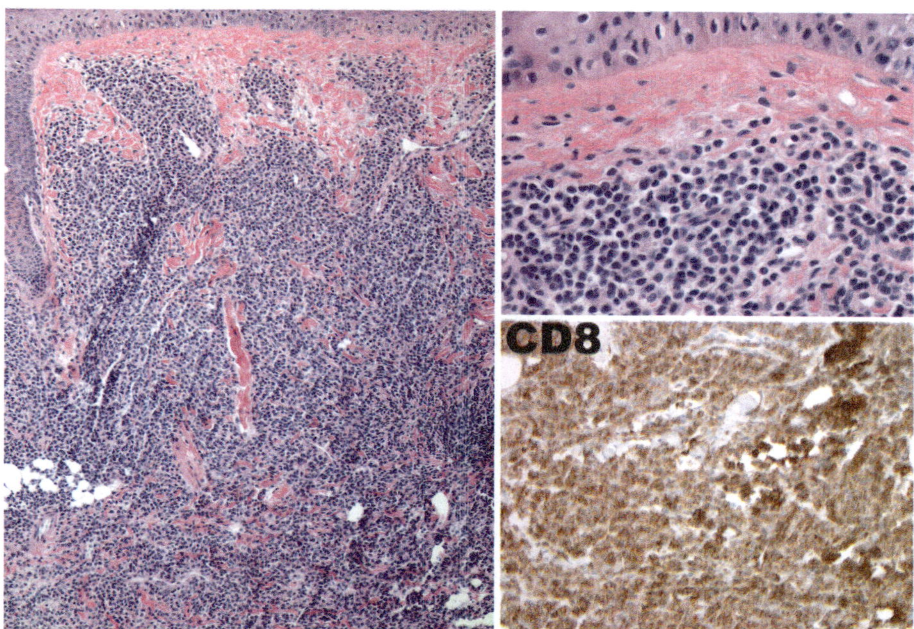

Fig. 16.4 Primary cutaneous acral CD8-positive T-cell lymphoma (indolent CD8-positive lymphoid proliferation of the ear). This case presented with a solitary nodular lesion on the ear. The biopsy showed a dense dermal infiltrate of CD8-positive blastoid cells without epitheliotropism

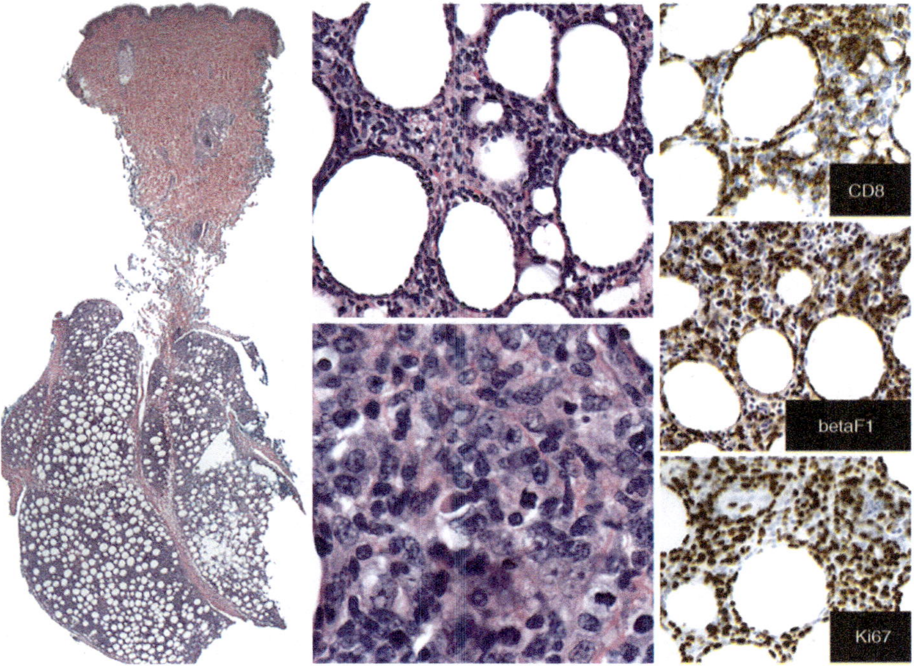

Fig. 16.5 Subcutaneous panniculitis-like T-cell lymphoma. Pannicular-based infiltrate of atypical lymphocytes with rimming of adipocytes. Mitotic figures and apoptosis are common. The infiltrate is composed of cytotoxic alpha-beta CD8-positive T cells. There is a high proliferation rate with Ki-67 stain

The majority of cutaneous lymphoid infiltrates demonstrates a significant predominance of CD4 expression. While less common, a CD8-predominant infiltrate (Fig. 16.1) raises an important differential diagnosis, including several aggressive lymphomas. However, indolent processes must also be considered (Table 16.1).

Mycosis fungoides (MF) is the most common type of skin lymphoma and classically demonstrates a CD4-positive phenotype. However, a subset of otherwise classical MF cases is CD8-positive. Hypopigmented variant of MF frequently expresses CD8. In addition, many cases of pagetoid reticulosis (localized, Woringer-Kolopp) are CD8-positive.

Some aggressive cutaneous lymphomas are CD8-positive and must be differentiated from indolent processes, such as lymphomatoid papulosis (LyP) type D (Fig. 16.2). While the histopathology of this variant of LyP appears very concerning (atypical cytotoxic CD8-positive T-cell infiltrate with marked epidermotropism and frequent ulceration), the clinical presentation and follow-up are benign (small, self-regressing papules). Cutaneous anaplastic large cell lymphoma (ALCL) is also part of the spectrum of primary cutaneous CD30-positive lymphoproliferative disorders. Similar to LyP, some cases of ALCL may also express CD8.

Primary cutaneous CD8-positive aggressive epidermotropic cytotoxic T-cell lymphoma (Fig. 16.3) is a rare skin lymphoma with poor prognosis. The clinical presentation is variable but is often associated with the development of ulcerated lesions and fast progression. The dense atypical lymphoid infiltrate generally shows prominent epidermotropism as well as infiltration of hair follicles (folliculotropism). Comprehensive immunophenotyping can be helpful, since the infiltrate is composed of immature CD8-positive T cells (CD2−, CD7+, CD45RA+, CD45RO−). Mycosis fungoides is usually CD2+, CD7−, CD45RA−, and CD45RO+.

Indolent CD8-positive lymphoid proliferation of the ear (Fig. 16.4) is a rare lymphoproliferative disorder classically presenting with a solitary nodular lesion on the ear (occasionally bilateral). While the histopathology appears concerning (dense dermal infiltrate of CD8-positive blastoid cells), the clinical behavior and follow-up are indolent. Both epitheliotropism and ulceration are absent. This entity is now included in the 2016 WHO classification under provisional status and has been renamed primary cutaneous acral CD8-positive T-cell lymphoma, since it may occasionally involve other acral sites.

Subcutaneous panniculitis-like T-cell lymphoma (Fig. 16.5) demonstrates a pannicul" based infiltrate of atypical lymphocytes with rimming of adipocytes. The infiltrate is composed of cytotoxic alpha-beta CD8-positive T cells. Gamma-delta T-cell lymphoma may also involve the panniculus but is composed of cytotoxic gamma-delta T cells with frequent CD56 expression (either CD4−/CD8+ or CD4−/CD8−).

Cutaneous pseudolymphomas should also be considered in the differential diagnosis of a CD8-positive T-cell infiltrate. CD8-positive infiltrates in the setting of advanced AIDS may mimic cutaneous T-cell lymphoma. In addition, many cases of pityriasis lichenoides exhibit a CD8-predominant lymphocytic infiltrate. In summary, the identification of CD8 expression in a cutaneous lymphoid infiltrate is not enough to make a diagnosis. Additional immunophenotyping and clinical correlation are necessary for proper classification.

Table 16.1 Differential diagnosis of CD8-positive cutaneous lymphoid infiltrate

Some cases of otherwise classical or hypopigmented mycosis fungoides
Many cases of localized pagetoid reticulosis
Lymphomatoid papulosis (LyP), type D
Some cases of anaplastic large cell lymphoma (ALCL)
Primary cutaneous CD8+ aggressive epidermotropic cytotoxic T-cell lymphoma
Many cases of cutaneous gamma-delta T-cell lymphoma
Subcutaneous panniculitis-like T-cell lymphoma
Indolent CD8+ lymphoid proliferation of the ear (primary cutaneous acral CD8+ T-cell lymphoma)
Cutaneous pseudolymphoma: CD8-positive infiltrates in the setting of advanced AIDS, many cases of pityriasis lichenoides

Pearls and Pitfalls

1. It is not uncommon for a CD8-positive skin lymphoma to have a false-negative result with PCR for T-cell receptor gene rearrangement. The absence of a T-cell clone by PCR does not exclude the possibility of lymphoma.

Suggested Reading

Berti E, Tomasini D, Vermeer MH, et al. Primary cutaneous CD8-positive epidermotropic cytotoxic T cell lymphomas. A distinct clinicopathological entity with an aggressive clinical behavior. Am J Pathol. 1999;155:483–92.

Petrella T, Maubec E, Cornillet-Lefebvre P, et al. Indolent CD8-positive lymphoid proliferation of the ear. A distinct primary cutaneous T-cell lymphoma. Am J Surg Pathol. 2007;31:1887–92.

Saggini A, Gulia A, Argenyi Z, et al. A variant of lymphomatoid papulosis simulating primary cutaneous aggressive epidermotropic CD8+ cytotoxic T-cell lymphoma. Description of 9 cases. Am J Surg Pathol. 2010 Aug;34(8):1168–75.

Swerdlow SH, Campo E, Pileri SA, et al. The 2016 revision of the WHO classification of lymphoid neoplasms. Blood. 2016;127(20):2375–90.

Fig. 17.1 This cutaneous lymphoid infiltrate shows significant CD30 expression. What is the differential diagnosis?

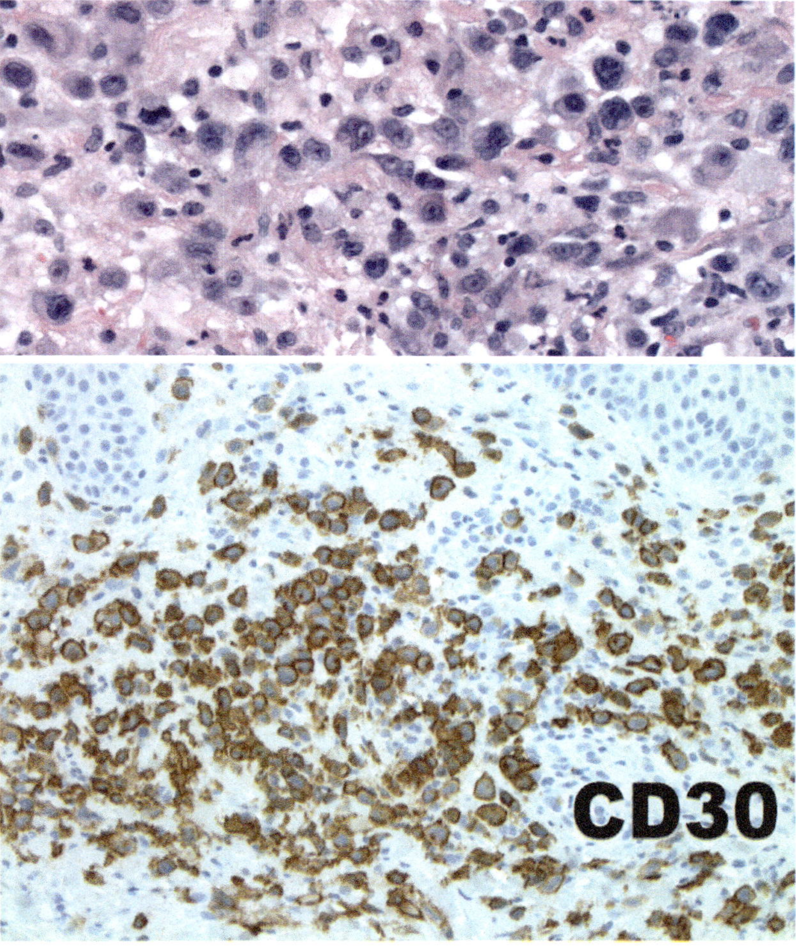

© Springer Nature Switzerland AG 2019
A. Subtil, *Diagnosis of Cutaneous Lymphoid Infiltrates*,
https://doi.org/10.1007/978-3-030-11654-5_17

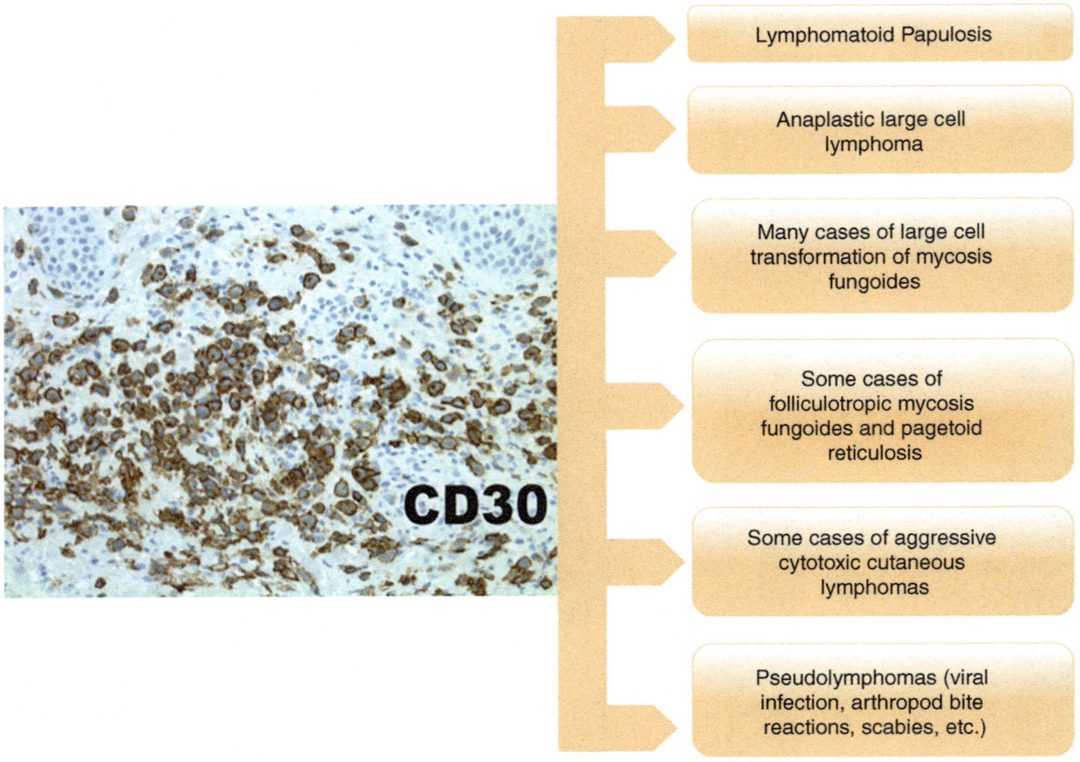

Fig. 17.2 Differential diagnosis of CD30 expression

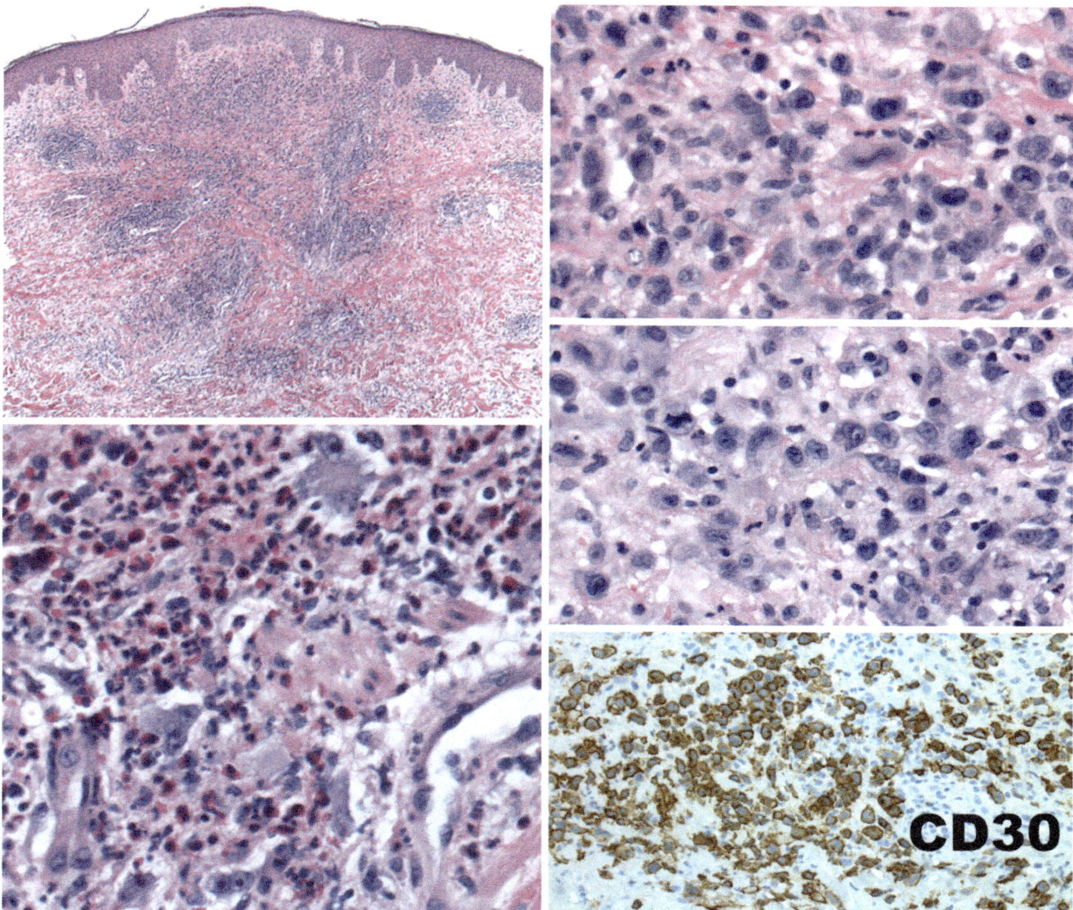

Fig. 17.3 Lymphomatoid papulosis (type A). Moderately dense, wedge-shaped mixed dermal infiltrate composed of large atypical lymphocytes (arranged as single cells and in small clusters) admixed with an inflammatory infiltrate of neutrophils, eosinophils, small lymphocytes, and histiocytes. The atypical lymphocytes exhibit large nuclear size, hyperchromasia, irregular nuclear membrane, and moderately abundant cytoplasm. Occasional lymphocytes show binucleation and prominent nucleolus resembling Reed-Sternberg cells. CD30 immunohistochemical stain marks scattered and clustered CD30-positive large cells

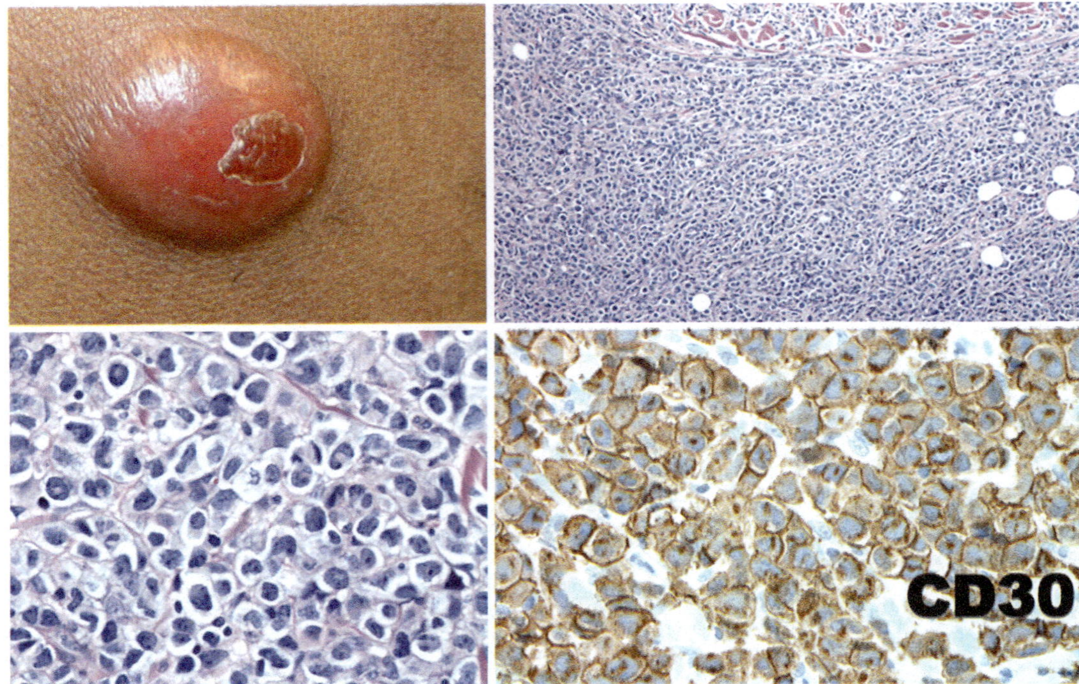

Fig. 17.4 Primary cutaneous anaplastic large cell lymphoma. Persistent large skin tumor. Dense diffuse dermal infiltrate composed of large atypical lymphocytes with strong CD30 expression (>75%). A significant mixed inflammatory infiltrate is not seen

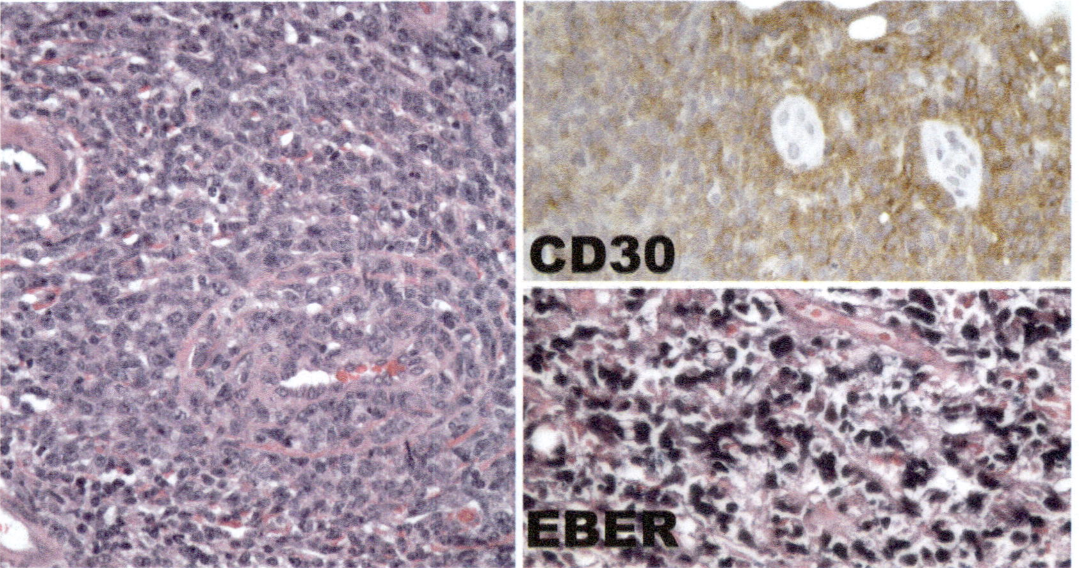

Fig. 17.5 Extranodal NK/T-cell lymphoma, nasal type. Some cases of aggressive cytotoxic cutaneous lymphomas may exhibit variable CD30 expression. Subtle infiltration of the walls of a blood vessel (angiocentrism) is present in the lower half of the figure. EBV in situ hybridization (EBER) is positive

CD30 is an activation marker that is characteristically expressed by cutaneous CD30-positive lymphoproliferative disorders (Fig. 17.1). However, CD30 is not specific for these entities and may show significant expression in a variety of benign and malignant cutaneous lymphoid infiltrates (Fig. 17.2 and Table 17.1).

Lymphomatoid papulosis and anaplastic large cell lymphoma are part of the spectrum of cutaneous CD30-positive lymphoproliferative disorders, which also includes borderline lesions. Lymphomatoid papulosis (LyP) generally presents with solitary or multiple, small, self-regressing papules. While the histopathology resembles that of a lymphoma (i.e., "lymphomatoid"), the clinical course is benign (i.e., "papulosis"). There are several histopathologic variants. LyP type A shows a wedge-shaped, mixed dermal infiltrate composed of large atypical lymphocytes (arranged as single cells and in small clusters) admixed with an inflammatory infiltrate of neutrophils, eosinophils, small lymphocytes, and histiocytes. The atypical lymphocytes exhibit large nuclear size, hyperchromasia, irregular nuclear membrane, and moderately abundant cytoplasm. Atypical lymphocytes may also show binucleation and prominent nucleolus resembling Reed-Sternberg cells. CD30 stain marks scattered and clustered CD30-positive large cells (Fig. 17.3). Other variants resemble different types of lymphoma: mycosis fungoides (type B), anaplastic large cell lymphoma (type C), aggressive epidermotropic CD8-positive cytotoxic T-cell lymphoma (type D), and angiocentric lymphoma (type E).

Cutaneous anaplastic large cell lymphoma (ALCL) generally presents with persistent, large skin tumors. Microscopically, dense diffuse dermal infiltrates composed of large atypical lymphocytes exhibit strong CD30 expression. In general, a significant mixed inflammatory infiltrate is not seen (Fig. 17.4). Since the differential diagnosis for primary cutaneous ALCL would include secondary skin involvement by systemic ALCL (ALK-positive or ALK-negative), correlation with staging results and ALK staining would be helpful. In addition, LyP type C can mimic ALCL in the biopsy. Therefore, careful clinicopathologic correlation and/or close follow-up is generally necessary to correctly distinguish between these two ends of the CD30-positive lymphoproliferative spectrum.

Some variants of mycosis fungoides may show variable CD30 expression, particularly folliculotropic mycosis fungoides and pagetoid reticulosis (Woringer-Kolopp). Large cell transformation of mycosis fungoides (LCT-MF) requires at least 25% of large atypical cells in the infiltrate or the formation of microscopic nodules of large cells. Once the histomorphologic criteria have been met, some cases express CD30 while other cases do not. It is important to emphasize that the definition of LCT-MF is based on H&E findings (not on the level of CD30 expression). LyP in association with MF must be excluded on clinical grounds for the CD30-positive cases. ALCL is not an option in this setting since absence of MF is part of the diagnostic criteria for cutaneous ALCL.

Pseudolymphomas may also exhibit significant CD30 expression, including reactive lymphoid hyperplasia in the setting of viral infection, persistent arthropod bite reactions, some drug reactions, and scabies. Identification of additional histopathologic findings (e.g., viral cytopathic effect, portions of an arthropod) and careful clinical correlation would be helpful to prevent overdiagnosis of lymphomatoid papulosis.

Cutaneous CD30-positive lymphoproliferative disorders (LyP and ALCL) and pseudolymphomas are indolent, and CD30 expression is generally associated with a good prognosis. However, some cases of aggressive cytotoxic cutaneous lymphomas (such as extranodal NK/T-cell lymphoma, nasal type; Fig. 17.5) may demonstrate variable CD30 expression. It is important to include them in the differential diagnosis of CD30-positive infiltrates. Since large cell morphology may occur in cytotoxic lymphomas, these aggressive conditions may be misdiagnosed as anaplastic large cell lymphoma (an indolent process).

In summary, the identification of CD30 expression in a cutaneous lymphoid infiltrate is not enough to make a diagnosis. Additional immunophenotyping, identification of other histopathologic findings, and clinical correlation are necessary for proper classification.

Pearls and Pitfalls

1. The degree of CD30 expression is important. For example, for anaplastic large cell lymphoma (ALCL), CD30 must be positive in at least 75% of atypical cells (i.e., even if 60% of a lymphoid infiltrate marks with CD30, that level of staining is not sufficient for ALCL, and other entities should be considered in the differential diagnosis).

Table 17.1 Differential diagnosis of CD30 expression

Lymphomatoid papulosis (LyP)
Anaplastic large cell lymphoma (primary cutaneous ALCL or secondary skin involvement by systemic ALCL)
Many (but not all) cases of large cell transformation of mycosis fungoides
Some cases of folliculotropic mycosis fungoides and pagetoid reticulosis
Some cases of aggressive cytotoxic cutaneous lymphomas
Pseudolymphomas: reactive lymphoid hyperplasia in the setting of viral infection, persistent arthropod bite reactions, some drug reactions, and scabies

Suggested Reading

Kempf W. Cutaneous CD30-positive lymphoproliferative disorders. Surg Pathol Clin. 2014;7(2):203–28.

Swerdlow SH, et al., editors. WHO classification of tumors of hematopoietic and lymphoid tissues. Lyon: IARC; 2008.

Werner B, Massone C, Kerl H, et al. Large CD30-positive cells in benign, atypical lymphoid infiltrates of the skin. J Cutan Pathol. 2008;35(12):1100–7.

Willemze R, Jaffe ES, Burg G, et al. WHO-EORTC classification for cutaneous lymphomas. Blood. 2005;105(10):3768–85.

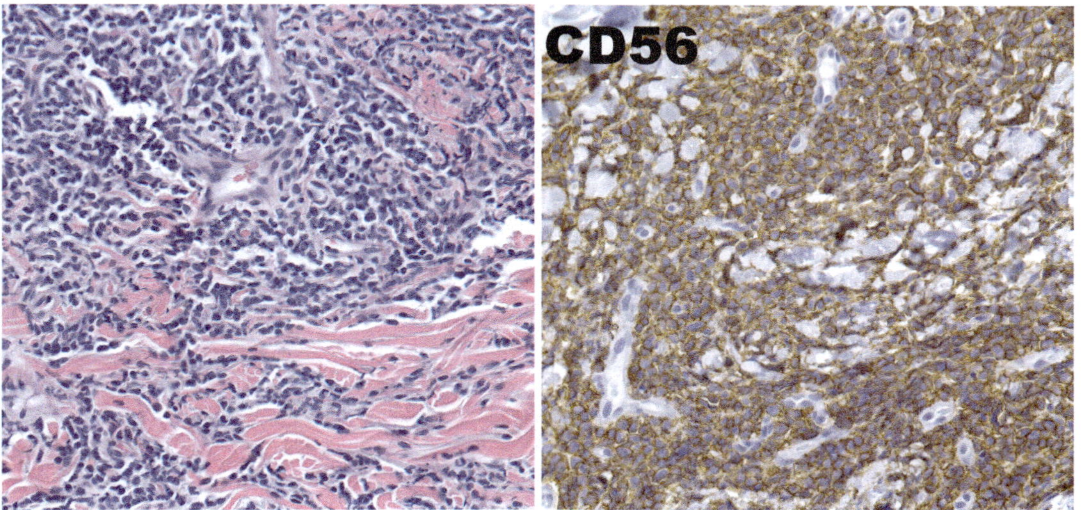

Fig. 18.1 What is the differential diagnosis of CD56 expression in the skin?

© Springer Nature Switzerland AG 2019
A. Subtil, *Diagnosis of Cutaneous Lymphoid Infiltrates*,
https://doi.org/10.1007/978-3-030-11654-5_18

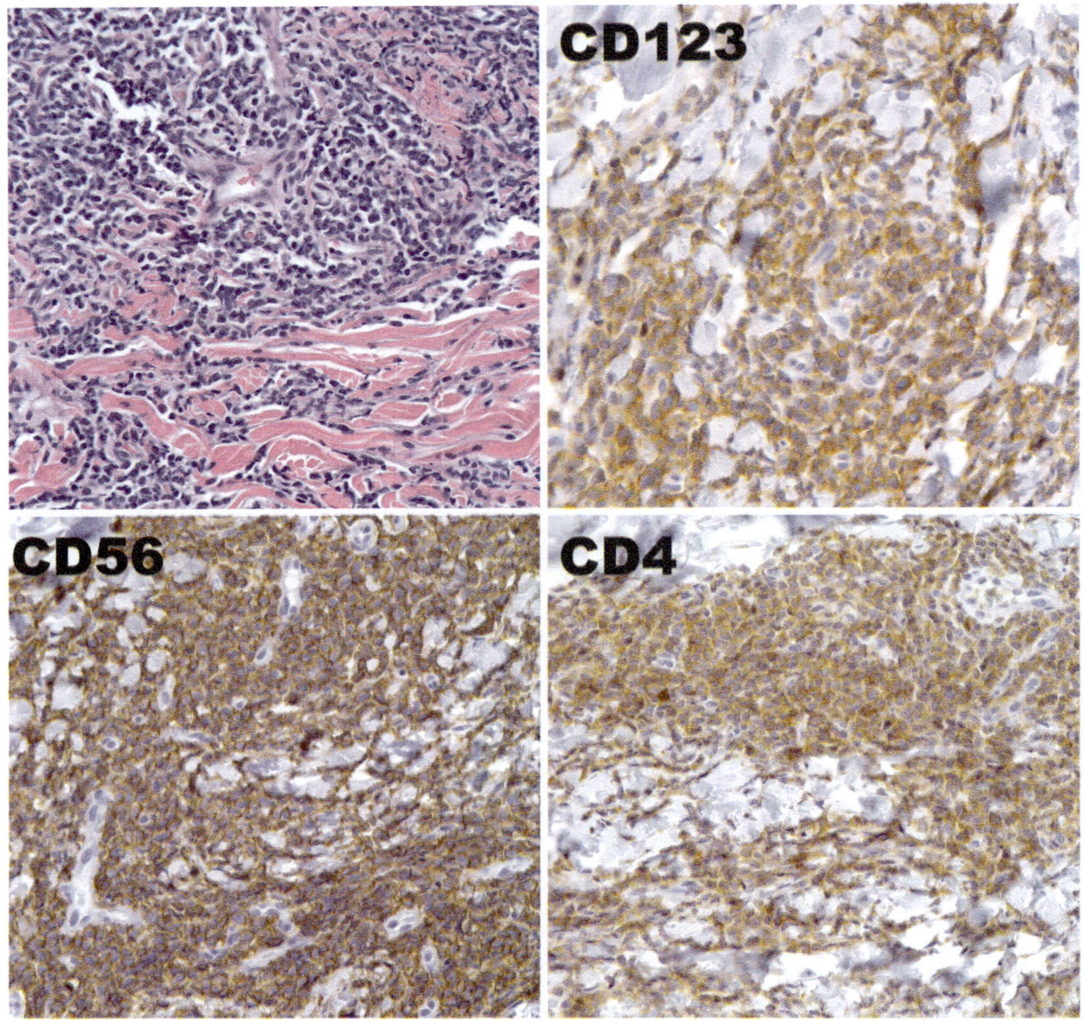

Fig. 18.2 Blastic plasmacytoid dendritic cell neoplasm. This aggressive hematopoietic neoplasm was previously known as CD4+/CD56+ hematodermic neoplasm and classically involves skin and bone marrow. In addition to CD4 and CD56, plasmacytoid dendritic cell markers such as CD123 are expressed

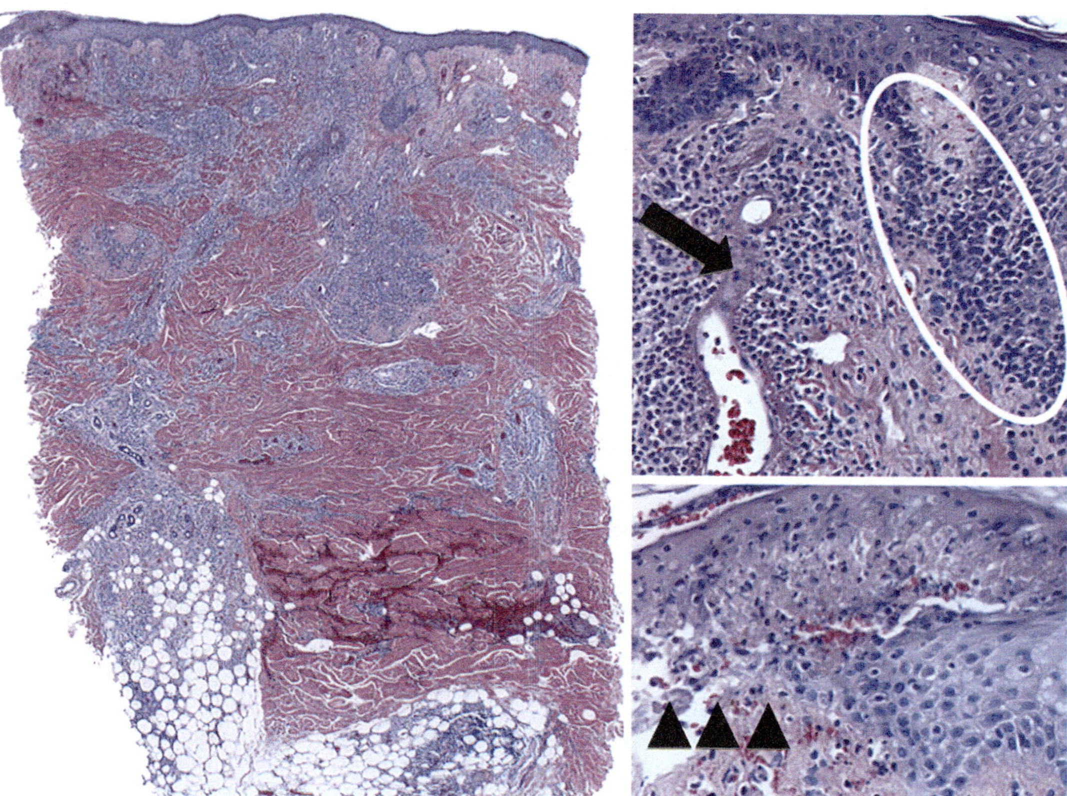

Fig. 18.3 Cutaneous gamma-delta T-cell lymphoma. Involvement of all layers of the skin (epidermis, dermis, and panniculus) may occur. The epidermis shows intraepi-thelial atypical lymphocytes (circle) and ulceration (arrowheads). Vasculitic changes with fibrin deposition are present (arrow). Most cases express CD56

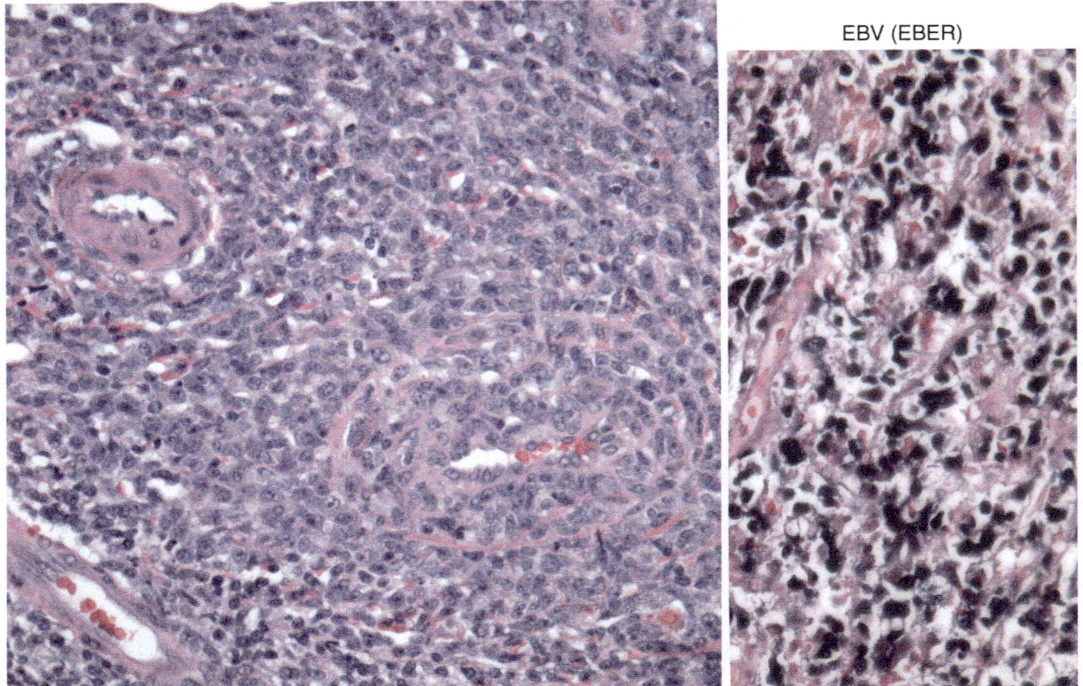

Fig. 18.4 Extranodal NK/T-cell lymphoma, nasal type. CD56 expression is frequent in this aggressive cytotoxic lymphoma. Subtle infiltration of the walls of a blood ves- sel (angioinvasion) is present in the lower half of the fig- ure. EBV in situ hybridization (EBER) is positive

CD56 is a useful marker for neural/neuroendo- crine differentiation and also marks certain hematopoietic populations, such as natural killer (NK) cells and a subset of cytotoxic T cells. CD56 plays an important role in the diagnosis of cytotoxic lymphomas, such as extranodal NK/T- cell lymphoma nasal type and gamma-delta T-cell lymphoma. Despite its seemingly restricted distribution, several conditions may unexpect- edly show CD56 expression, including metastatic renal cell carcinoma and most cases of plasma cell myeloma (Fig. 18.1, Table 18.1).

Mycosis fungoides (MF) is the most common type of skin lymphoma and classically demon- strates a CD4-positive phenotype. However, MF may rarely exhibit a CD56-positive immunophe- notype (generally in younger patients). These rare CD56-positive MF cases largely behave in a manner similar to that predicted for MF with classic phenotype. Rare cases of CD56-positive lymphomatoid papulosis (LyP) have also been reported. Since several aggressive cutaneous lymphomas are CD56-positive, careful clinical pathologic correlation and close follow-up are critical for the correct diagnosis of phenotypic variants of indolent conditions such as MF and LyP.

Blastic plasmacytoid dendritic cell neoplasm (BPDCN) is an aggressive hematopoietic neo- plasm of immature plasmacytoid dendritic cells that usually involves skin and bone marrow. It was previously known as "CD4+/CD56+ hema- todermic neoplasm" and "blastic NK cell lym- phoma." The blastic cytomorphology and CD56 expression initially suggested an NK precursor origin. In addition to CD4 and CD56, plasmacy- toid dendritic cell-associated antigens (such as CD123, TCL1, and CD303) are expressed (Fig. 18.2). A comprehensive immunohistochem- ical panel is necessary to differentiate BPDCN from myeloid leukemia cutis, which may occa- sionally express CD56.

Cutaneous gamma-delta T-cell lymphoma (GDTCL) is an important differential diagnosis in an atypical CD56-positive lymphoid infiltrate. GDTCL is an aggressive cytotoxic cutaneous lymphoma of gamma-delta T cells (betaF1-, CD3+, CD5-, CD4-, CD8−/+, CD56+, TIA1+) that may involve any or all layers of the skin (epidermis, dermis, and/or panniculus; Fig. 18.3). Ulceration and angiocentrism may also occur.

Extranodal NK/T-cell lymphoma, nasal type most commonly involves the upper aerodigestive tract but frequently presents in the skin (Fig. 18.4). This aggressive EBV-positive angiodestructive malignant process is designated "NK/T" because the immunophenotype can be NK cell or cytotoxic T cell. While CD56 expression is generally present, some cases of cytotoxic T cell origin may be CD56-negative. Therefore, in the setting of angiocentrism and cytotoxic phenotype, EBV in situ hybridization (EBER) should be obtained.

In summary, the identification of CD56 expression in a cutaneous lymphoid infiltrate is not enough to make a diagnosis. Additional immunophenotyping and clinical correlation are necessary for proper classification.

Table 18.1 Differential diagnosis of CD56 expression in the skin

Lymphoid/hematopoietic	Non-lymphoid
Rare cases of mycosis fungoides	Merkel cell carcinoma
Rare cases of CD30-positive lymphoproliferative disorders	Schwannoma
Cutaneous gamma-delta T-cell lymphoma	Neuroblastoma
Extranodal NK/T-cell lymphoma, nasal type	Cellular neurothekeoma
Blastic plasmacytoid dendritic cell neoplasm (CD4+/CD56+ hematodermic neoplasm)	Plexiform fibrohistiocytic tumor
Some cases of myeloid leukemia cutis	Metastatic renal cell carcinoma
Most cases of plasma cell myeloma	Damaged muscle fibers

Pearls and Pitfalls

1. Merkel cell carcinoma (MCC) is immunoreactive with CD56. While most cases would not resemble a lymphoma, some cases of MCC may be discohesive, poorly fixed, and/or partially obscured by inflammation and may resemble a CD56-positive lymphoma.
2. Damaged and/or regenerating muscle fibers exhibit strong CD56 expression. This phenomenon may be observed in the skin and panniculus after trauma or in association with lymphoid infiltrates.

Suggested Reading

Flann S, Orchard GE, Wain EM, et al. Three cases of lymphomatoid papulosis with a CD56+ phenotype. J Am Acad Dermatol. 2006 Nov;55(5):903–6.

Hodak E, David M, Maron L, et al. CD4/CD8 double-negative epidermotropic cutaneous T-cell lymphoma: an immunohistochemical variant of mycosis fungoides. J Am Acad Dermatol. 2006;55:276–84.

Mckay K, McNiff J, Subtil A. Prominent CD56 expression by damaged and regenerating muscle fibers in the skin. J Cutan Pathol. 2012;39:425–30.

McNiff JM, Cowper SE, Lazova R, et al. CD56 staining in Merkel cell carcinoma and natural killer-cell lymphoma: magic bullet, diagnostic pitfall, or both? J Cutan Pathol. 2005;32(8):541–5.

Swerdlow SH, Campo E, Harris NL, et al. WHO classification of tumors of hematopoietic and lymphoid tissues. Lyon: IARC; 2008.

Wain EM, Orchard GE, Mayou S, et al. Mycosis fungoides with a CD56+ immunophenotype. J Am Acad Dermatol. 2005;53(1):158–63.

Fig. 19.1 What is the differential
diagnosis of an EBV-positive
lymphoid infiltrate?

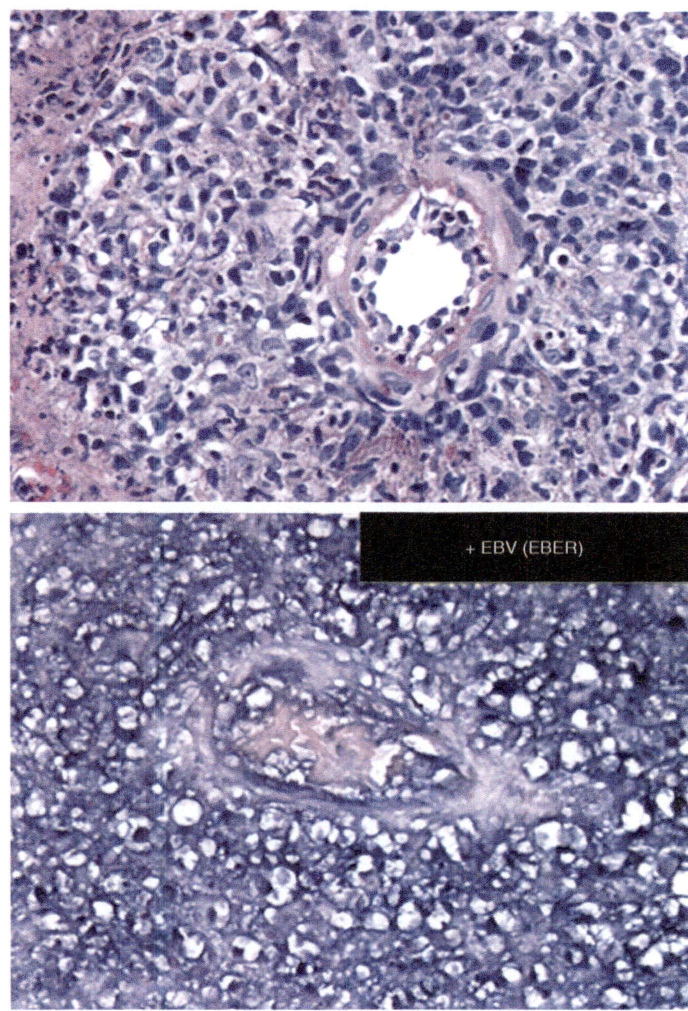

© Springer Nature Switzerland AG 2019
A. Subtil, *Diagnosis of Cutaneous Lymphoid Infiltrates*,
https://doi.org/10.1007/978-3-030-11654-5_19

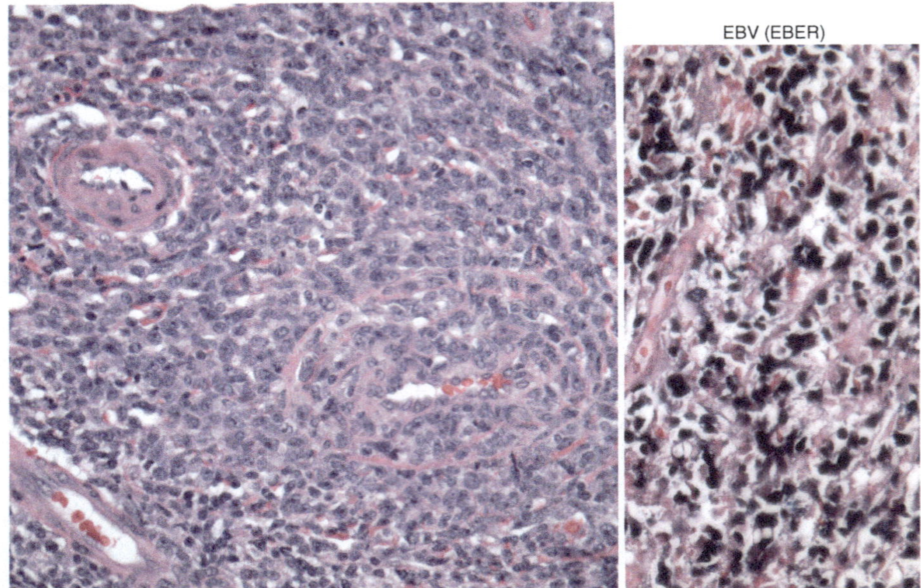

Fig. 19.2 Extranodal NK/T-cell lymphoma, nasal type. Subtle infiltration of the walls of a blood vessel (angiocentrism) is present in the lower half of the figure. EBV in situ hybridization (EBER) is positive

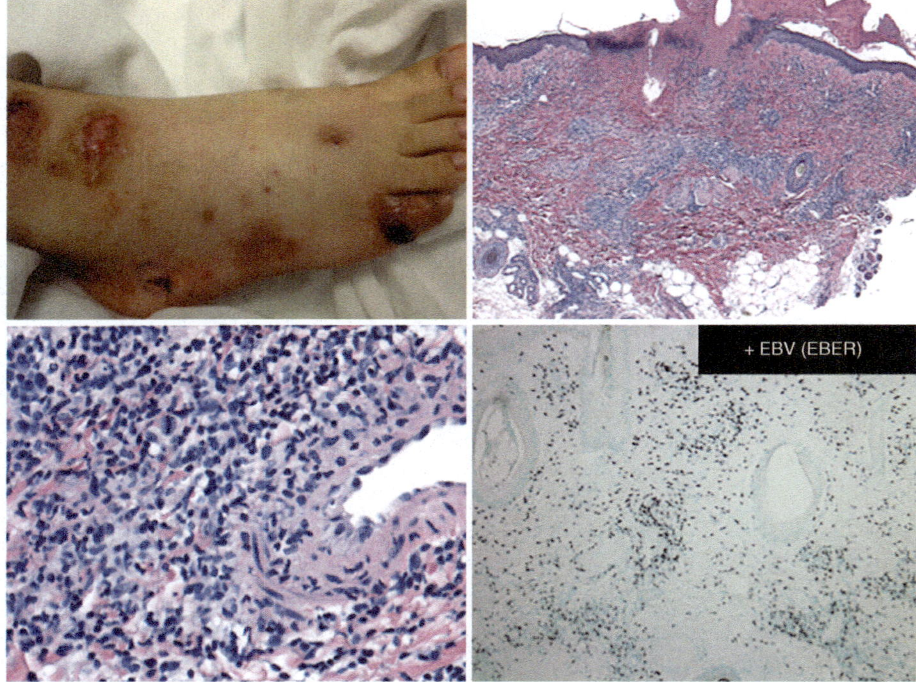

Fig. 19.3 Hydroa vacciniforme-like lymphoproliferative disorder. This child initially presented with edema and ulcerated, necrotic lesions on sun-exposed skin. Biopsy showed abrupt necrosis of both epidermis and dermis in association with an atypical EBV-positive lymphoid infiltrate with angiocentrism

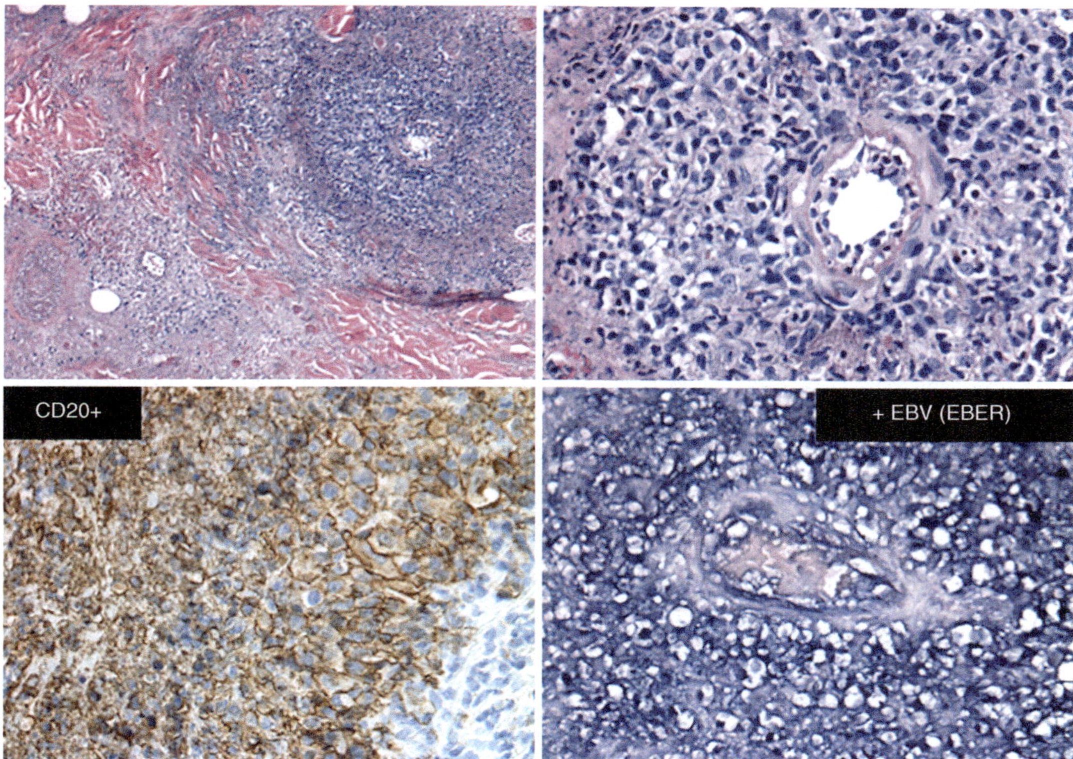

Fig. 19.4 Lymphomatoid granulomatosis (LYG). This skin biopsy shows an atypical lymphoid infiltrate with angiocentrism and necrosis. The large atypical lympho-cytes infiltrating the blood vessel walls are predominantly CD20-positive B cells. EBV in situ hybridization is positive

A cutaneous lymphoid infiltrate may occasionally be associated with Epstein-Barr virus (EBV). Angiodestruction and prominent necrosis are often present in this setting (Fig. 19.1, Table 19.1). The identification of EBV in an atypical lymphoid infiltrate would raise the possibility of several disorders, many of which are associated with poor prognosis (Table 19.2).

Since EBV expression is an uncommon finding in most geographic regions, most laboratories do not routinely check EBV in situ hybridization (EBER). Therefore, it is important to determine scenarios to consider EBV testing (Table 19.3). As mentioned, the identification of angiodestruction in a lymphoid infiltrate would be a clue for an EBV-positive lymphoproliferative disorder. While angiocentrism is not always present in a biopsy of an angioinvasive lymphoid process, the presence of infarct-like necrosis or a cytotoxic and/or CD56-positive immunophenotype should also prompt EBV testing. In addition, there are also clinical indications, such as history of immunosuppression (transplant, congenital or acquired immunodeficiency, advanced age) and clinical clues for certain diagnoses (presence of both skin and lung lesions for lymphomatoid granulomatosis; young patients with facial edema and lesions on sun-exposed skin for hydroa vacciniforme-like lymphoproliferative disorder).

Extranodal NK/T-cell lymphoma nasal type most commonly involves the upper aerodigestive tract but frequently presents in the skin (Fig. 19.2). This EBV-positive angiodestructive malignant process is designated "NK/T" because the immunophenotype can be NK cell or cytotoxic T cell. Another EBV-positive condition with NK- or T-cell phenotype is hydroa vacciniforme-like lymphoproliferative disorder. This rare entity affects children and usually presents with ulcerated necrotic lesions on sun-exposed skin.

Angiocentrism and necrosis are usually present (Fig. 19.3).

While an EBV-positive angiocentric process in the skin would generally be associated with a NK- or T-cell immunophenotype, it may also occur in a B-cell process, such as lymphomatoid granulomatosis (LYG, Fig. 19.4). LYG is an angiocentric lymphoproliferative disease involving extranodal sites (particularly lung and skin) composed of EBV-positive B cells admixed with reactive T cells. There is a spectrum of histopathologic grade and clinical aggressiveness, which are related to the proportion of large B cells.

Considering the wide variety and different prognoses of the entities with EBV expression, it is critical to obtain comprehensive immunophenotyping and careful clinical correlation for accurate classification.

Table 19.1 Differential diagnosis of an atypical angiocentric lymphoid infiltrate in relation to Epstein-Barr virus (EBV) and immunophenotype

EBV	Angiocentric process	Immunophenotype
Positive (+)	Extranodal NK/T-cell lymphoma nasal type	T cell or NK cell
	Hydroa vacciniforme-like lymphoproliferative disorder	T cell or NK cell
	Lymphomatoid granulomatosis (LYG)	B cell
Negative (−)	Cutaneous gamma-delta T-cell lymphoma	Gamma-delta T cell
	Lymphomatoid papulosis (LyP type E)	CD30-positive T cell

Table 19.2 Lymphoproliferative diseases with frequent EBV expression

Extranodal NK/T-cell lymphoma, nasal type
EBV+ diffuse large B-cell lymphoma
Systemic EBV+ T-cell lymphoma of childhood
Hydroa vacciniforme-like lymphoproliferative disorder
Lymphomatoid granulomatosis (LYG)
EBV+ mucocutaneous ulcer
Aggressive NK-cell leukemia
Posttransplant lymphoproliferative disorders
Plasmablastic lymphoma
Primary effusion lymphoma
Diffuse large B-cell lymphoma associated with chronic inflammation
Angioimmunoblastic T-cell lymphoma
Classical Hodgkin lymphoma
Burkitt lymphoma

Table 19.3 When to check EBV in situ hybridization (EBER)

Presence of angioinvasion/ angiodestruction
Presence of extensive, infarct-like necrosis
Infiltrate with prominent CD56 expression
Infiltrate with cytotoxic immunophenotype
Patient with both skin and lung lesions
Young patients with facial edema and lesions on sun-exposed skin
Elderly patients
History of congenital or acquired immunodeficiency
History of transplant

Pearls and Pitfalls

1. While several lymphomas may express EBV, the identification of EBV may or may not be part of the minimum diagnostic criteria for a particular lymphoma. For example, Burkitt lymphoma is frequently EBV-positive, but if a case of Burkitt lymphoma were EBV-negative, this would not change the diagnosis. In contrast, a nasal T-cell lymphoma that is CD3-positive and CD56-negative but negative for EBV would not be classified as extranodal NK/T-cell lymphoma nasal type.

2. In situ hybridization for Epstein-Barr encoded RNA (EBER) is the most reliable method to demonstrate the presence of EBV. Immunohistochemical stains for EBV yield variable and inconsistent results.

Suggested Reading

Li S, Feng X, Li T, et al. Extranodal NK/T-cell lymphoma, nasal type: a report of 73 cases at MD Anderson Cancer Center. Am J Surg Pathol. 2013 Jan;37(1):14–23.

Song JY, Pittaluga S, Dunleavy K, et al. Lymphomatoid granulomatosis. A single institution experience: pathologic findings and clinical correlations. Am J Surg Pathol. 2015;39(2):141–56.

Swerdlow SH, et al., editors. WHO classification of tumors of hematopoietic and lymphoid tissues. Lyon: IARC; 2008.

Swerdlow SH, Campo E, Pileri SA, et al. The 2016 revision of the WHO classification of lymphoid neoplasms. Blood. 2016;127(20):2375–90.

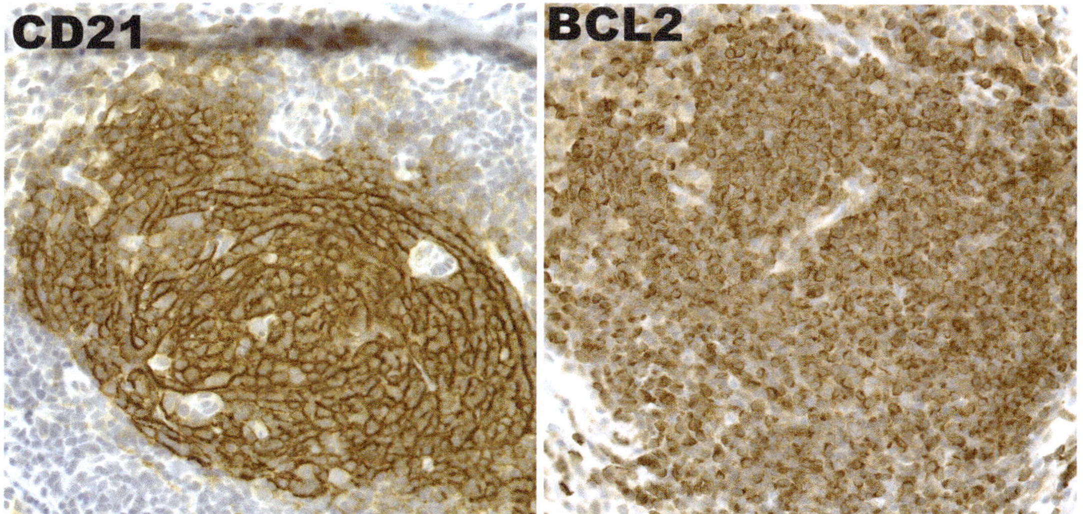

Fig. 20.1 CD21 stain highlights a lymphoid follicle. While the germinal center is usually negative with BCL2 stain, this follicle shows diffuse positivity. What is the differential diagnosis of BCL2-positive lymphoid follicles?

© Springer Nature Switzerland AG 2019

A. Subtil, *Diagnosis of Cutaneous Lymphoid Infiltrates*,

https://doi.org/10.1007/978-3-030-11654-5_20

Mantle zone
Germinal Center

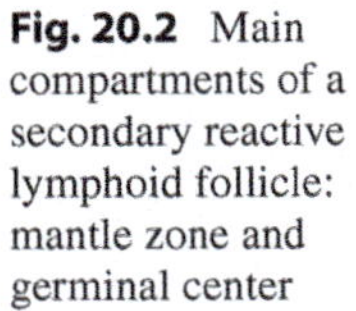

Fig. 20.2 Main compartments of a secondary reactive lymphoid follicle: mantle zone and germinal center

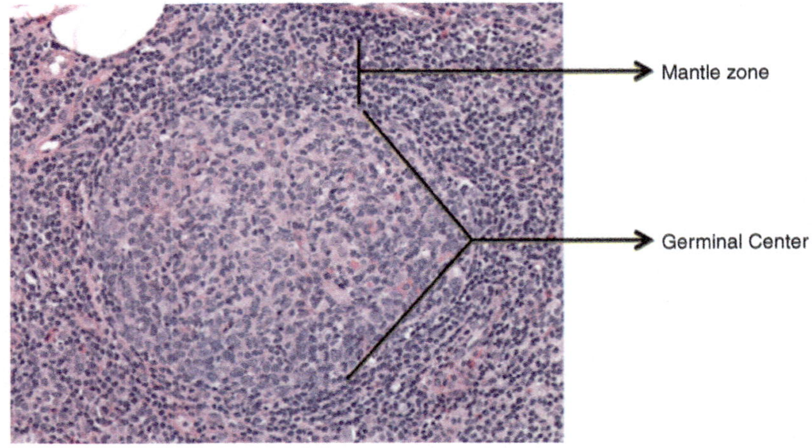

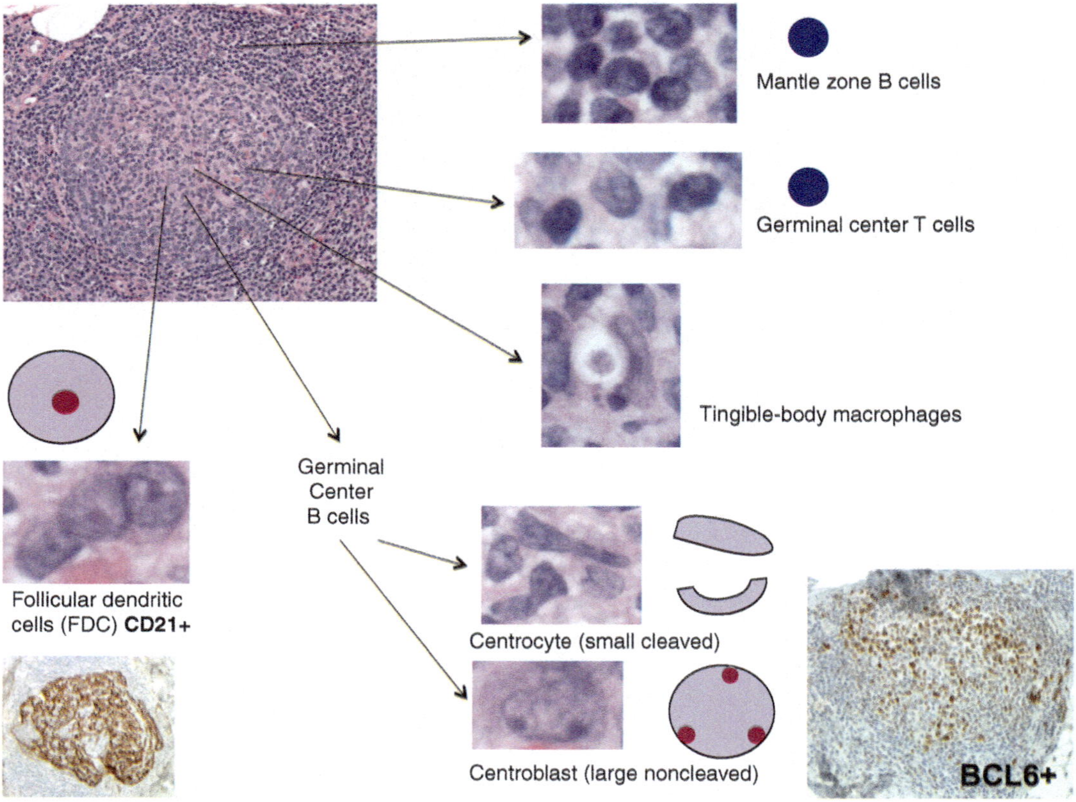

Mantle zone B cells
Germinal center T cells
Tingible-body macrophages
Germinal Center B cells
Follicular dendritic cells (FDC) CD21+
Centrocyte (small cleaved)
Centroblast (large noncleaved)
BCL6+

Fig. 20.3 Cellular components of the compartments of the lymphoid follicle

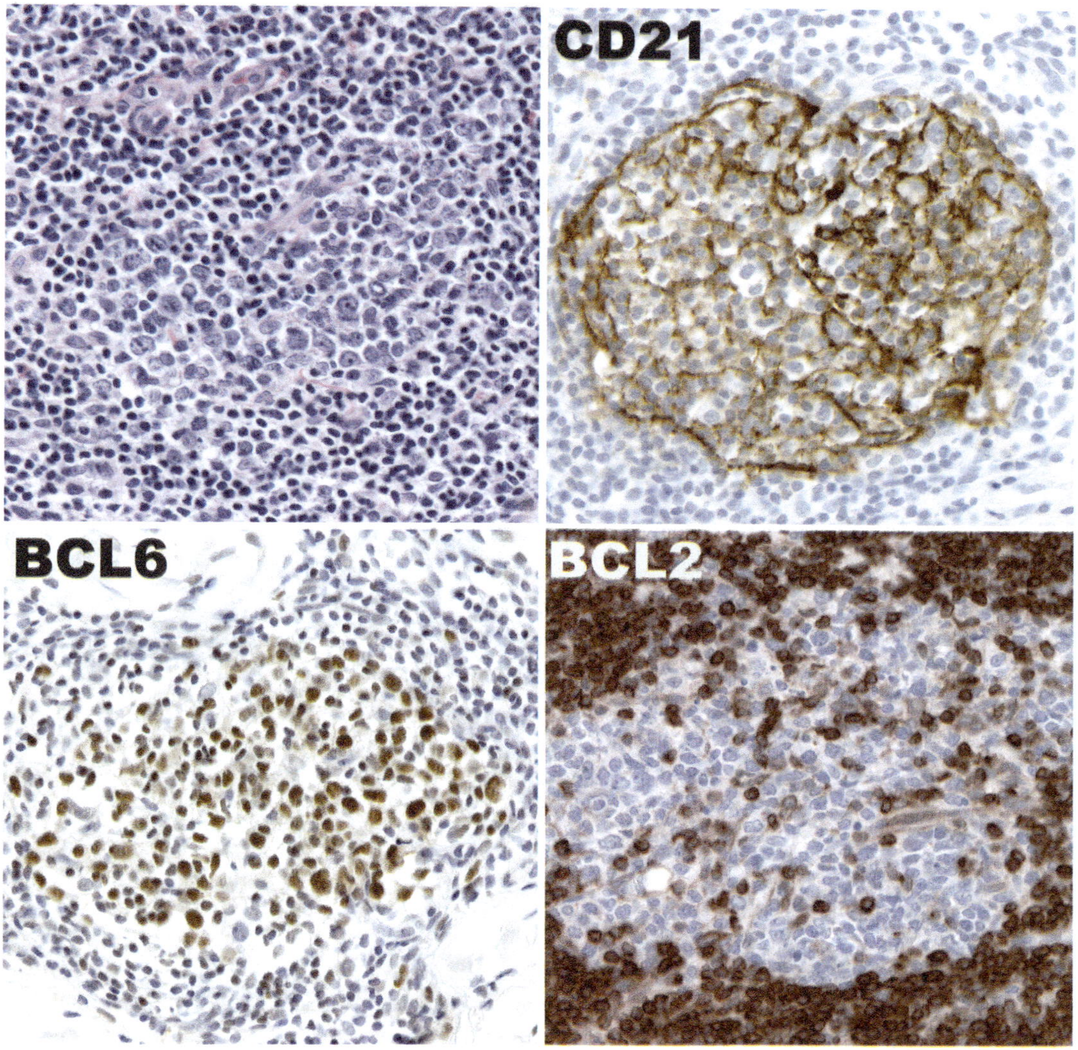

Fig. 20.4 BCL2-negative reactive lymphoid follicle in cutaneous reactive lymphoid hyperplasia (pseudolymphoma). The mantle zones are preserved, and the germinal centers are well spaced. CD21 stain highlights the follicular dendritic cell meshwork of the follicle. Centrocytes and centroblasts are the main cellular component of the germinal center and are highlighted by a positive BCL6 stain. BCL2 stain marks the mantle zone B cells and the follicular helper T cells in the germinal center, while the reactive centrocytes and centroblasts are negative

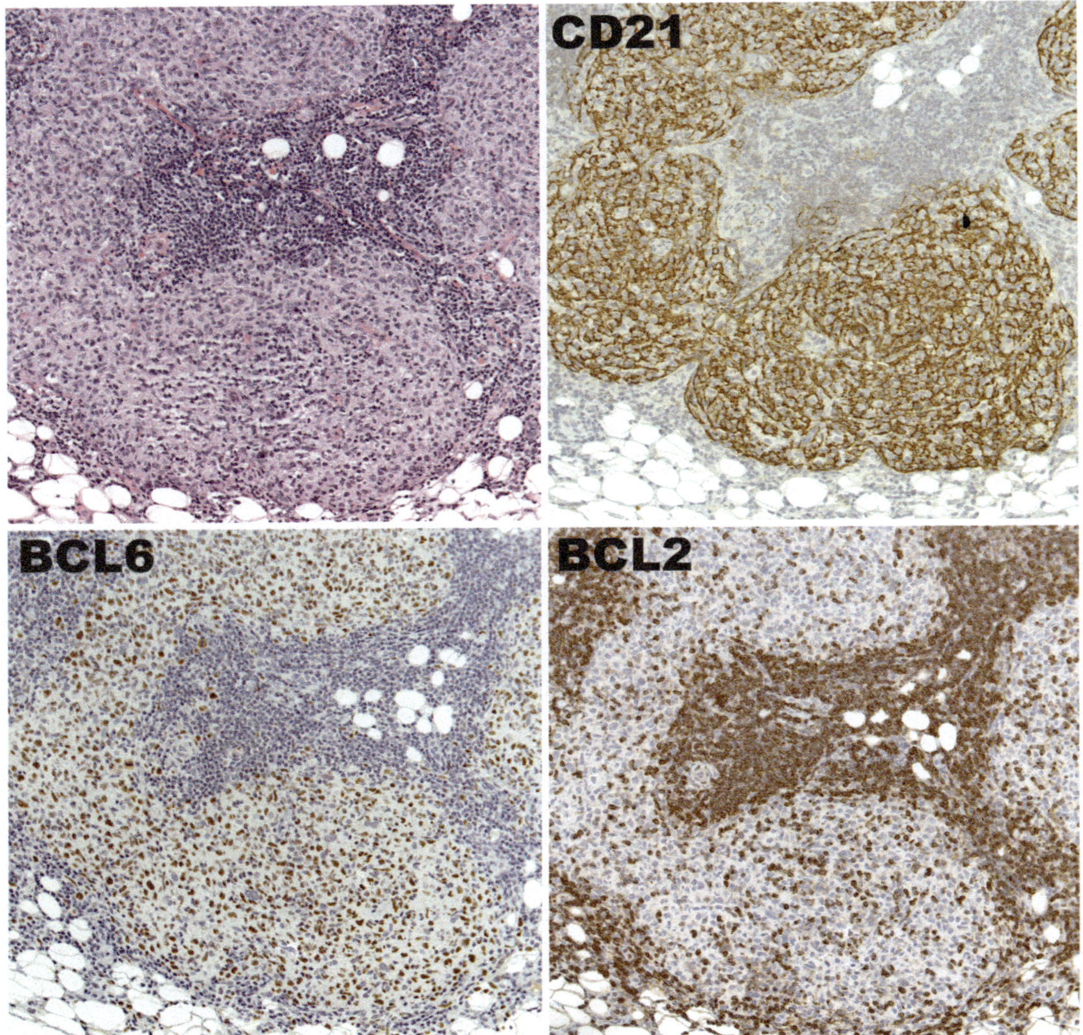

Fig. 20.5 BCL2-negative lymphoid follicles in primary cutaneous follicle center lymphoma. The mantle zones are diminished to absent, and the germinal centers are crowded. CD21 stain highlights the follicular dendritic cell meshworks of crowded follicles. Centrocytes and centroblasts are the main cellular component of the germinal centers and are highlighted by prominent BCL6 staining. BCL2 stain marks the mantle zone B cells and the follicular helper T cells in the germinal centers, while the neoplastic centrocytes and centroblasts are negative

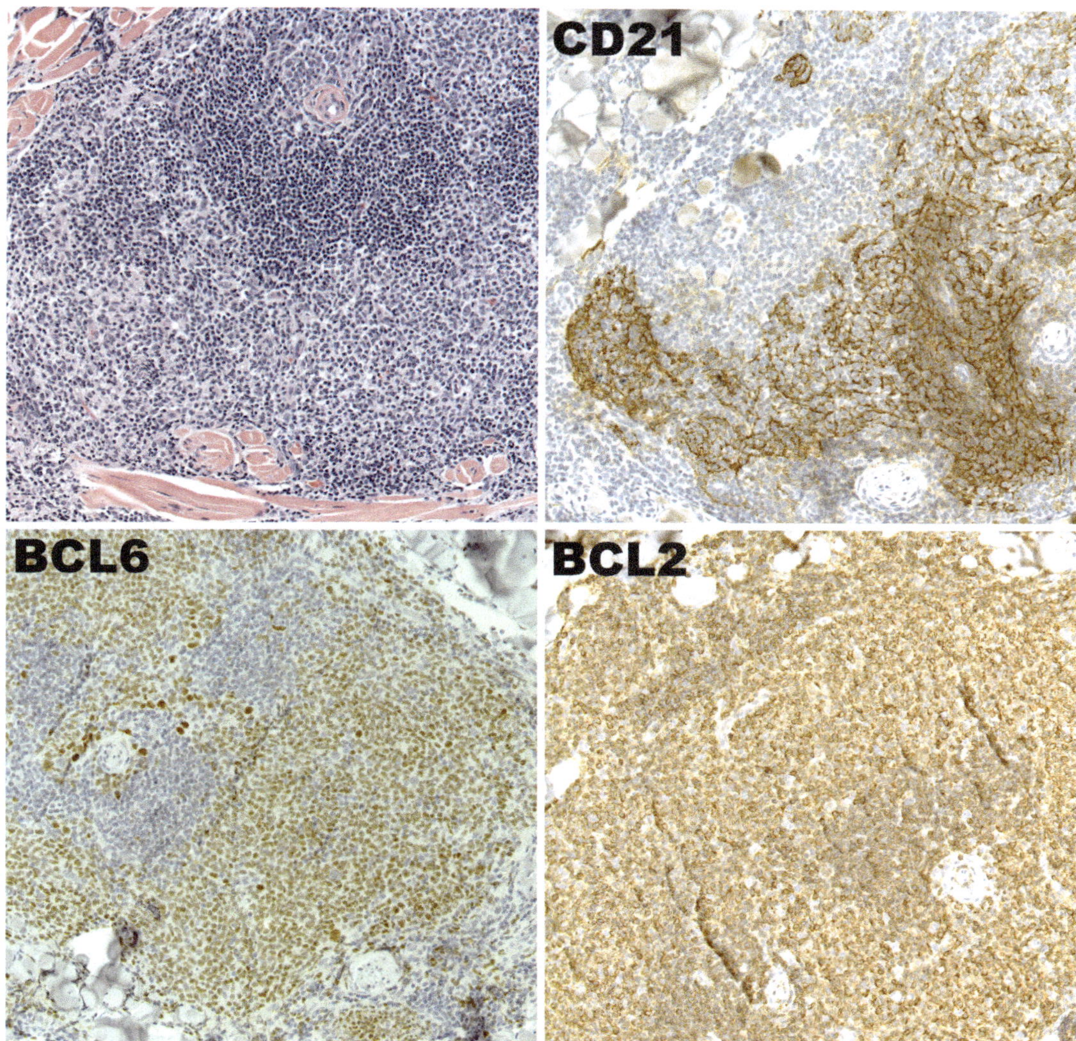

Fig. 20.6 BCL2-positive lymphoid follicles in primary cutaneous follicle center lymphoma. The mantle zones are diminished to absent, and the germinal centers are crowded. CD21 stain highlights the follicular dendritic cell meshworks of crowded follicles. Centrocytes and centroblasts are the main cellular component of the germi-nal centers and are highlighted by prominent BCL6 staining. BCL2 stain marks all cellular components, including the reactive mantle zone B cells and follicular helper T cells. The neoplastic centrocytes and centroblasts show aberrant expression of BCL2

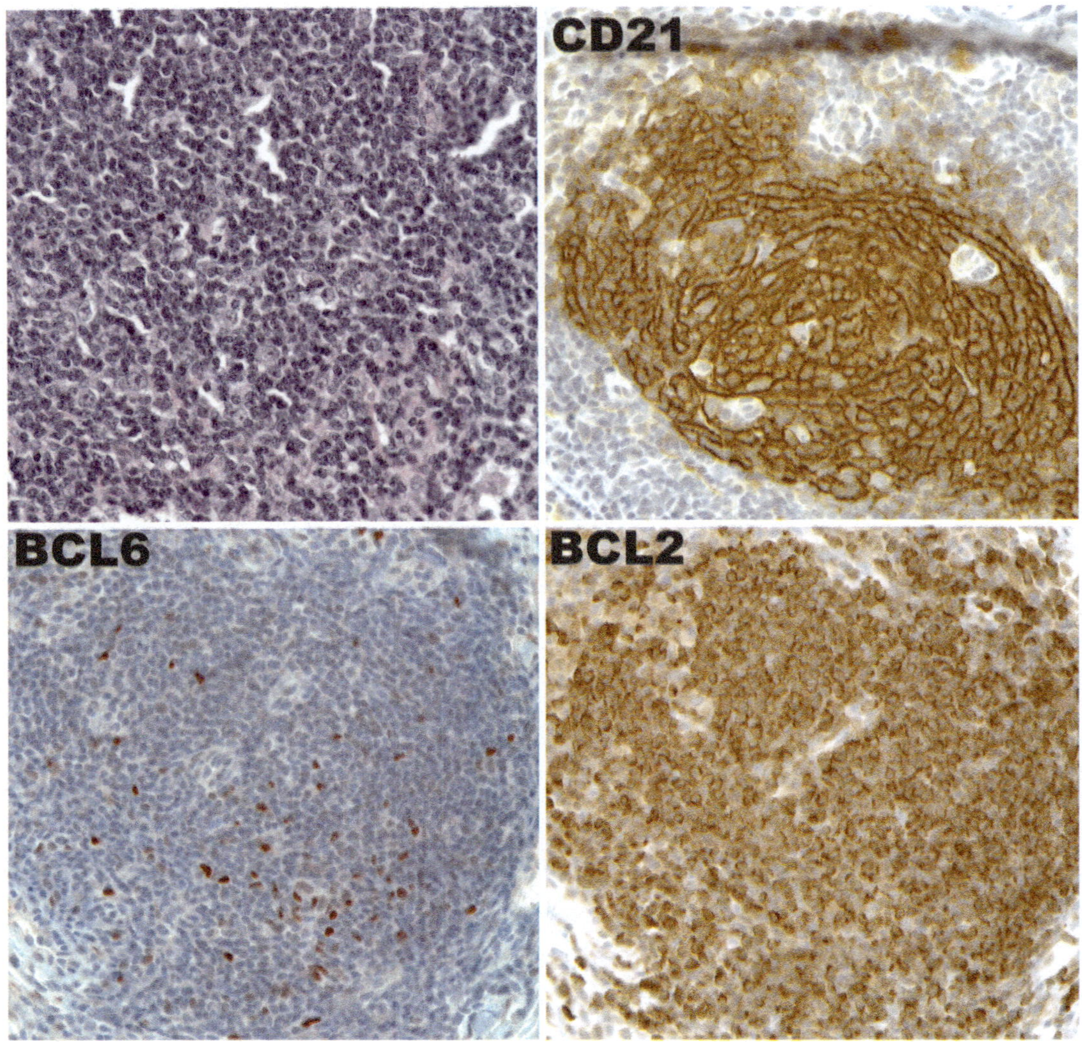

Fig. 20.7 BCL2-positive, colonized lymphoid follicle in cutaneous marginal zone lymphoma. Follicles are difficult to visualize but are highlighted by CD21 staining of the follicular dendritic cell meshwork of the germinal center. Centrocytes and centroblasts are rare, and there is minimal BCL6 staining. BCL2 stain marks the reactive mantle zone B cells and follicular helper T cells, as well as the small noncleaved marginal zone B cells colonizing the germinal center

The presence of lymphoid follicles in a skin biopsy is always a pathologic finding and may occur in several conditions, such as reactive lymphoid hyperplasia (e.g., secondary to vaccinations, arthropod bites, medications, and spirochetal infections), cutaneous Rosai-Dorfman disease, lupus panniculitis, cutaneous IgG4-related disease, low-grade cutaneous B-cell lymphomas (marginal zone lymphoma and follicle center lymphoma), and occasionally tumor-stage mycosis fungoides. In most instances, the germinal center of lymphoid follicles is negative with BCL2 immunostain. BCL2-positive lymphoid follicles (Fig. 20.1) can be a source of confusion, and the differential diagnosis for this finding is discussed here.

Reactive secondary lymphoid follicles show two main compartments: the mantle zone and the germinal center (Fig. 20.2). The *mantle zone* is located at the periphery of the follicle and consists predominantly of mantle zone B cells (BCL2-positive, small noncleaved lymphocytes with dense chromatin, inconspicuous nucleoli, and scant cytoplasm). The other cell types are located within the *germinal center* and include (a) *centrocytes* (BCL2-negative, small germinal center B cells with cleaved nuclei and inconspicuous nucleoli), (b) *centroblasts* (BCL2-negative, large germinal center B cells with round, noncleaved nuclei and multiple conspicuous peripheral nucleoli), (c) *follicular helper T cells* (BCL2-positive, small noncleaved lymphocytes with dense chromatin, inconspicuous nucleoli, and scant cytoplasm), (d) *follicular dendritic cells* (CD21-positive, single or clustered large cells with round, noncleaved nuclei and single central nucleolus), and (e) *tingible-body macrophages* (CD68-positive, histiocytes with reniform, elongated nucleus and abundant cytoplasm with apoptotic fragments) (see Fig. 20.3). The immunophenotype of these cell types is listed in Table 20.1.

Lymphoid follicles can be reactive (benign) or neoplastic (malignant). While reactive primary lymphoid follicles lack germinal centers, reactive secondary follicles show well-defined mantle zones and well-spaced germinal centers. Centrocytes and centroblasts are the main cellular component of the germinal center and are highlighted by BCL6 stain. BCL2 protein is normally expressed in memory lymphocytes and has an antiapoptotic function. In a reactive lymphoid follicle, BCL2 stain marks the mantle zone B cells and the follicular helper T cells in the germinal center. Reactive centrocytes and centroblasts downregulate BCL2, and therefore most cells in the germinal center are negative with BCL2 immunostain (Fig. 20.4).

In pseudolymphomas (reactive lymphoid hyperplasia) and in marginal zone lymphoma, lymphoid follicles are reactive, while in follicle center (follicular) lymphoma, lymphoid follicles are malignant and are composed of an admixture of neoplastic centrocytes and centroblasts (generally with a diminished component of the other cellular elements of the follicle). Most cases of primary cutaneous follicle center lymphoma (PCFCL) are BCL2-negative (Fig. 20.5). However, a significant subset of PCFCL and most cases of systemic/nodal follicular lymphoma are positive with BCL2 immunohistochemistry (Fig. 20.6). Staging workup would demonstrate whether a follicular lymphoma in the skin is primary cutaneous or secondary cutaneous involvement by systemic/nodal follicular lymphoma.

Lymphoid follicles in marginal zone lymphoma (MZL) can be colonized by BCL2-positive neoplastic B cells and mimic BCL2-positive follicular lymphoma. In this differential, it is important to analyze the predominant cytomorphology (admixture of small cleaved/large noncleaved vs. predominantly small noncleaved) and the degree of BCL6 expression. Colonized follicles in MZL are often difficult to visualize but are highlighted by CD21 staining of the follicular dendritic cell meshwork of the germinal center. Centrocytes (small cleaved) and centroblasts (large noncleaved) are rare, and there is minimal to absent BCL6 staining. BCL2 stain marks the reactive mantle zone B cells and follicular helper T cells, as well as the small noncleaved marginal zone B cells colonizing the germinal center. (Fig. 20.7).

Table 20.1 Cellular components of reactive lymphoid follicles and immunophenotype

Cell type	Location in lymphoid follicle	Cytomorphologic features	Immunophenotype
Follicular dendritic cell (FDC)	Germinal center	Large round noncleaved nucleus with single central nucleolus	CD21+ (immunohistochemical stain highlights the meshwork of the dendritic processes)
Germinal center B cells (centrocytes and centroblasts)	Germinal center	Small cleaved (centrocytes) and large noncleaved (centroblasts) with scant cytoplasm	CD20+, BCL6+, BCL2−
(Tingible-body) macrophages	Germinal center	Reniform, elongated nucleus and abundant cytoplasm with apoptotic debris	CD68+
Follicular helper T cells	Germinal center	Small noncleaved nuclei and scant cytoplasm	CD3+, CD20−, BCL2+
Mantle zone B cells	Mantle zone	Small noncleaved nuclei and scant cytoplasm	CD20+, BCL6−, BCL2+

Pearls and Pitfalls

1. Lymphoid follicles are often smaller in skin than in tonsils or lymph nodes. Deeper sections quickly cut through follicles in a skin biopsy. When comparing different immunostains, it is important to remember that the germinal center of a given follicle may be present in some but absent in other sections. For example, a tangentially sectioned follicle would only show the mantle zone (normally BCL2-positive) but not the germinal center (normally BCL2-negative).
2. Reactive primary lymphoid follicles lack germinal centers. Since only the mantle zone is present, the primary follicle is BCL2-positive.

Suggested Reading

Leinweber B, Colli C, Chott A, et al. Differential diagnosis of cutaneous infiltrates of B lymphocytes with follicular growth pattern. Am J Dermatopathol. 2004 Feb;26(1):4–13.

Orazi A, Weiss LM, Foucar K, Knowles DM. Knowles' neoplastic hematopathology. 3rd ed. Philadelphia: Lippincott Williams & Wilkins; 2014.

Swerdlow SH, Campo E, Harris NL, et al., editors. WHO classification of tumors of hematopoietic and lymphoid tissues. Lyon: IARC; 2008.

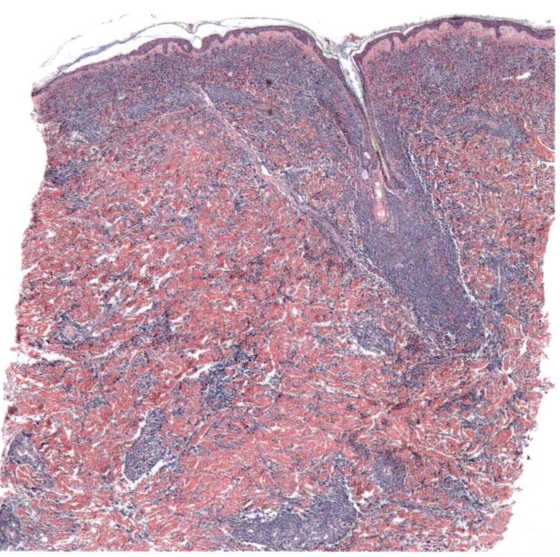

Fig. 21.1 Secondary skin involvement by mantle cell lymphoma showing a combination of perivascular, interstitial, and periadnexal patterns

Table 21.1 Key Facts

Definition
Primary skin lymphomas are cutaneous T-cell and B-cell lymphomas that present in the skin with no evidence of extracutaneous disease at the time of diagnosis. However, a wide variety of systemic/nodal lymphomas may affect the skin secondarily and may be the initial manifestation of underlying disease
Prototypic clinical presentation
Solitary/localized or generalized erythematous to violaceous papules, plaques, or tumors. Neoplastic infiltrates may be incidentally found at sites of cutaneous inflammation or epithelial neoplasms
Histopathologic findings
Variable density. Triple pattern of perivascular, interstitial, and periadnexal distribution of atypical lymphocytes is common. Epitheliotropism is infrequent
Immunophenotype: variable
Prognosis
Variable (depending on the type of lymphoma)

© Springer Nature Switzerland AG 2019
A. Subtil, *Diagnosis of Cutaneous Lymphoid Infiltrates*,
https://doi.org/10.1007/978-3-030-11654-5_21

Fig. 21.2 Secondary cutaneous involvement by nodal diffuse large B-cell lymphoma showing a combination of perivascular, interstitial, and periadnexal patterns

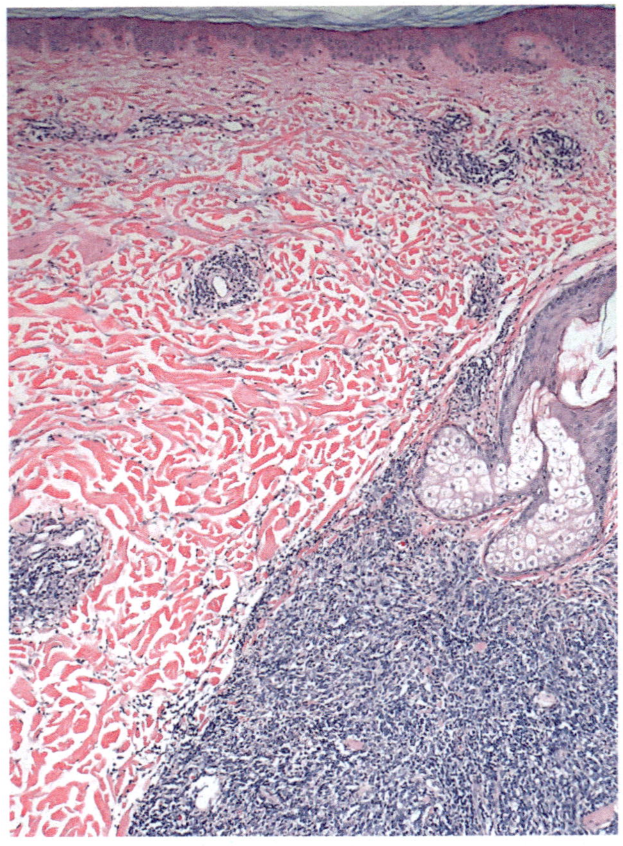

Fig. 21.3 The triple pattern of perivascular, interstitial, and periadnexal distribution of atypical lymphocytes is common in cases of systemic lymphoma involving the skin secondarily

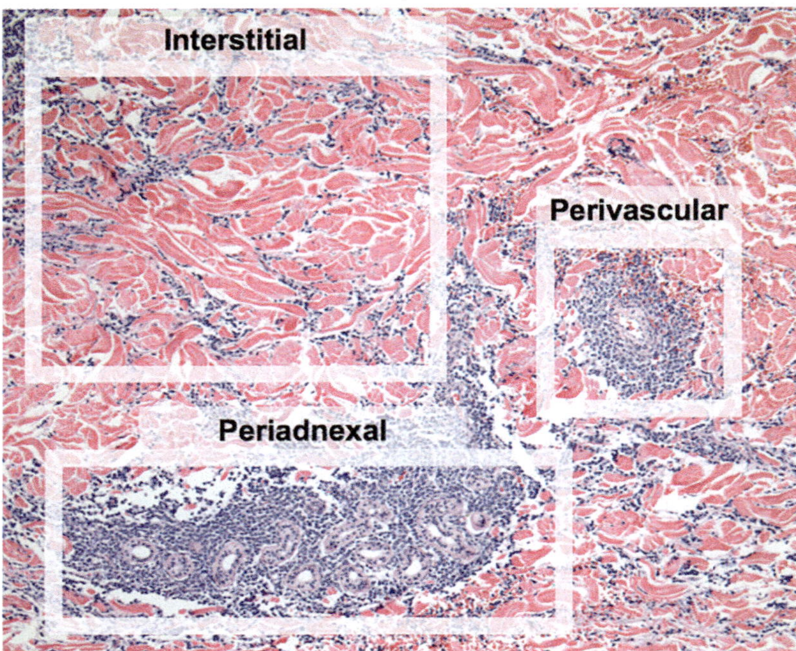

Fig. 21.4 Secondary cutaneous involvement by small lymphocytic lymphoma/chronic lymphocytic leukemia showing three cytomorphologic components (small lymphocytes, prolymphocytes, and paraimmunoblasts)

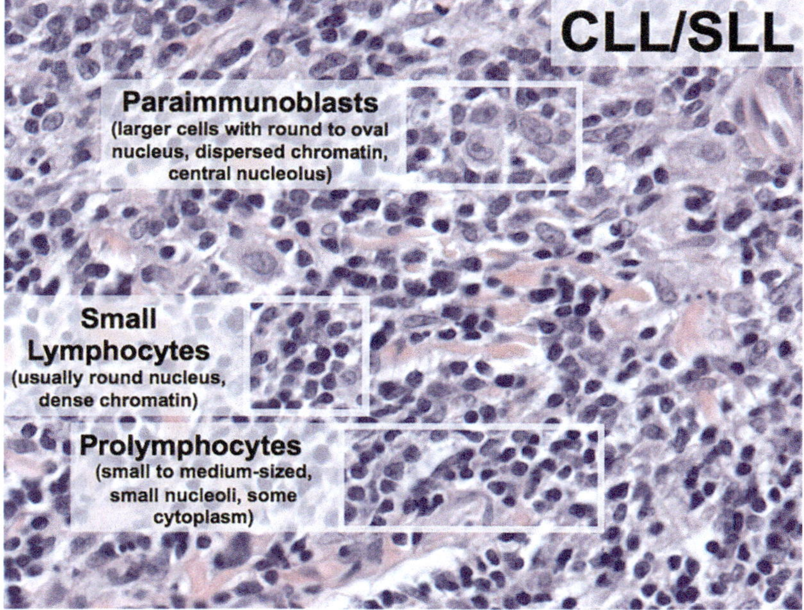

Fig. 21.5 Incidental small lymphocytic lymphoma/chronic lymphocytic leukemia in association with actinic keratosis. A dense infiltrate of CD20-positive B cells is present in the dermis

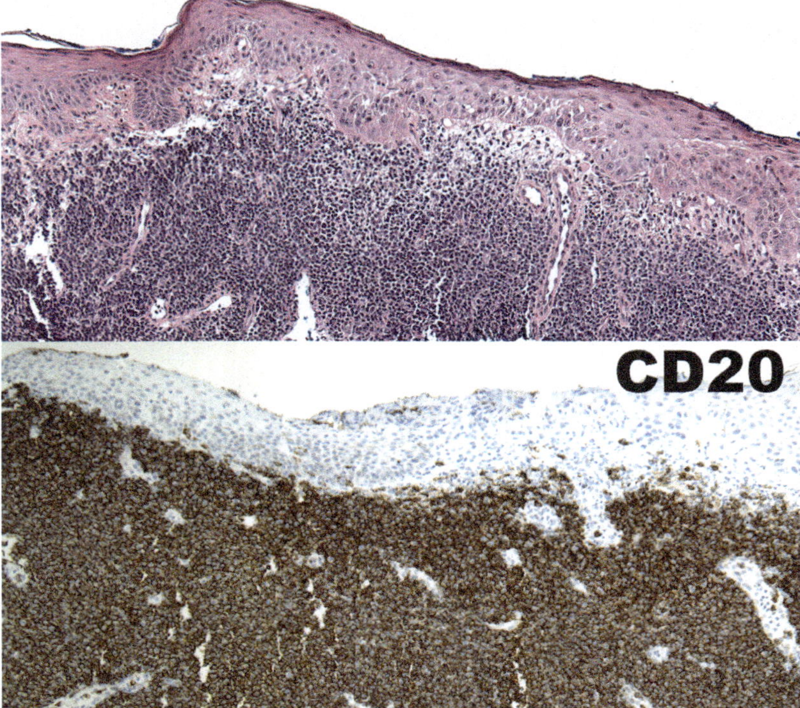

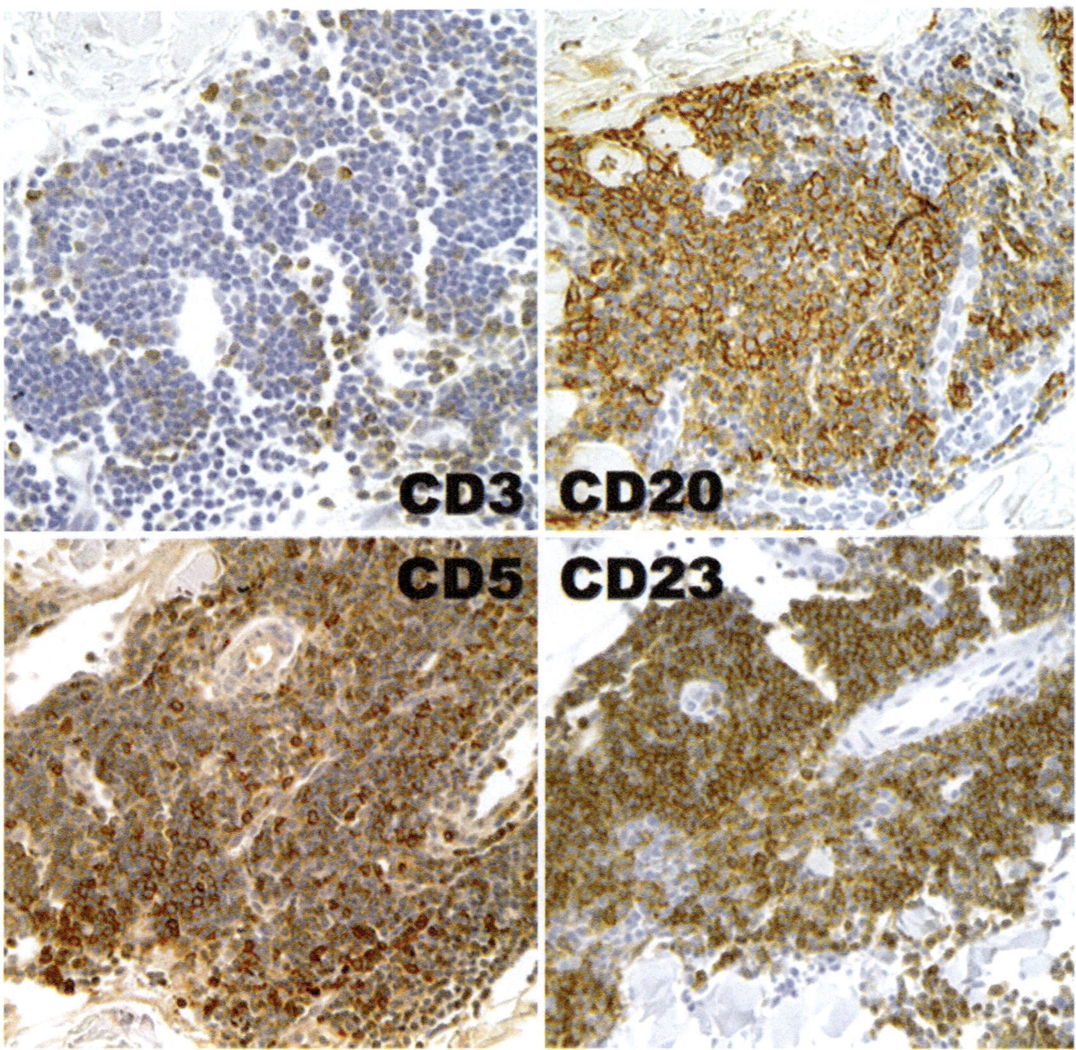

Fig. 21.6 Cutaneous involvement by small lymphocytic lymphoma/chronic lymphocytic leukemia. Skin biopsy shows a dermal CD3-/CD20+ B-cell infiltrate with coexpression of CD5 and CD23. CD5 is a T-cell marker and shows a biphasic pattern: strong staining in scattered T cells (similar to that seen with CD3) and weaker staining in neoplastic B cells

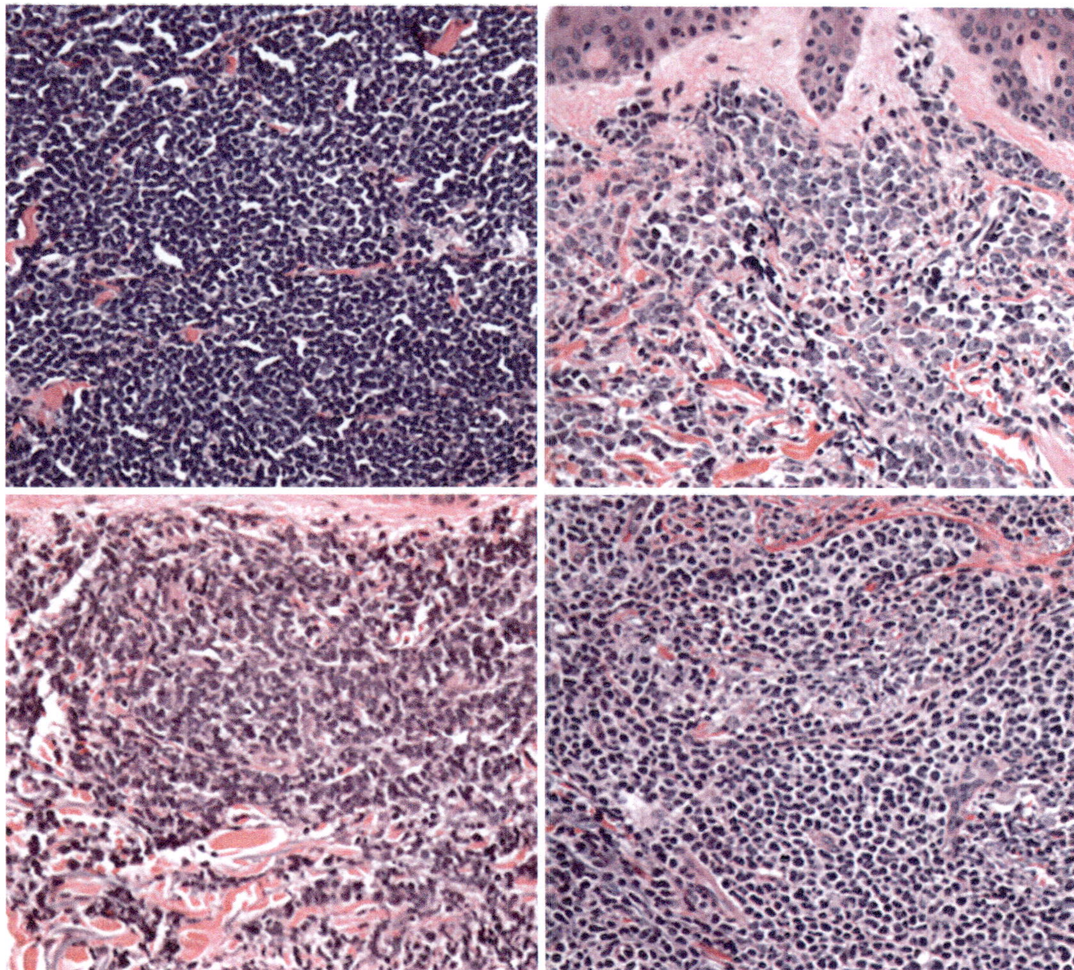

Fig. 21.7 Secondary skin involvement by different morphologic variants of mantle cell lymphoma (clockwise from top left: small cell, pleomorphic, marginal zone-like, blastoid)

Fig. 21.8 Secondary cutaneous involvement by mantle cell lymphoma showing positive nuclear staining with cyclin D1

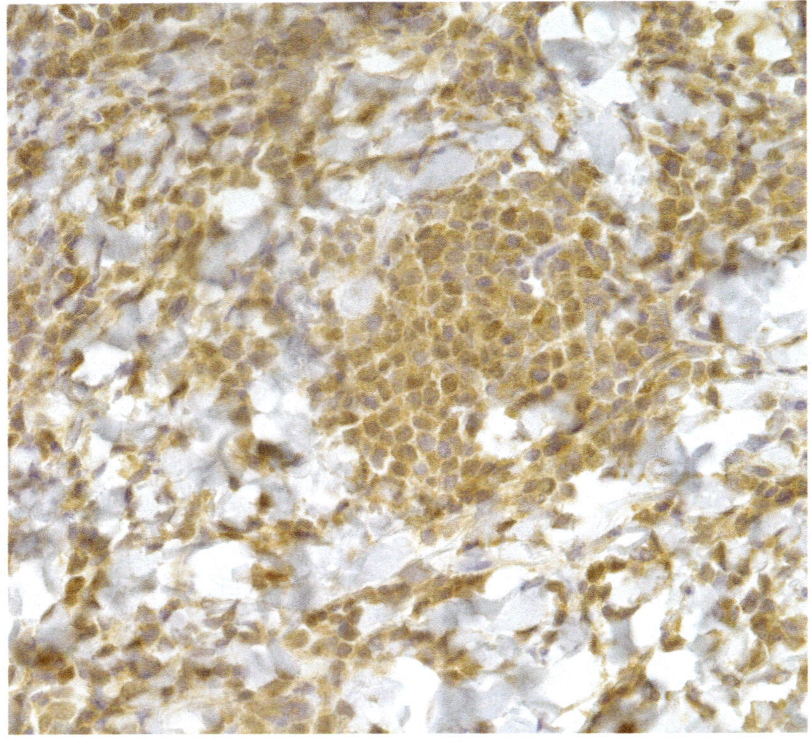

Fig. 21.9 Secondary skin involvement by systemic ALK-positive anaplastic large cell lymphoma

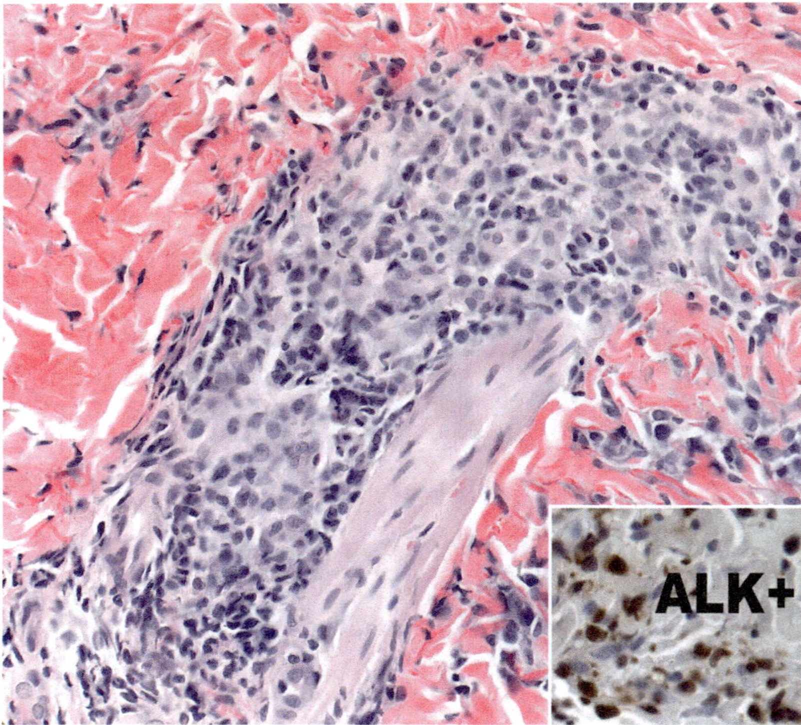

Fig. 21.10 Secondary cutaneous involvement by plasma cell myeloma showing atypical plasma cells

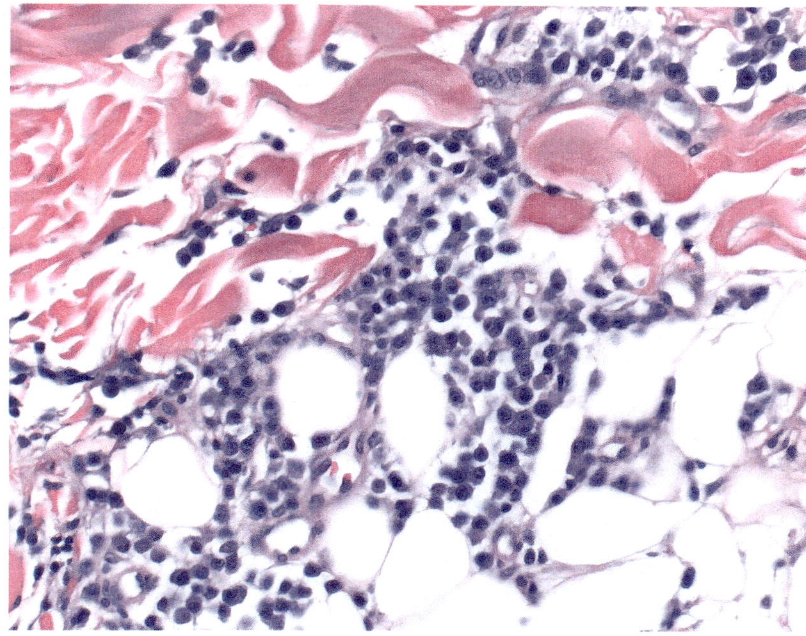

Disease Definition

- Primary skin lymphomas are cutaneous T-cell and B-cell lymphomas that present in the skin with no evidence of extracutaneous disease at the time of diagnosis. However, a wide variety of systemic/nodal lymphomas may affect the skin secondarily. Secondary cutaneous involvement by systemic/nodal lymphomas may be the initial manifestation of disease. In addition to immunophenotyping, careful correlation with cytomorphologic features, clinical findings, and staging results are critical for proper classification (Table 21.1).

Epidemiology

- The skin is a relatively common extranodal site of involvement by systemic/nodal lymphomas.
- Usually adults and elderly patients.

Preferential Sites of Involvement

- Head and neck region, trunk and/or extremities.

Clinical Features

- Solitary/localized or generalized erythematous to violaceous papules, plaques, or tumors, usually without ulceration.
- Neoplastic infiltrates may be incidentally found at sites of cutaneous inflammation (including arthropod bites) or skin tumors (predominantly epithelial, such as squamous cell carcinoma and basal cell carcinoma).
- A wide range of cutaneous manifestations may occur in patients with small lymphocytic lymphoma/chronic lymphocytic leukemia and may predate the hematologic diagnosis (Table 21.2).
- *Less common presentations*: leonine facies, purpuric lesions, erythroderma, ulcerated lesions.

Histomorphology

- *Pattern*: variable density, from sparse to dense diffuse dermal infiltrates with variable pannicular extension. Combination of perivascular, interstitial, and periadnexal patterns is common (Figs. 21.1, 21.2, and 21.3).

Table 21.2 Cutaneous manifestations of small lymphocytic lymphoma/chronic lymphocytic leukemia (SLL/CLL)

1. Incidental SLL/CLL in association with cutaneous epithelial lesions (invasive squamous cell carcinoma, squamous cell carcinoma in situ, actinic keratosis, basal cell carcinoma, and lichenoid keratosis)
2. Specific skin involvement by SLL/CLL (absence of an associated cutaneous lesion)
3. SLL/CLL with transformation (Richter's large cell transformation may occur in the skin or at an extracutaneous site)
4. SLL/CLL in association with another lymphoproliferative process (aggressive cytotoxic lymphomas are rare neoplasms but are overrepresented in this patient population)
5. Cutaneous hypersensitivity reaction in the absence of neoplastic cells in the skin (exaggerated arthropod bite-like reaction/eosinophilic dermatosis of myeloproliferative disease)

Table 21.3 Immunophenotype of low-grade B-cell neoplasms

	CD5	CD10	BCL2	IgD	BCL6	MUM1	CD43	Cyclin D1	CD23
Mantle cell lymphoma	+	−	+	+	−	−	+	+	−
Chronic lymphocytic leukemia/small lymphocytic lymphoma	+	−	+	+	−	+/−	+	− (may be + in proliferation centers)	+
Follicular lymphoma	−	+	+/−	−/+	+	−	−	−	−/+
MALT lymphoma	−	−	+	−	−	+/−	+/−	−	−
Plasma cell myeloma	−	−	+	+/−	−	+	+/−	+/−	−

- *Less common patterns*: epidermotropism may occasionally occur.
- *Neoplastic cells*: variable cytomorphology, depending on the type of lymphoma. While infiltrates of small lymphocytic lymphoma/chronic lymphocytic leukemia appear monotonous at low magnification, three cytomorphologic components are present: small lymphocytes, prolymphocytes, and paraimmunoblasts (Figs. 21.4, 21.5, and 21.6). Mantle cell lymphoma shows highly variable cytomorphology (small cell, pleomorphic, blastoid, or marginal zone-like) (Fig. 21.7).
- *Reactive cells*: usually small lymphocytes and scattered histiocytes. There may be prominent inflammation if the neoplastic infiltrate is associated with an epithelial neoplasm.

Immunophenotype

- Variable phenotype, depending on the type of lymphoma (Table 21.3). In addition, aberrant staining patterns are fairly common.
- Since mantle cell lymphoma shows variable cytomorphology (and may even resemble marginal zone lymphoma), cyclin D1 (and occasionally SOX11) is recommended in the evaluation of all cutaneous B-cell infiltrates (Figs. 21.7 and 21.8).
- Systemic anaplastic large cell lymphoma may be ALK-positive or ALK-negative and may involve the skin secondarily (Fig. 21.9). Staging is usually the best method to rule out this possibility, since there have been rare reports of ALK-positive cutaneous anaplastic large cell lymphoma.

Genetics

- Variable, depending on the type of lymphoma.
- Genetic markers may be diagnostically helpful in some cases.

Prognosis

- Variable, depending on the type of lymphoma.
- The prognosis of small lymphocytic lymphoma/chronic lymphocytic leukemia does not appear to be affected by cutaneous involvement.
- Adverse risk factors: large cell transformation of low-grade lymphoma.

Pearls and Pitfalls

1. Primary cutaneous lymphomas often exhibit different clinical behavior and prognosis from histologically similar systemic lymphomas.
2. While some lymphomas have systemic/nodal and primary cutaneous counterparts (e.g., nodal follicular and cutaneous follicle center lymphoma, nodal and extranodal marginal zone lymphoma, systemic and cutaneous anaplastic large cell lymphoma), several are by definition systemic (e.g., small lymphocytic lymphoma/chronic lymphocytic leukemia, mantle cell lymphoma). If the latter are found in a skin biopsy, the diagnosis is secondary cutaneous involvement by systemic lymphoma (i.e., there is no primary cutaneous mantle cell lymphoma).
3. Staging should be performed after a lymphoma diagnosis (in any organ).
4. Tissue immunohistochemistry results often do not perfectly match flow cytometry results. This frequent mismatch may be multifactorial (e.g., greater sensitivity of flow cytometry in detecting dim expression, the use of different antibodies with different epitope targets, downregulation of certain proteins during the process of extranodal infiltration).
5. The more stains are performed, the higher the probability that a given stain might not have worked (and would need to be repeated). Recognition of technical problems is critically important in the interpretation of special stains.
6. Systemic T-cell lymphomas (which may have T follicular helper phenotype) may occasionally present in the skin and may closely mimic primary cutaneous CD4-positive small/medium T-cell lymphoproliferative disorder. Therefore, adequate staging at the time of initial diagnosis and/or close follow-up would be judicious to exclude this possibility. This differential is important because of the significantly worse prognosis of systemic T-cell lymphoma.
7. B-cell lymphomas are associated with light chain restriction. While this is easily identifiable with flow cytometry, demonstration of light chain restriction via tissue immunohistochemistry (of formalin-fixed, paraffin-embedded tissue) would generally require significant cytoplasmic immunoglobulin (i.e., plasmacytic differentiation in a substantial subset of the neoplastic B cells).
8. The plasmacytic variant of cutaneous marginal zone lymphoma (skin-only infiltrates composed almost exclusively of monotypic plasma cells) may resemble plasma cell myeloma, which can involve the skin secondarily (Fig. 21.10). If the initial skin biopsy shows an infiltrate composed exclusively of monotypic plasma cells, staging workup is necessary to rule out the possibility of a systemic plasma cell dyscrasia.
9. Rituximab, which targets the B-cell marker CD20, is commonly used for the treatment of systemic B-cell lymphoma. If secondary cutaneous involvement occurs in these patients, the neoplastic infiltrates are often (though not always) CD20-negative. CD79a stain is a better option in these cases.

Suggested Reading

Byrd JA, Scherschun L, Chaffins ML, Fivenson DP. Eosinophilic dermatosis of myeloproliferative disease: characterization of a unique eruption in patients with hematologic disorders. Arch Dermatol. 2001;137(10):1378–80.

Higgins RA, Blankenship JE, Kinney MC. Application of immunohistochemistry in the diagnosis of non-Hodgkin and Hodgkin lymphoma. Arch Pathol Lab Med. 2008;132:441–61.

Orazi A, Weiss LM, Foucar K, Knowles DM. Knowles' neoplastic hematopathology. 3rd ed. Philadelphia: Lippincott Williams & Wilkins; 2014.

Swerdlow SH, Campo E, Harris NL, Jaffe ES, Pileri SA, Stein H, Thiele J, editors. WHO classification of tumours of haematopoietic and lymphoid tissues (revised 4th ed). Lyon: IARC; 2017.

Classic Mycosis Fungoides

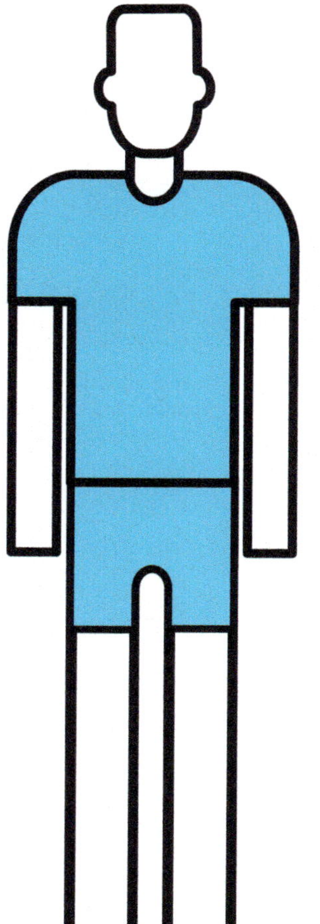

Fig. 22.1 Classic mycosis fungoides preferentially involves sun-protected areas

Table 22.1 Key facts

Definition

Mycosis fungoides is a primary cutaneous T-cell lymphoma composed of epidermotropic cerebriform lymphocytes and a clinical pattern of chronic patches/plaques, which evolve in some patients to tumors

Prototypic clinical presentation

Chronic lesions on sun-protected sites (back, buttocks, abdomen, breasts, axilla, inguinal, proximal extremities). Patches/plaques may be annular, atrophic, erythematous, and/or scaly. Lesions are usually >5 cm in diameter. Slow progression

Histopathologic findings

Epidermotropism by atypical small- to medium-sized lymphocytes and fibrosis. Variable additional findings depending on the stage of disease (see text)

Most common immunophenotype: CD3+, CD4+, CD8−, CD2+, CD5+, CD7−, betaF1+

Prognosis

Indolent

© Springer Nature Switzerland AG 2019

A. Subtil, *Diagnosis of Cutaneous Lymphoid Infiltrates*,

https://doi.org/10.1007/978-3-030-11654-5_22

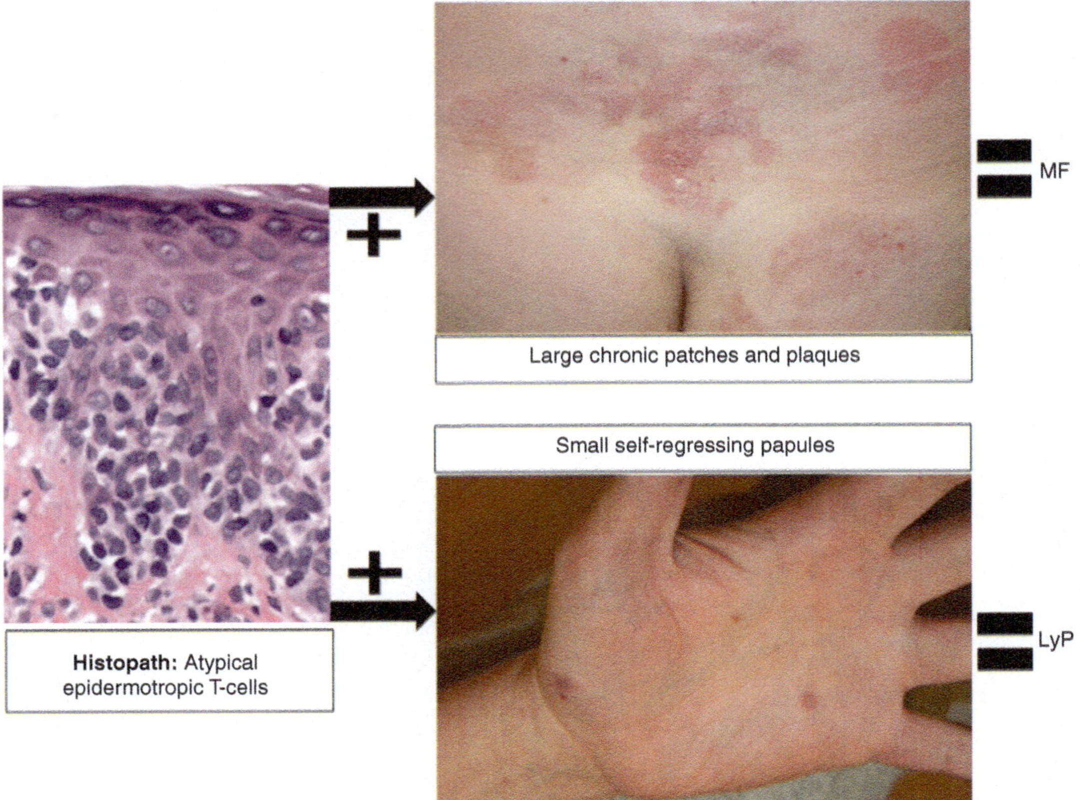

Fig. 22.2 Since the same histopathologic pattern may occur in several entities, clinical pathologic correlation and/or immunophenotyping is necessary to correctly classify cutaneous lymphoid infiltrates. An epidermotropic histopathologic pattern will result in different diagnoses depending on the clinical picture: large, chronic patches and/or plaques on sun-protected skin for classic mycosis fungoides vs. small, self-regressing papules for lymphomatoid papulosis

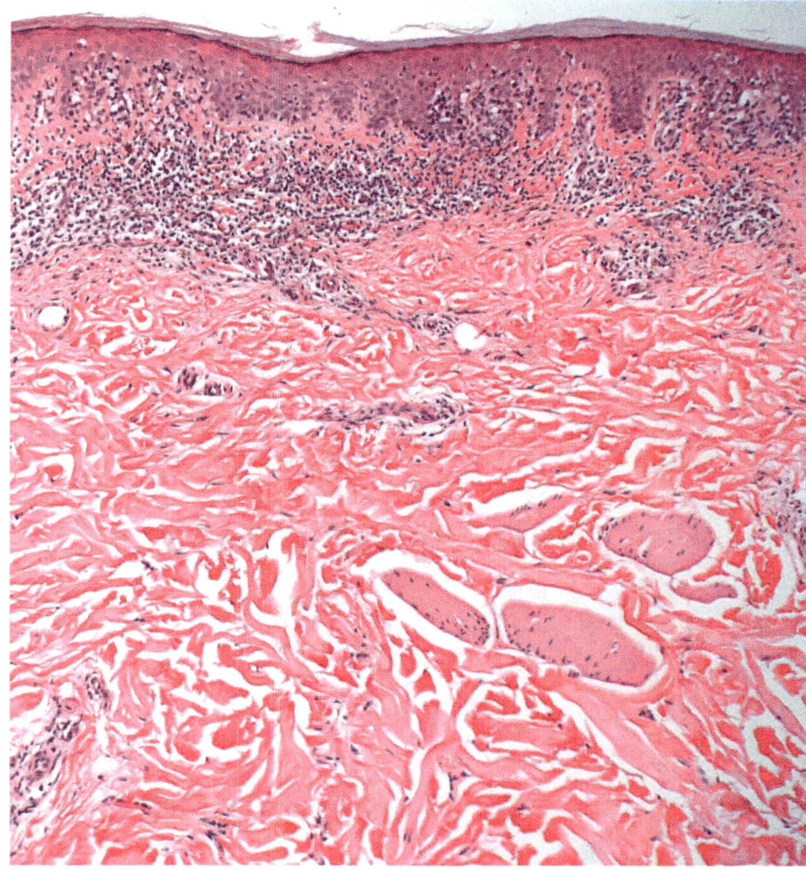

Fig. 22.3 Low-power magnification of patch-stage classic mycosis fungoides. Mild patchy superficial dermal lymphocytic infiltrate

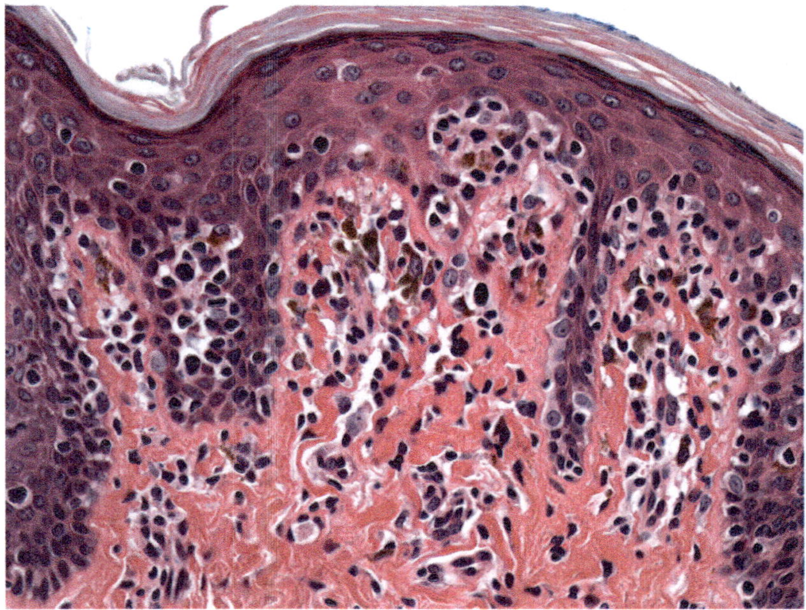

Fig. 22.4 High-power magnification of patch-stage classic mycosis fungoides. Mild superficial dermal lymphocytic infiltrate with atypical intraepidermal cells

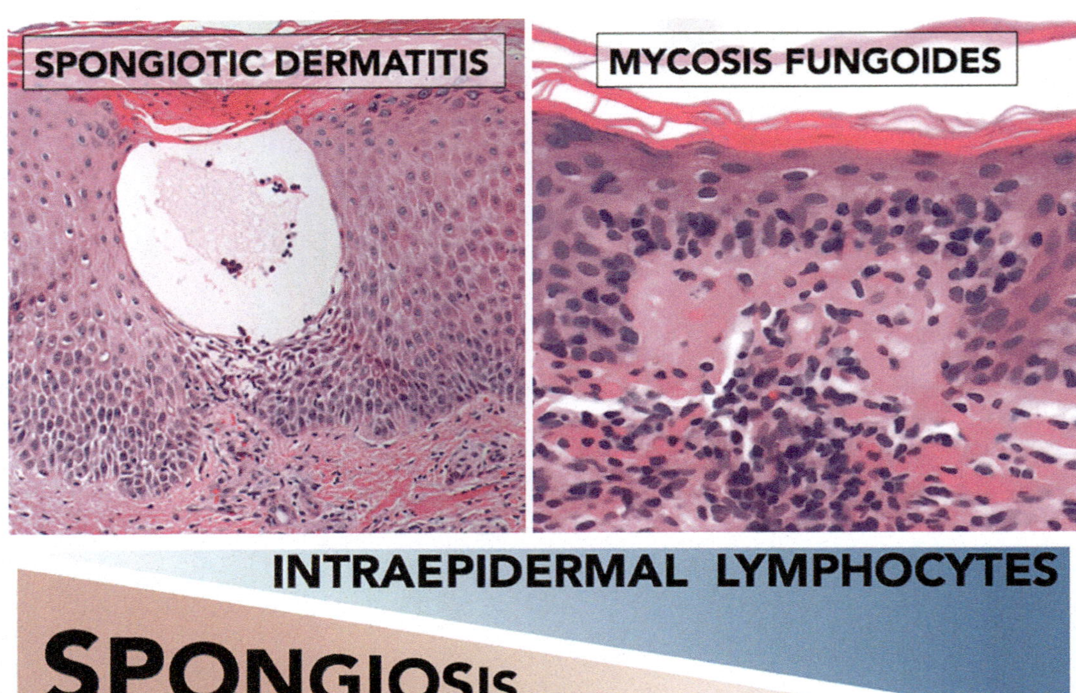

Fig. 22.5 MF tends to have frequent intraepidermal lymphocytes and relatively scant spongiosis (disproportionate exocytosis), while the opposite proportion of lymphocytes versus spongiosis is seen in spongiotic/eczematous dermatitis

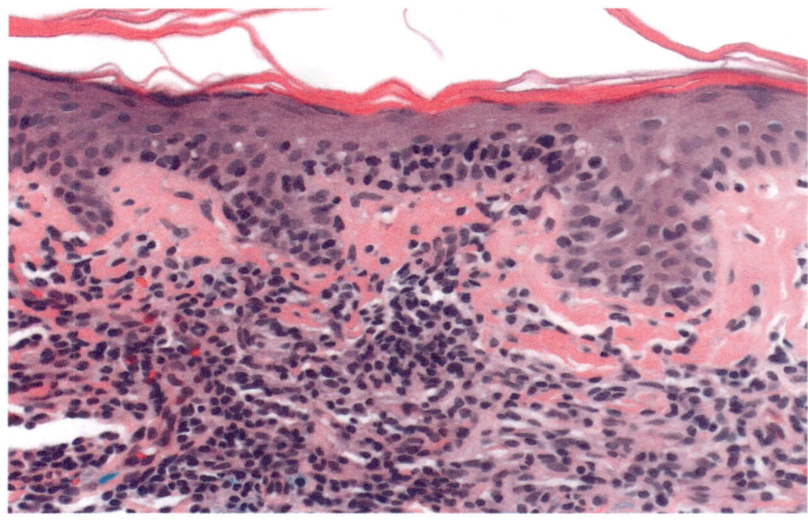

Fig. 22.6 High-power magnification of plaque-stage classic mycosis fungoides. Band-like superficial dermal lymphocytic infiltrate with epidermotropism and fibrosis

Fig. 22.7 Epidermotropism is present in this skin biopsy of classic mycosis fungoides. Intraepidermal lymphocytes are highlighted by arrowheads (single) and circles (clusters or Pautrier microabscesses). Prominent spongiosis is not seen

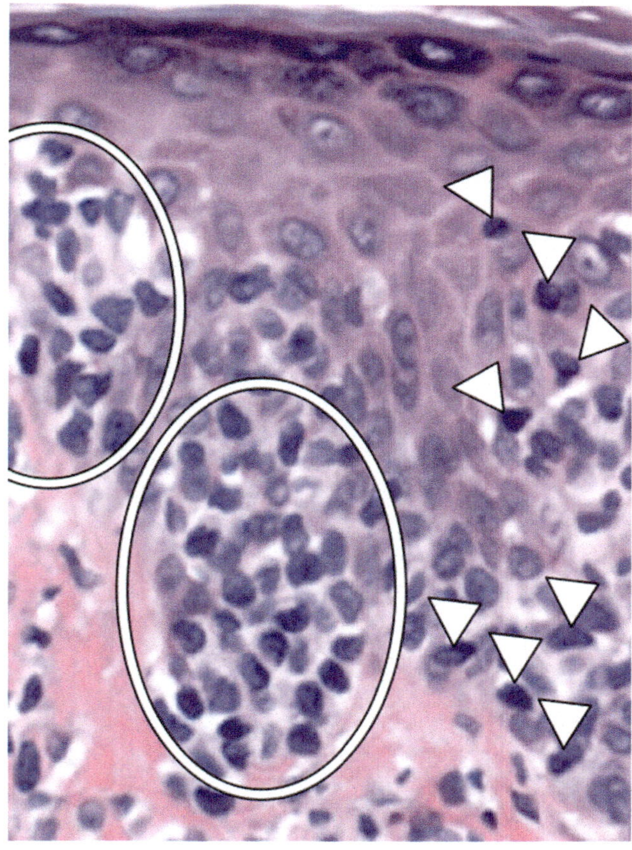

Fig. 22.8 Low-power magnification of classic mycosis fungoides in a patient who progressed to tumor stage after several years of patch/plaque disease. Epidermotropism has been lost, and ulceration is present

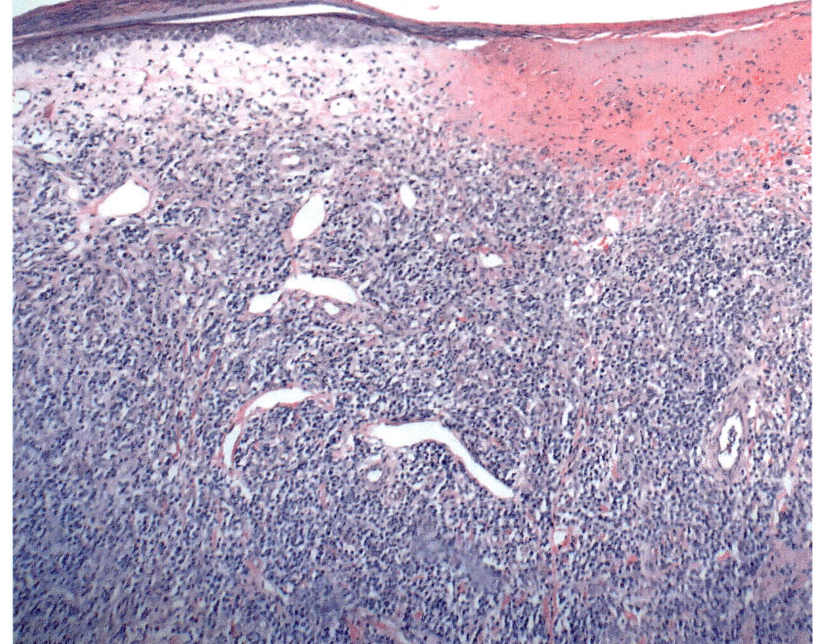

Fig. 22.9 High-power magnification of classic mycosis fungoides. Intraepidermal neoplastic cells are haloed and slightly larger than reactive dermal lymphocytes

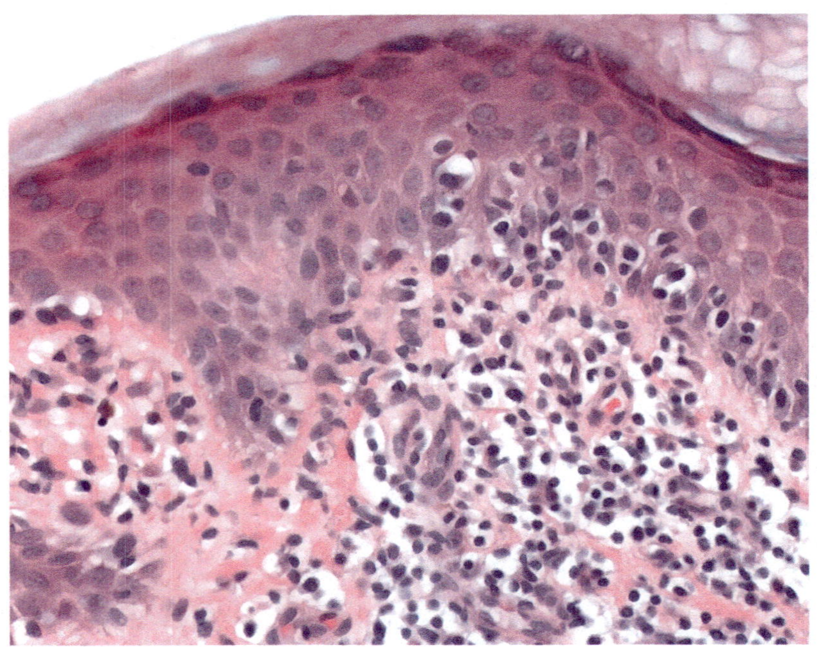

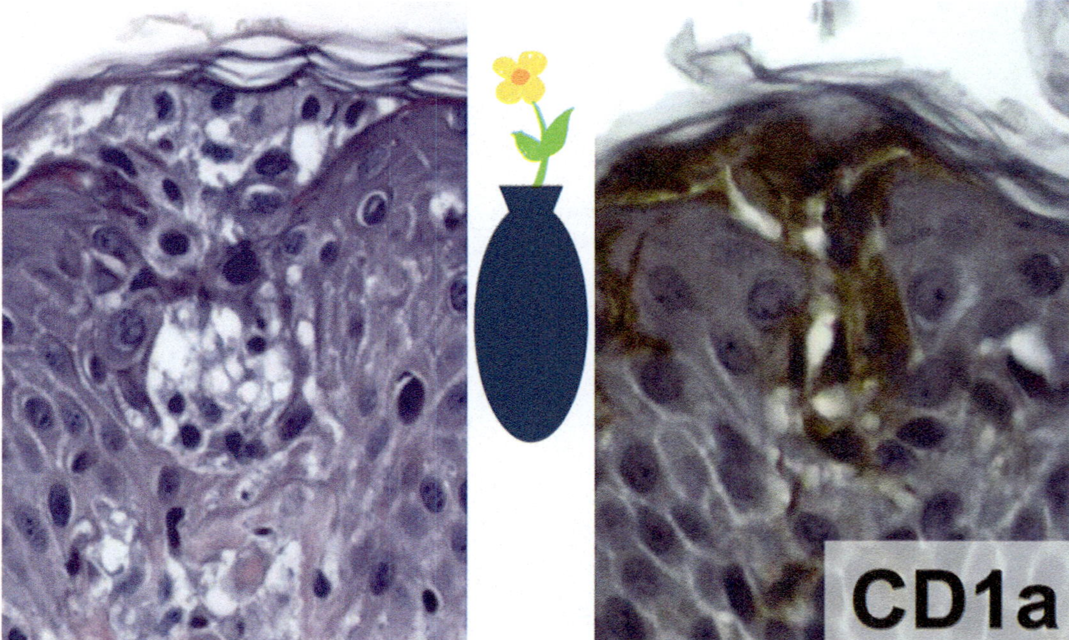

Fig. 22.10 Intraepidermal Langerhans cell microabscesses show a vaselike shape and are highlighted by CD1a stain. They are common in spongiotic/eczematous dermatitis and should not be confused with Pautrier microabscesses (intraepidermal aggregates of atypical lymphocytes)

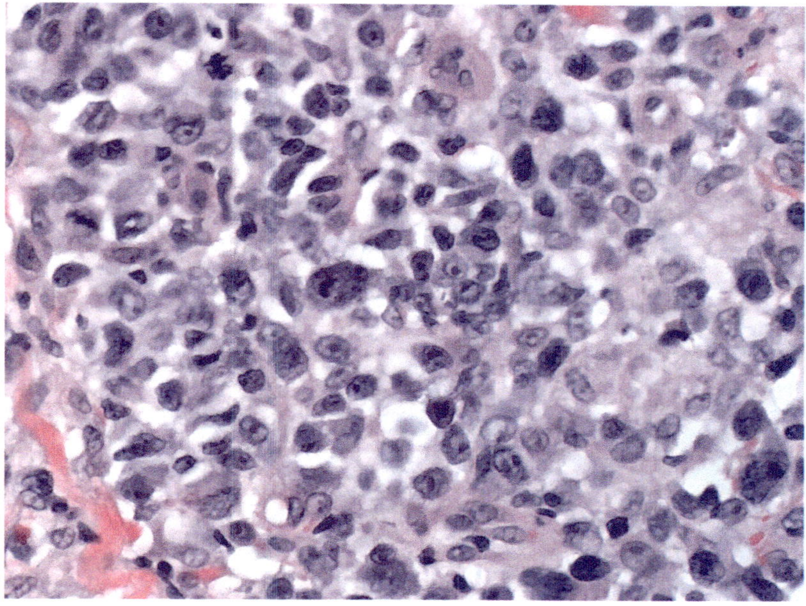

Fig. 22.11 Large cell transformation in a tumor of mycosis fungoides. There should be at least 25% of large atypical cells or formation of microscopic nodules of large cells in the infiltrate

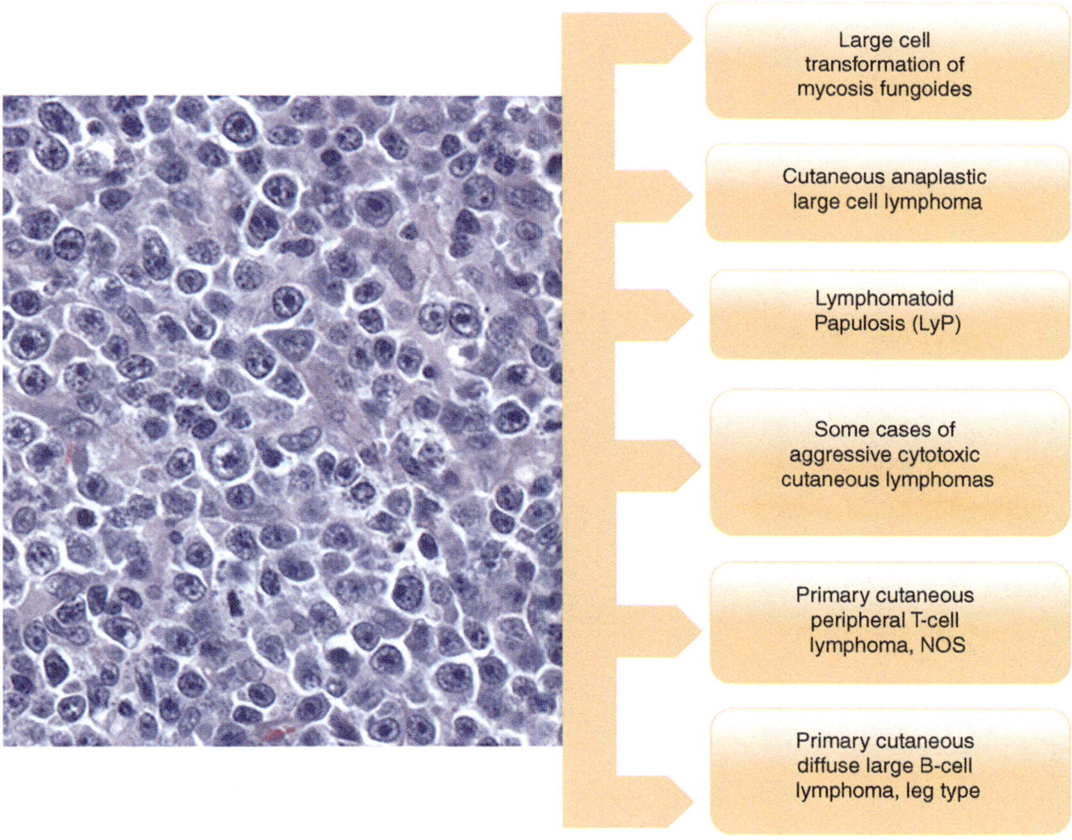

Fig. 22.12 Differential diagnosis of atypical large cell lymphoid infiltrate (>25% large cells)

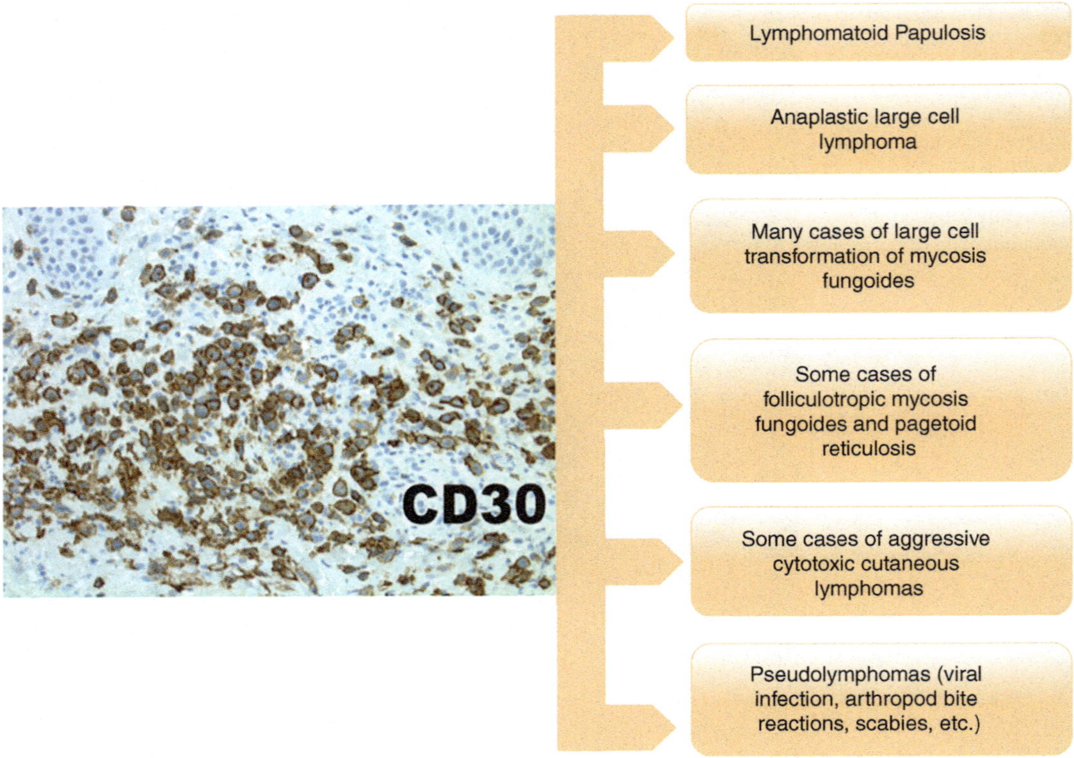

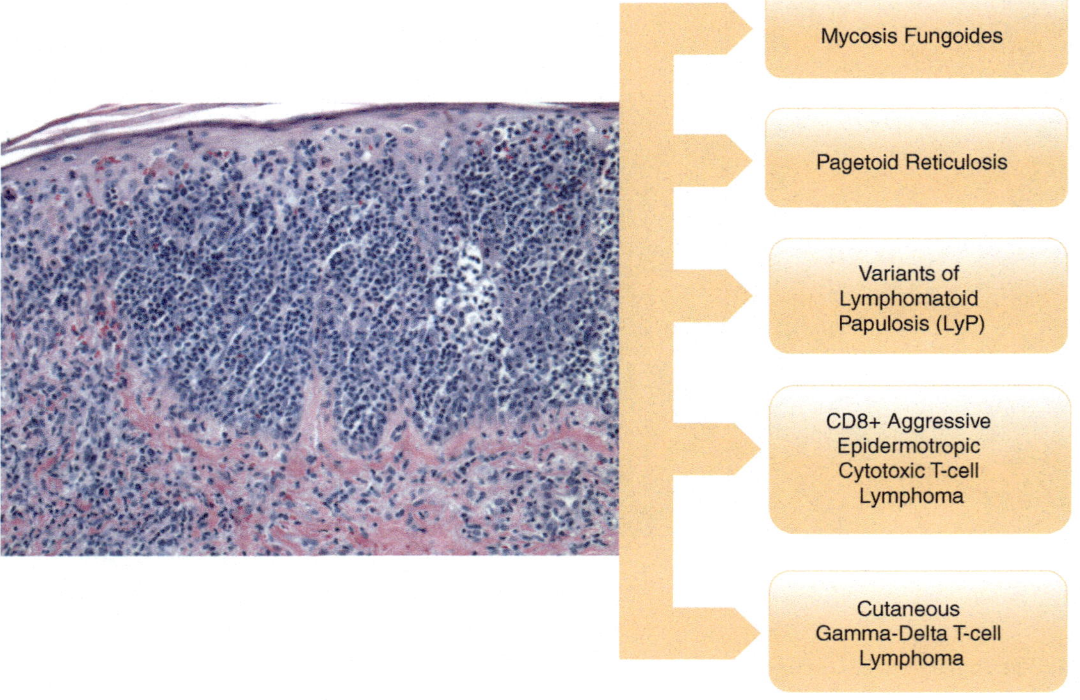

Fig. 22.13 Differential diagnosis of CD30 expression

Fig. 22.14 Differential diagnosis of epidermotropism. Several entities besides mycosis fungoides may exhibit prominent intraepidermal lymphocytes

Disease Definition

- Mycosis fungoides (MF) is a primary cutaneous T-cell lymphoma composed of epidermotropic cerebriform lymphocytes. Classic MF should only be considered for cases with the conventional clinical evolution of patches, plaques, and (in some patients) tumors ("Alibert-Bazin" type) (Table 22.1).
- MF variants with a similar clinical course are included under classic MF, while variants with distinct clinicopathologic features and prognosis are considered separately (folliculotropic MF, pagetoid reticulosis, and granulomatous slack skin; Chaps. 23, 24, and 25).

Epidemiology

- The most common type of skin lymphoma (approximately 50% of all primary cutaneous lymphomas)
- Male predominance
- Usually adults and elderly patients but may occur in childhood
- Higher incidence in patients of African descent

Preferential Sites of Involvement

- Sun-protected sites (back, buttocks, abdomen, breasts, axilla, inguinal, proximal lower extremities/upper thighs) (Fig. 22.1).
- Generally restricted to the skin but may show limited involvement of peripheral blood.
- Involvement of head and neck region and extracutaneous dissemination may occur in advanced disease (oral cavity, lymph nodes, visceral organs).
- Enlarged lymph nodes in MF patients may show dermatopathic lymphadenopathy as well as early (no architectural effacement) to overt (partial or complete architectural effacement) involvement by the disease.

Clinical Features

- Indolent course with very slow progression over several years from chronic patches to plaques and, in some patients, to tumors.

- Patches/plaques may be annular, atrophic, erythematous, and/or scaly (Fig. 22.2). Lesions are usually large (>5 cm in diameter). May cover <10% (skin stage T1) or ≥10% (T2) of the skin surface.
- Tumors (skin stage T3) may ulcerate.
- *Less common presentations*: slow evolution of some persistent cases of parapsoriasis and pigmented purpuric dermatosis to MF.
- Clinical variants of classic MF: hypopigmented, hyperpigmented, MF palmaris et plantaris, ichthyosiform, erythrodermic, bullous, vegetating, unilesional, purpuric, poikilodermatous.

Histomorphology

- *Pattern*: variable depending on the stage of disease. While there are histologic differences for each stage, final classification of lesion type (patch versus plaque versus tumor) is best made clinically.

Patch stage: mild patchy superficial dermal lymphocytic infiltrate with variable degrees of epidermotropism (Fig. 22.3). Reactive lymphocytes may predominate over atypical cells. Since MF lesions are chronic, papillary dermal fibrosis must be present and is often composed of thin, wiry collagen fibers (Fig. 22.4). Fibrosis may expand dermal papillae. Limited to absent spongiosis/intercellular edema: MF tends to have frequent intraepidermal lymphocytes and relatively scant spongiosis (disproportionate exocytosis), while the opposite proportion of lymphocytes versus spongiosis is seen in spongiotic/eczematous dermatitis (Fig. 22.5).

Plaque stage: moderate band-like superficial dermal lymphocytic infiltrate with prominent epidermotropism (Figs. 22.6 and 22.7). Epidermis may show psoriasiform hyperplasia. Since MF lesions are chronic, dermal fibrosis must be present. There may be some extension of the infiltrate into the reticular dermis.

Tumor stage: dense diffuse superficial and deep dermal lymphocytic infiltrate with variable pannicular extension. Epidermotropism may be lost in progression to tumor-stage disease. Ulceration may occur (Fig. 22.8).

- *Neoplastic cells*: generally small- to intermediate-sized lymphocytes with convoluted, cerebriform, hyperchromatic nuclei with dense chromatin and scant cytoplasm. Clear halos may be seen within the epidermis (Fig. 22.9). Epidermotropism may be composed of single and/or clustered cells (Pautrier microabscesses) (Fig. 22.7). Pautrier microabscesses are present in less than half of MF cases (more common in plaque stage) and should not be confused with vaselike Langerhans cell microabscesses, which are common in spongiotic/eczematous dermatitis (Fig. 22.10). Intraepidermal neoplastic cells may be slightly larger than reactive dermal lymphocytes (Fig. 22.9). Epidermotropic cells may be predominantly located in the basal layer in a linear pattern (basilar epidermotropism) or may involve all epidermal layers (pagetoid pattern).
- *Reactive cells*: variable admixture of small lymphocytes (tend to be more dermal than intraepidermal, except in early lesions) and histiocytes (usually sparse and scattered, but prominent in granulomatous variant). While eosinophils and plasma cells are generally rare in patch-stage lesions, both can be fairly prominent in MF plaques and tumors.
- Less common patterns: (a) rare cases may show interstitial infiltrates in the reticular dermis that may resemble interstitial inflammatory dermatoses. Pseudo vascular clefts with "free-floating" collagen fibers surrounded by neoplastic T cells may be seen. (b) Rare cases show incidental granulomatous/ histiocyte-rich infiltrates but with clinical features of classic MF (as opposed to the pendulous flexural skinfolds of granulomatous slack skin). (c) Some cases of tumor-stage MF may show reactive lymphoid follicles (preferentially located at the base of the infiltrate). (d) Apoptotic keratinocytes and interface change (usually focal and limited). (e) Large cell transformation of MF is defined by the presence at least 25% of large atypical cells or formation of microscopic nodules of large cells (Figs. 22.11 and 22.12). It is important not to overcall hyperchromatic medium-sized cells with dense chromatin as large cells, which are defined as at least four times the size of a small lymphocyte and generally exhibit vesicular chromatin and conspicuous nucleoli. Large cell transformation usually occurs in tumor-stage disease (occasionally in plaque stage).

Immunophenotype

- *Neoplastic cells*: most cases are CD3+, CD4+, CD8−, CD2+, CD5+, CD7−, CD45RO+, and betaF1+. Some CD30 expression may be seen (usually <75% of the infiltrate). CD4 to CD8 ratios are often nondiagnostic in early disease due to the abundance of reactive lymphocytes at that stage.
- *Less common patterns*: (a) while MF characteristically demonstrates a CD4-positive phenotype, a subset of otherwise classic MF cases is CD4-negative/CD8-positive or CD4-negative/CD8-negative (alpha-beta or gamma-delta) and shows a similarly indolent behavior. Cytotoxic phenotype is common in the hypopigmented and hyperpigmented variants as well as in pediatric MF (the latter may also express CD56). (b) Cytotoxic protein (TIA1, granzyme B) expression in CD4+ MF may occasionally be seen and is more common in advanced disease. (c) Rare aberrant CD20 expression (more common in tumor-stage disease). (d) T follicular helper (TFH) phenotype in a subset of cases (PD1+, BCL6+, CD10+, CXCL13+). (e) Loss of additional T-cell markers in tumor-stage disease. (f) Large cell transformation of MF is defined by the cytomorphology on H&E (not by CD30 expression). The large cells may be CD30-negative or CD30-positive (Fig. 22.13). The differential diagnosis for CD30-positive large cell transformation of MF includes lymphomatoid papulosis (LyP) types C and with DUSP22-IRF4 rearrangement. This is an important differential, since LyP is not rare in MF patients and the prognosis is quite different. The distinction is best made clinically (small self-regressing

papules in all variants of LyP versus persistent/progressive disease in advanced MF); however, molecular testing for DUSP22-IRF4 rearrangement may prove helpful in select cases.

- *Reactive cells*: small predominantly CD8+ lymphocytes, CD68+ histiocytes, polytypic plasma cells, CD1a + Langerhans cells.

Genetics

- Monoclonal rearrangement of T-cell receptor genes in the majority of cases.
- Dual PCR or next-generation sequencing may prove helpful since T-cell clones may be identified in some inflammatory dermatoses (e.g., pityriasis lichenoides, lichen sclerosus, lichen planus). Identification of identical T-cell clones at two different sites or intervals would favor cutaneous T-cell lymphoma over the possibility of an inflammatory mimic.

Prognosis

- Indolent lymphoma with slow progression
- Excellent prognosis in limited disease. Worse prognosis in tumor-stage MF and extracutaneous dissemination
- 5-year survival: 88%
- Adverse risk factors: advancing stage of disease, large cell transformation, nodal or visceral involvement

Differential Diagnosis

- The presence of atypical epidermotropic T cells is not specific for mycosis fungoides and may occur in other lymphoproliferative disorders and lymphomas (Fig. 21.14). There are variants of lymphomatoid papulosis (LyP) with epidermotropic T cells. Type B LyP shows a predominantly intraepidermal lymphocytic infiltrate mimicking MF. Type D LyP is a CD8-positive cytotoxic T-cell variant

with prominent epidermotropism. LyP with 6p25.3 (DUSP22-IRF4) rearrangement shows a biphasic growth pattern, with small cerebriform lymphocytes in the epidermis and large lymphocytes in the dermis (thus resembling tumor-stage MF with CD30-positive large cell transformation). Both indolent and aggressive non-MF cutaneous lymphomas may exhibit epidermotropism. Pagetoid reticulosis (localized type, Woringer-Kolopp) is a variant of MF with excellent prognosis and generally presents with localized patches or plaques on distal extremities. Aggressive epidermotropic CD8-positive cytotoxic T-cell lymphoma is a rare cytotoxic cutaneous lymphoma with poor prognosis and is associated with marked epitheliotropism. Gamma-delta T-cell lymphoma is an aggressive cutaneous lymphoma and may variably involve one or several layers of the skin (epidermis, dermis, and/or panniculus). Careful clinical pathologic correlation is essential to correctly classify epidermotropic lymphoid infiltrates (Fig. 22.2).
- Prominent exocytosis of lymphocytes in the epidermis is not definitively diagnostic of lymphoma and may be observed in several benign dermatoses, such as inflammatory stage of vitiligo, pityriasis lichenoides, lymphomatoid lichenoid keratosis, early lichen sclerosus, pigmented purpuric dermatoses, lymphomatoid drug reaction, pseudolymphomatous tattoo reaction, digitate dermatosis/chronic superficial dermatitis, and CD8-positive cutaneous infiltrates in the setting of acquired immunodeficiency syndrome (AIDS) (Table 22.2). Identification of other diagnostic histopathologic findings as well as clinical correlation will prove helpful to prevent misdiagnosis.
- The intraepidermal infiltrate in hypopigmented MF is often relatively sparse and may overlap with that seen in the inflammatory stage of vitiligo, particularly in young patients. This differential diagnosis is generally difficult and may require careful correlation with clinical (including lesional size and border, symmetric versus asymmetric distribution,

and hypopigmentation versus depigmentation) and molecular findings. Complete destruction of melanocytes is not usually found in hypopigmented MF, though they may be diminished in number. Close follow-up with additional biopsies over time may prove helpful in indeterminate cases.

– While mycosis fungoides classically demonstrates a CD4-positive phenotype, a subset of otherwise classic MF cases is CD8-positive and shows a similarly indolent behavior. However, some aggressive lymphomas are CD8-positive and must be differentiated from indolent processes, such as lymphomatoid papulosis type D (Table 22.3).

– Large cell transformation of mycosis fungoides (LCT-MF) requires at least 25% of large atypical cells in the infiltrate or the formation of microscopic nodules of large cells. It is important to emphasize that the definition of LCT-MF is based on H&E findings (not on the level of CD30 expression). Once this histomorphologic criterion has been met, some cases express CD30, while other cases do not. LyP in association with MF must be excluded on clinical grounds for the CD30-positive cases. Anaplastic large cell lymphoma (ALCL) is not a diagnostic option in this setting since absence of MF is part of the diagnostic criteria for cutaneous ALCL.

Table 22.2 Differential diagnosis of frequent intraepidermal lymphocytes

Lymphomas/lymphoproliferative disorders	Benign dermatoses
Mycosis fungoides	Inflammatory stage of vitiligo
Pagetoid reticulosis	Pityriasis lichenoides
Lymphomatoid papulosis (LyP types B, D, and with 6p25.3 rearrangement)	Lymphomatoid lichenoid keratosis
Primary cutaneous aggressive epidermotropic CD8-positive cytotoxic T-cell lymphoma	Early lichen sclerosus
Cutaneous gamma-delta T-cell lymphoma	Pigmented purpuric dermatoses
	Lymphomatoid drug reaction
	Pseudolymphomatous tattoo reaction
	CD8-positive cutaneous infiltrates in the setting of acquired immunodeficiency syndrome

Table 22.3 Differential diagnosis of CD8-positive cutaneous lymphoid infiltrate

Some cases of otherwise classical or hypopigmented mycosis fungoides
Many cases of localized pagetoid reticulosis
Lymphomatoid papulosis (LyP), type D
Some cases of anaplastic large cell lymphoma (ALCL)
Primary cutaneous CD8+ aggressive epidermotropic cytotoxic T-cell lymphoma
Many cases of cutaneous gamma-delta T-cell lymphoma
Subcutaneous panniculitis-like T-cell lymphoma
Indolent CD8+ lymphoid proliferation of the ear (primary cutaneous acral CD8+ T-cell lymphoma)
Cutaneous pseudolymphoma: CD8-positive infiltrates in the setting of advanced AIDS, many cases of pityriasis lichenoides

Table 22.4 Differential diagnosis of ulceration

Lymphomas/lymphoproliferative disorders	Benign dermatoses/pseudolymphomas
Tumor-stage mycosis fungoides	Pityriasis lichenoides et varioliformis acuta (PLEVA)
CD30-positive lymphoproliferative disorders: lymphomatoid papulosis, cutaneous anaplastic large cell lymphoma	Inflamed molluscum contagiosum
Primary cutaneous aggressive epidermotropic CD8-positive cytotoxic T-cell lymphoma	Herpesvirus infection
Cutaneous gamma-delta T-cell lymphoma	Primary syphilis
Extranodal NK/T-cell lymphoma, nasal type	Leishmania infection

Pearls and Pitfalls

1. Normal human skin lacks inflammatory cells within the epidermis, except for Langerhans cells in the stratum spinosum. Exocytosis is the process of migration of inflammatory cells into the epidermis and occurs in a variety of benign dermatoses. In spongiotic/eczematous dermatitis, exocytosis of a relatively small number of lymphocytes is associated with prominent intercellular edema (spongiosis). The presence of atypical lymphocytes within the epidermis is described as epidermotropism and is usually associated with scant spongiosis (Fig. 22.5).

2. Too much epidermotropism would actually be unusual for classic mycosis fungoides and would raise the possibility of another epidermotropic process, including type D lymphomatoid papulosis (LyP), pagetoid reticulosis, and aggressive epidermotropic CD8-positive cytotoxic T-cell lymphoma (Fig. 22.14).

3. Epidermotropism is often absent in tumor-stage mycosis fungoides and in folliculotropic mycosis fungoides.

4. The presence of epidermal destruction is an important histopathologic finding in the evaluation of skin biopsies with lymphoid infiltrates. Ulceration is generally absent in MF, except for advanced tumor-stage disease, which only occurs in a small subset of patients after several years. Therefore, the presence of ulceration at an early onset would raise the possibility of a non-MF cutaneous lymphoproliferative process. Some pseudolymphomas may also demonstrate ulceration (Table 22.4).

5. The identification of CD30 expression by itself in a cutaneous lymphoid infiltrate is not enough to make any diagnosis. Additional immunophenotyping and clinical correlation are necessary for proper classification (Fig. 22.13).

6. While Sézary syndrome and mycosis fungoides are closely related, they are distinct entities. Sézary syndrome is associated with a significantly worse prognosis as well as marked immunosuppression.

7. A few patients with mycosis fungoides may progress from the conventional clinical picture of chronic patches/plaques into erythroderma during the course of their disease (erythrodermic mycosis fungoides). In contrast, Sézary syndrome starts with erythroderma.

8. Rare MF patients may be diagnosed late in the course of their disease (tumor-stage, large cell transformation, or even nodal involvement). In such cases, there should be a combination of skin lesions consistent with MF (patches, plaques, and tumors). Lack of current or previous patches/plaques should indicate another lymphoma rather than MF.

9. If the initial skin lesion in a patient is a tumor (in the absence of prior patches or plaques), other lymphomas other than MF should be considered. The possibility of MF should only be entertained for cases with the conventional slow clinical progression of patches to plaques and (in some patients) to tumors. Historic aggressive cases previously called "rapidly progressive MF" or "mycosis fungoides d'emblee" are currently classified as other lymphomas.

10. Since MF lesions are chronic, superficial dermal fibrosis must be present. An intraepidermal lymphocytic infiltrate (particularly if predominantly basilar) lacking associated dermal fibrosis should raise the possibility of a mimic (including epidermotropic

variants of lymphomatoid papulosis and inflammatory stage of vitiligo).

11. The most common cutaneous lymphoma in children is MF.

12. Epidermotropism may be absent in biopsies of treated lesions of MF, which could lead to nonspecific histopathologic findings in early-stage disease. Rebiopsy of an untreated lesion may prove helpful.

13. Large shave biopsies provide more epidermis for examination than a punch biopsy. Since epidermotropism in early-stage MF can be patchy, a large shave specimen may be more advantageous in chronic patches that are clinically suspicious for MF. However, a punch biopsy provides deeper sampling of the dermis and is recommended for nodules/tumors or follicular-based lesions (including cases with associated alopecia). Two skin biopsies would also increase diagnostic yield and would allow dual PCR (if necessary).

14. Loss of CD2 and presence of CD7 is a very unusual combination for MF and would raise the possibility of primary cutaneous CD8-positive aggressive epidermotropic cytotoxic T-cell lymphoma. Comprehensive immunophenotyping can be helpful, since MF is usually CD2+, CD7−, CD45RA−, and CD45RO+ as opposed to the immature T-cell phenotype of this aggressive lymphoma (CD2−, CD7+, CD45RA+, CD45RO−). Clinical correlation is essential, since fast progression and ulceration early in the clinical course would also indicate an aggressive cytotoxic lymphoma.

Suggested Reading

Elder DE, Massi D, Scolyer RA, Willemze R, editors. WHO classification of skin tumors. 4th ed. Lyon: IARC; 2018.

Ferrara G, Di Blasi A, Zalaudek I, Argenziano G, Cerroni L. Regarding the algorithm for the diagnosis of early mycosis fungoides proposed by the International Society for Cutaneous Lymphomas: suggestions from routine histopathology practice. J Cutan Pathol. 2008;35(6):549–53.

Hodak E, David M, Maron L, et al. CD4/CD8 double-negative epidermotropic cutaneous T-cell lymphoma: an immunohistochemical variant of mycosis fungoides. J Am Acad Dermatol. 2006;55:276–84.

Pimpinelli N, Olsen EA, Santucci M, et al. Defining early mycosis fungoides. J Am Acad Dermatol. 2005;53(6):1053–63.

Pincus LB. Mycosis fungoides. Surg Pathol Clin. 2014;7(2):143–67.

Saggini A, Gulia A, Argenyi Z, et al. A variant of lymphomatoid papulosis simulating primary cutaneous aggressive epidermotropic CD8+ cytotoxic T-cell lymphoma. Description of 9 cases. Am J Surg Pathol. 2010;34(8):1168–75.

Shapiro PE, Pinto FJ. The histologic spectrum of mycosis fungoides/Sézary syndrome (cutaneous T-cell lymphoma). A review of 222 biopsies, including newly described patterns and the earliest pathologic changes. Am J Surg Pathol. 1994;18(7):645–67.

Suchak R, Verdolini R, Robson A, Stefanato CM. Extragenital lichen sclerosus et atrophicus mimicking cutaneous T-cell lymphoma: report of a case. J Cutan Pathol. 2010;37(9):982–6.

Swerdlow SH, Campo E, Harris NL, Jaffe ES, Pileri SA, Stein H, Thiele J, editors. WHO classification of tumours of haematopoietic and lymphoid tissues (revised 4th ed). Lyon: IARC; 2017.

Wain EM, Orchard GE, Mayou S, et al. Mycosis fungoides with a CD56+ immunophenotype. J Am Acad Dermatol. 2005;53(1):158–63.

Willemze R, Jaffe ES, Burg G, et al. WHO-EORTC classification for cutaneous lymphomas. Blood. 2005;105(10):3768–85.

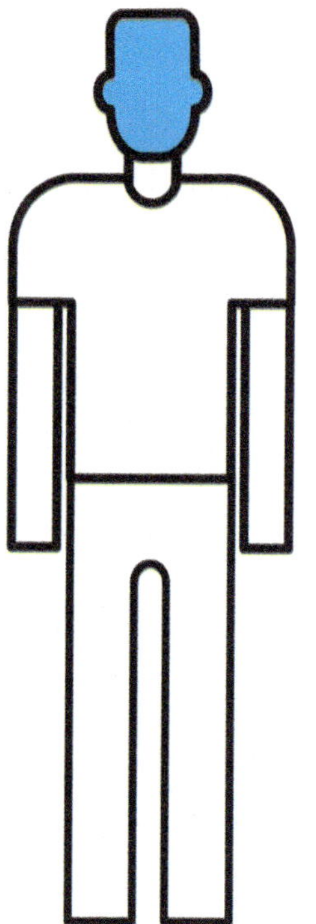

Fig. 23.1 Folliculotropic mycosis fungoides preferentially involves the scalp and face

Table 23.1 Key facts

Definition	
Folliculotropic mycosis fungoides is a variant of mycosis fungoides characterized by tropism for hair follicles and preferential involvement of the head and neck region	
Prototypic clinical presentation	
Grouped follicular papules and plaques with alopecia	
Histopathologic findings	
Folliculotropism (infiltration of hair follicles by lymphocytes with architectural disruption and diminished sebaceous glands). A subset of cases is associated with follicular mucinosis Most common immunophenotype: CD3+, CD4+, CD8−, and variable loss of pan-T-cell markers. CD30 expression is common	
Prognosis	
Indolent	

© Springer Nature Switzerland AG 2019

A. Subtil, *Diagnosis of Cutaneous Lymphoid Infiltrates*,

https://doi.org/10.1007/978-3-030-11654-5_23

Fig. 23.2 Folliculotropic mycosis fungoides with plaques and tumors on the face. There is hair loss within the lesions

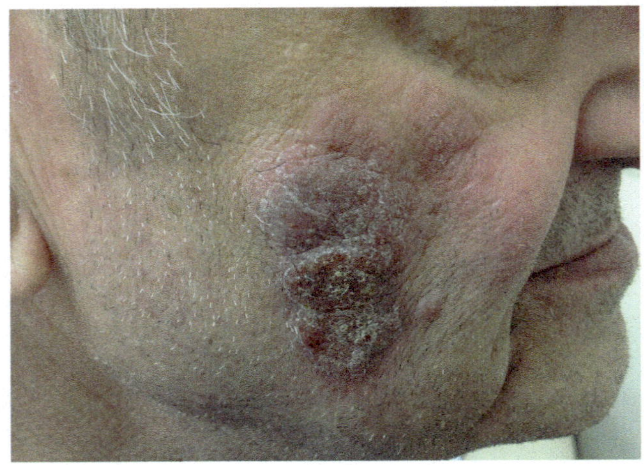

Fig. 23.3 Low-power magnification of folliculotropic mycosis fungoides. The lymphocytic infiltrate targets the hair follicles. In addition to epithelial infiltration by lymphocytes, there is architectural disruption of the hair follicles and diminished sebaceous glands

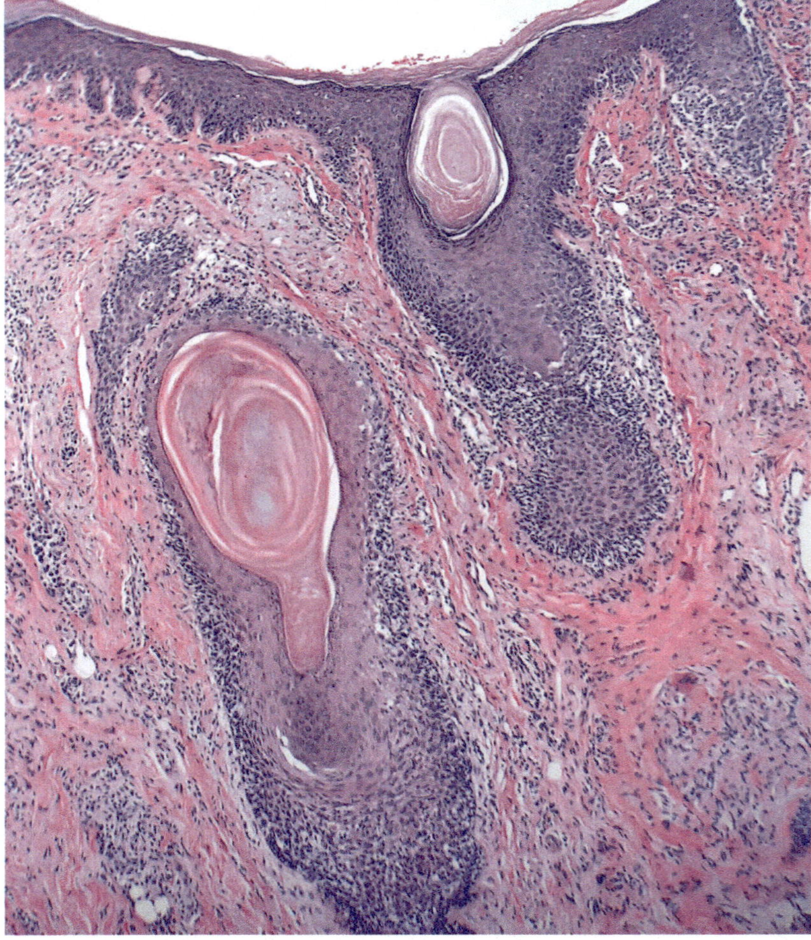

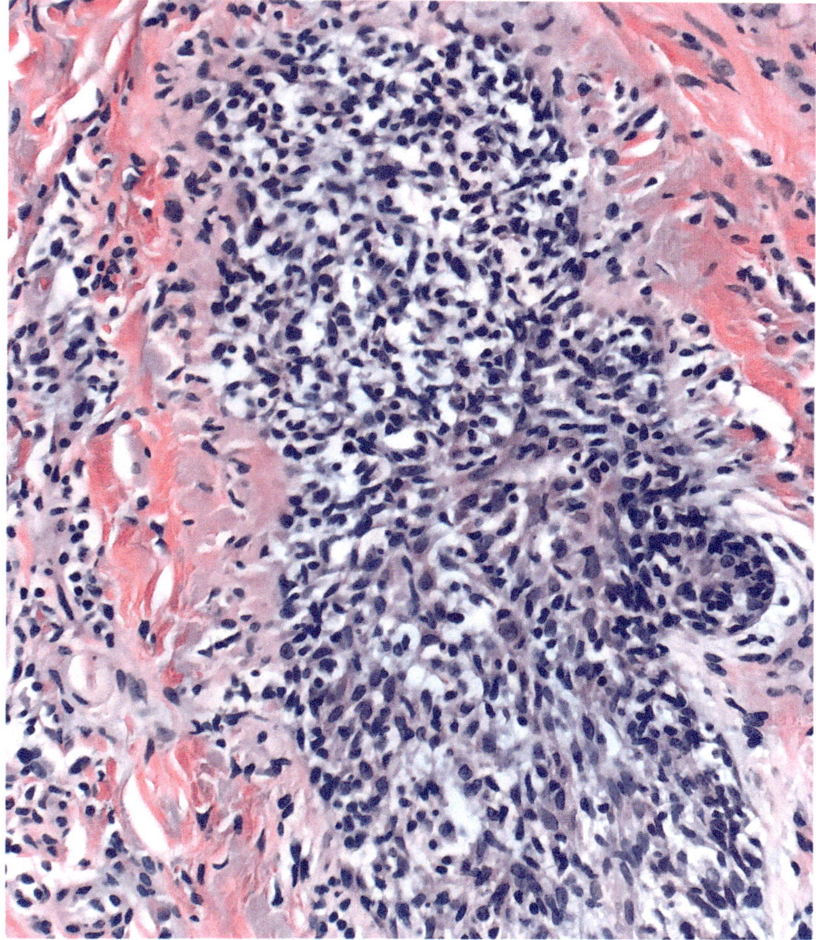

Fig. 23.4 High-power magnification of folliculotropic mycosis fungoides. Hair follicle showing prominent epithelial infiltration and disruption by lymphocytes

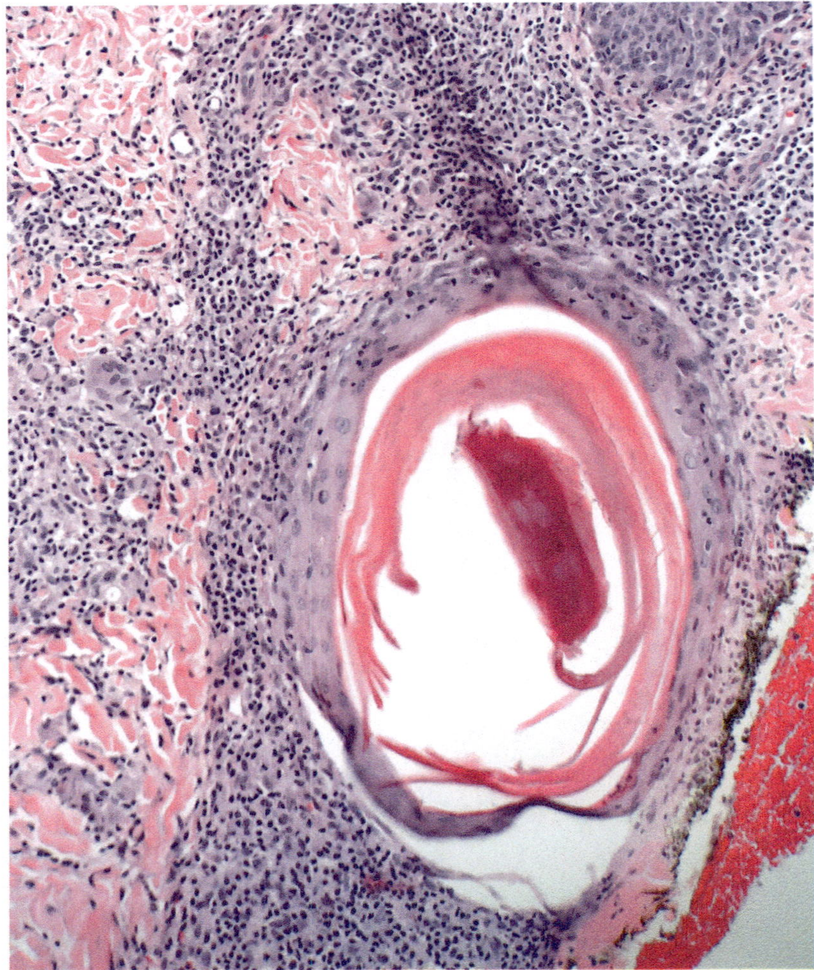

Fig. 23.5 Folliculotropic mycosis fungoides with cystic follicular dilatation. There are histiocytes and multinucleated giant cells in the dermis, suggestive of adjacent follicular rupture and destruction

Fig. 23.6 Folliculotropic mycosis fungoides with mucin deposition (follicular mucinosis)

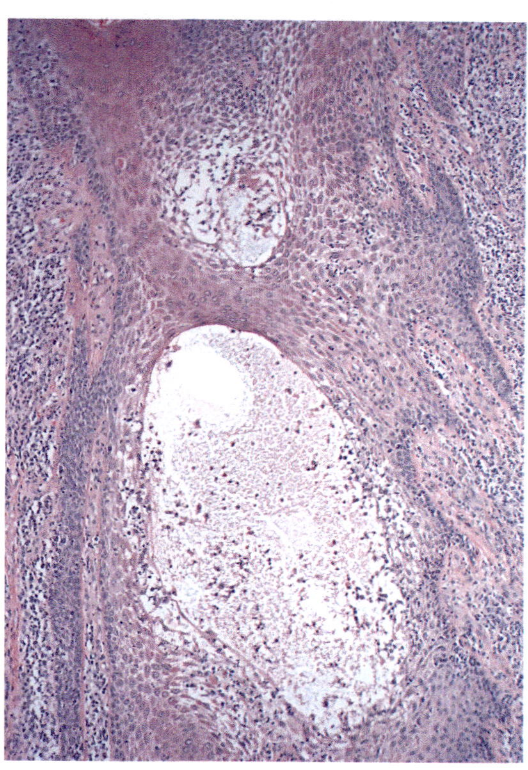

Fig. 23.7
Folliculotropic mycosis fungoides with follicular mucinosis

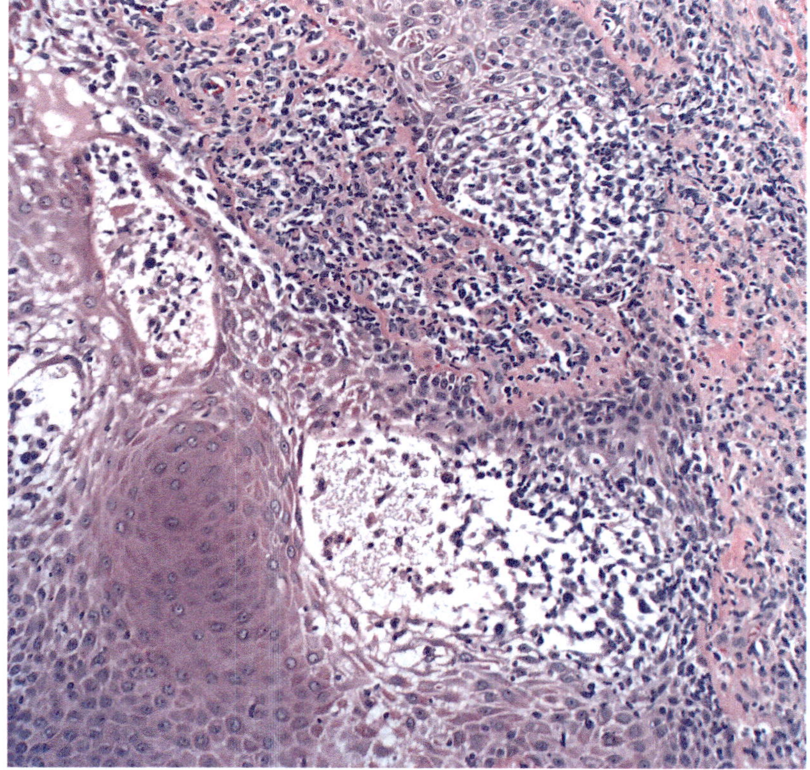

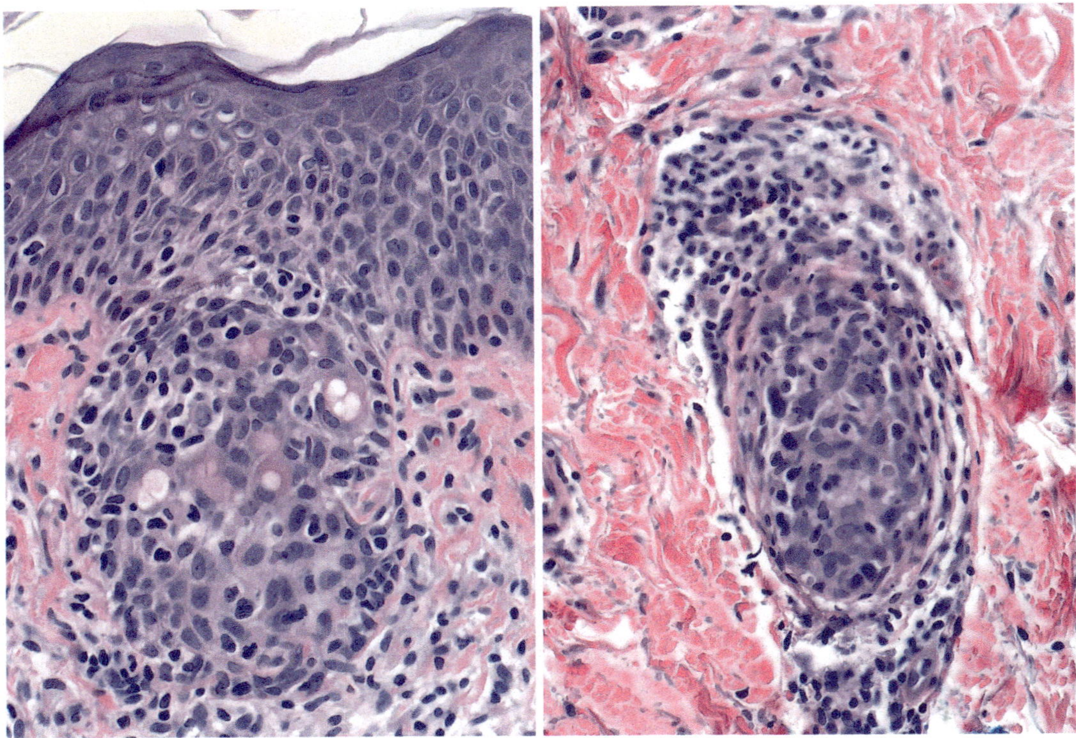

Fig. 23.8 Folliculotropic mycosis fungoides with syringotropism (i.e., adnexotropic mycosis fungoides). Sweat gland ducts are infiltrated by lymphocytes and show hyperplasia of the epithelium

Fig. 23.9 Primary cutaneous aggressive epidermotropic CD8-positive cytotoxic T-cell lymphoma. Involvement of hair follicles is a common finding in this lymphoma

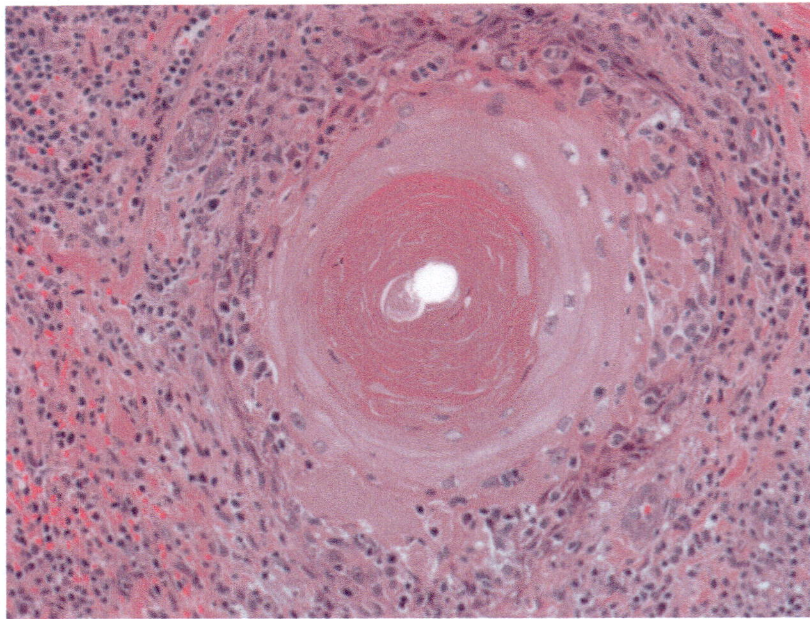

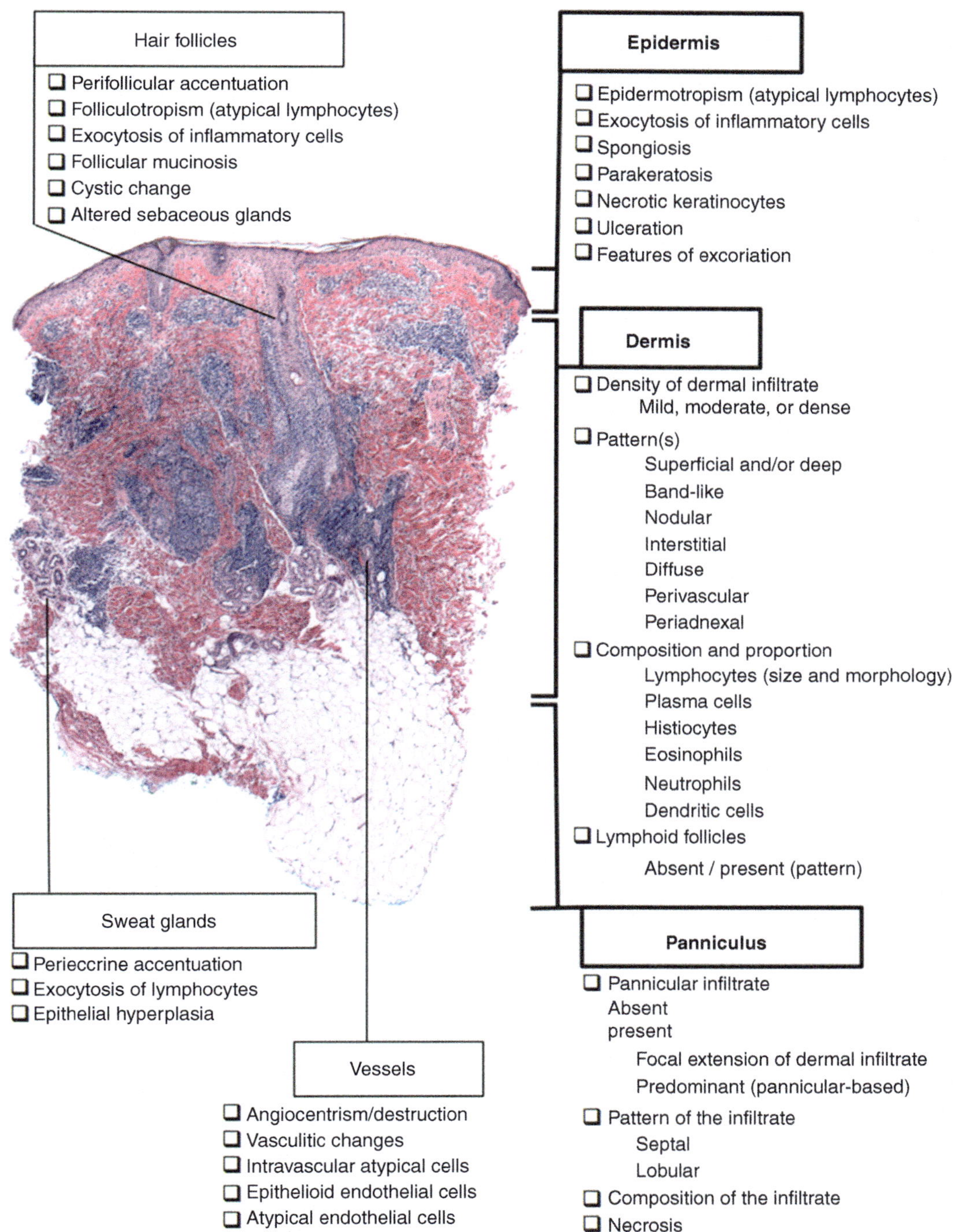

Fig. 23.10 Checklist of possible histomorphologic findings in the evaluation of cutaneous lymphoid infiltrates

Disease Definition

- Folliculotropic mycosis fungoides (FMF) is a variant of mycosis fungoides characterized by tropism for hair follicles (folliculotropism) and preferential involvement of the head and neck region. Epidermotropism is variable, and hair loss is common (Table 23.1).

Epidemiology

- Usually adults
- Male predominance

Preferential Sites of Involvement

- Head and neck (Figs. 23.1 and 23.2).
- Lesions may occasionally be present on the extremities or trunk.

Clinical Features

- Grouped follicular papules and plaques, often associated with alopecia.
- Indurated plaques and tumors may be seen in more advanced disease.
- Grouped comedones and small follicular cysts, sometimes resembling milia en plaque.
- Acneiform and pustular lesions.
- Pruritus and secondary bacterial infection are common.
- Eyebrow alopecia in association with a plaque is a clue to the diagnosis.
- *Less common presentations*: small keratotic spines protruding from hair follicles resembling lichen spinulosus. Mucinorrhea.

Histomorphology

- *Pattern*: The infiltrate targets hair follicles. In addition to epithelial infiltration by lymphocytes, there is architectural disruption of the hair follicles and diminished sebaceous glands (Figs. 23.3 and 23.4). Cystic dilatation of hair follicles may occur (Fig. 23.5). A subset of cases of FMF is associated with follicular mucinosis (deposition of mucin within a disrupted hair follicle), which can be highlighted by Alcian Blue stain (Figs. 23.6 and 23.7).
- *Less common patterns*: (a) Affected follicles may sometimes show basaloid features ("basaloid folliculolymphoid hyperplasia"). (b) Dense dermal lymphocytic infiltrate in addition to infiltrated hair follicles ("tumor-type" infiltrate). (c) While sparing of the epidermis is common in FMF, a subset of cases may also show epidermotropism. (d) In addition to folliculotropism, some cases of FMF may show evidence of syringotropism (exocytosis of lymphocytes and epithelial hyperplasia in eccrine sweat glands) in the same lesion or in different lesions of the same patient (i.e., adnexotropic mycosis fungoides) (Fig. 23.8).
- *Neoplastic cells*: Small- to intermediate-sized lymphocytes with dense chromatin and generally scant cytoplasm. While nuclei may be convoluted and irregular, cytologic atypia is often minimal or absent.
- *Reactive cells*: Eosinophils, plasma cells, histiocytes, and/or multinucleated giant cells are common and may be prominent. Hair follicles are often destroyed by the neoplastic infiltrate, and some biopsies may only show foci of dermal granulomatous inflammation, sometimes in association with prominent eosinophils and/or mucin.

Immunophenotype

- *Neoplastic cells*: CD3+, CD4+, CD8−, and variable loss of pan-T-cell markers. CD30 expression is common (often around 50% of the infiltrate). CD4 to CD8 ratios are often more definitive in FMF than in classic mycosis fungoides.
- *Reactive cells*: frequent CD68 expression from reactive histiocytes. Polytypic plasma cells.

Genetics

- Monoclonal rearrangement of T-cell receptor genes in the majority of cases. However, false-negative results may occur if affected hair follicles are not included in the tissue sections taken for PCR.

Prognosis

- Indolent. Risk of disease progression is higher than in classic mycosis fungoides, particularly after 5–10 years.
- 5-year survival: 80%
- Adverse risk factors: advanced age and/or stage, large cell transformation

Differential Diagnosis (Table 23.2)

- Folliculotropism may also be identified in primary cutaneous aggressive epidermotropic CD8-positive cytotoxic T-cell lymphoma (Fig. 23.9). Correlation with clinical findings and identification of an immature cytotoxic alpha-beta CD8-positive T-cell phenotype would help distinguish this aggressive lymphoma from mycosis fungoides.
- The subset of cases of FMF associated with follicular mucinosis must be differentiated from benign idiopathic follicular mucinosis. While both conditions would show folliculotropism and follicular mucinosis, certain histopathologic features would strongly favor folliculotropic mycosis fungoides (e.g., associated epidermotropism and/or dense dermal infiltrate beyond hair follicles). However, most cases of FMF do not show these distinguishing histopathologic features. Therefore, this distinction is best made on clinical grounds (solitary lesion in a young patient would be classified as idiopathic follicular mucinosis). Close follow-up and additional biopsies over time may prove helpful in indeterminate cases.

- Another condition to consider in a folliculotropic pattern differential would be lymphomatoid papulosis (LyP), which may occasional demonstrate a follicular pattern and even follicular mucinosis. A clinical presentation of self-regressing papules would favor LyP.
- Pseudolymphomatous folliculitis (PF) is a clinicopathologic variant of cutaneous pseudolymphoma and generally presents with a solitary lesion showing a dense dermal lymphohistiocytic infiltrate with follicular architecture disruption. PF classically lacks T-cell clonality and does not recur after excision.
- Herpes folliculitis may show a dense dermal lymphocytic infiltrate with follicular involvement. The presence of sebaceous gland necrosis is a clue to the diagnosis and should elicit searching for herpetic viral cytopathic effect within hair follicles.
- Discoid lupus erythematosus and lichen planopilaris often involved the scalp and exhibit a lymphocytic interface inflammatory infiltrate (with perifollicular distribution and occasionally epidermal), but the density of the infiltrate and the lack of prominent epithelial infiltration are unlikely to raise the possibility of folliculotropic mycosis fungoides. Mucin deposition in lupus occurs in the dermis, not within hair follicles.
- Arthropod bite reactions are unlikely to raise the possibility of lymphoma; however, the density of the infiltrate may occasionally be denser than usual and appear lymphomatoid. Persistent nodular scabies may occasionally exhibit folliculotropism. Careful clinical correlation will be helpful to prevent misdiagnosis.

Table 23.2 Differential diagnosis of cutaneous lymphocytic infiltrates with perifollicular accentuation

Lymphomas/lymphoproliferative disorders	Benign dermatoses
Cutaneous marginal zone B-cell lymphoma	Lymphomatoid drug eruption
Folliculotropic mycosis fungoides	Pseudolymphomatous folliculitis
Follicular lymphomatoid papulosis	Primary follicular mucinosis
Primary cutaneous aggressive epidermotropic CD8-positive cytotoxic T-cell lymphoma	Arthropod bite reaction (including persistent nodular scabies)
	Herpes folliculitis
	Lichen striatus
	Lupus erythematosus
	Lichen planopilaris
	Alopecia areata
	Graft-versus-host disease
	Infundibulofolliculitis

Pearls and Pitfalls

1. Shave biopsies are generally too superficial for adequate examination of hair follicles and sweat glands. A deeper biopsy (punch or ellipse) is indicated for follicular-based lesions, alopecia, and lesions on the head/neck or acral areas.

2. The involved hair follicle may not be present in a particular histological section. Serial sections are generally necessary in conditions with follicular involvement.

3. An infiltrate with perifollicular accentuation may not necessarily be associated with folliculotropism (disruption of follicular architecture and infiltration of the follicular epithelium by atypical lymphocytes) (Table 23.2). For example, cutaneous marginal zone lymphoma is often perifollicular but generally lacks follicular epithelial infiltration.

4. Focal extension into occasional hair follicles may be observed in otherwise classic mycosis fungoides. In the presence of both epidermotropism and focal folliculotropism, careful clinical examination is recommended to determine whether follicular-based lesions, head and neck involvement, or unusual alopecia may be present.

5. The neoplastic cells in classic mycosis fungoides are superficially located (intraepidermal), in contrast to the deep (intrafollicular) localization in folliculotropic MF. Therefore, they may be less accessible to skin-targeted therapies.

6. Adnexal structures (hair follicles and sweat glands) are frequently overlooked in the evaluation of cutaneous lymphoid infiltrates but may show critical diagnostic features (Fig. 23.10). Multiple abnormalities may be found in hair follicles (e.g., folliculotropism of atypical lymphocytes, exocytosis of neutrophils or eosinophils, follicular mucinosis, disrupted architecture, cystic change, and/or necrotic or atrophic sebaceous glands).

Suggested Reading

Arai E, Okubo H, Tsuchida T, et al. Pseudolymphomatous folliculitis: a clinicopathologic study of 15 cases of cutaneous pseudolymphoma with follicular invasion. Am J Surg Pathol. 1999;23(11):1313–9.

Brown HA, Gibson LE, Pujol RM, et al. Primary follicular mucinosis: long-term follow-up of patients younger than 40 years with and without clonal T-cell receptor gene rearrangement. J Am Acad Dermatol. 2002;47(6):856–62.

Elder DE, Massi D, Scolyer RA, Willemze R, editors. WHO classification of skin tumors. 4th ed. Lyon: IARC; 2018.

Gerami P, Guitart J. The spectrum of histopathologic and immunohistochemical findings in folliculotropic mycosis fungoides. Am J Surg Pathol. 2007;31(9):1430–8.

Kempf W, Kazakov DV, Baumgartner HP, et al. Follicular lymphomatoid papulosis revisited: a study of 11 cases, with new histopathological findings. J Am Acad Dermatol. 2013;68(5):809–16.

Swerdlow SH, et al., editors. WHO Classification of tumors of hematopoietic and lymphoid tissues. Lyon: IARC; 2008.

Swerdlow SH, Campo E, Harris NL, Jaffe ES, Pileri SA, Stein H, Thiele J, editors. WHO classification of tumours of haematopoietic and lymphoid tissues (revised 4th ed). Lyon: IARC; 2017.

Willemze R, Jaffe ES, Burg G, et al. WHO-EORTC classification for cutaneous lymphomas. Blood. 2005;105(10):3768–85.

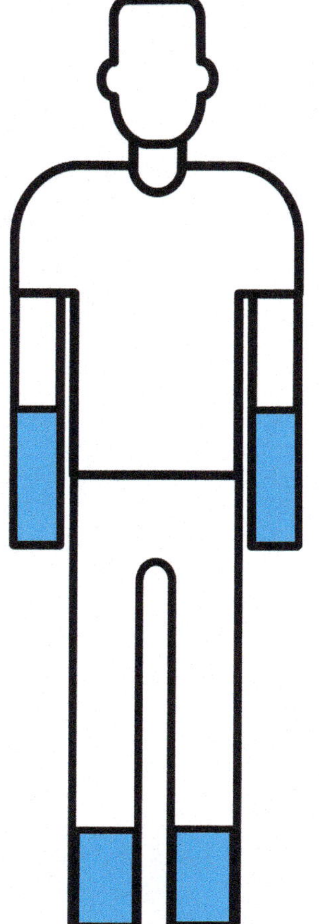

Fig. 24.1 Pagetoid reticulosis (localized, Woringer-Kolopp type) preferentially involves one acral (or near acral) site

Table 24.1 Key facts

Definition
Pagetoid reticulosis is a localized variant of mycosis fungoides characterized clinically by patches and/or plaques occurring mostly on acral sites and histologically by intraepidermal T cells
Prototypic clinical presentation
Solitary or localized, slow-growing patch(es) or plaque(s) on (or near) one acral site
Histopathologic findings
Prominent epidermotropism with numerous intraepidermal lymphocytes, often with a pagetoid pattern. Epidermal hyperplasia
Most common immunophenotype: The neoplastic CD3+ T cells may be CD4−/CD8+, CD4+/CD8− or CD4−/CD8−. CD30 expression is common
Prognosis
Excellent (5-year survival: 100%)

© Springer Nature Switzerland AG 2019
A. Subtil, *Diagnosis of Cutaneous Lymphoid Infiltrates*,
https://doi.org/10.1007/978-3-030-11654-5_24

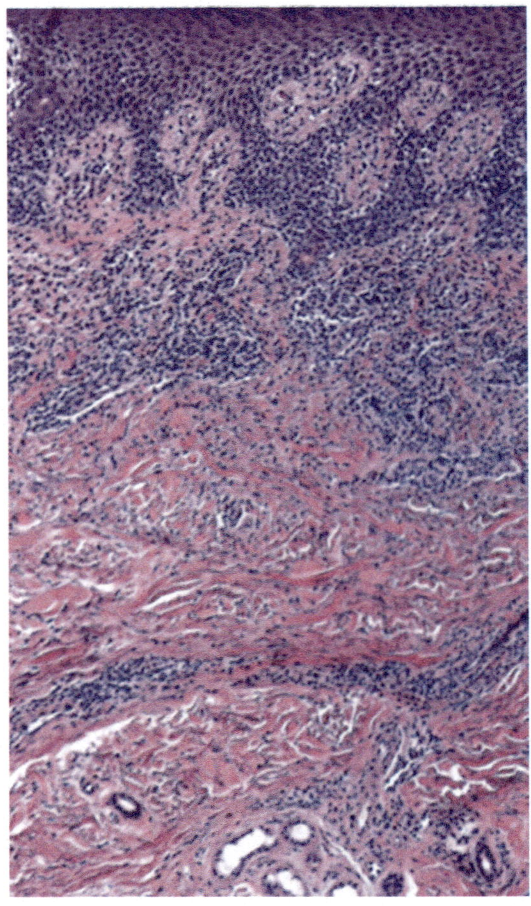

Fig. 24.2 Low-power magnification of pagetoid reticulosis. Acral skin with epidermal hyperplasia and superficial epidermotropic lymphocytic infiltrate

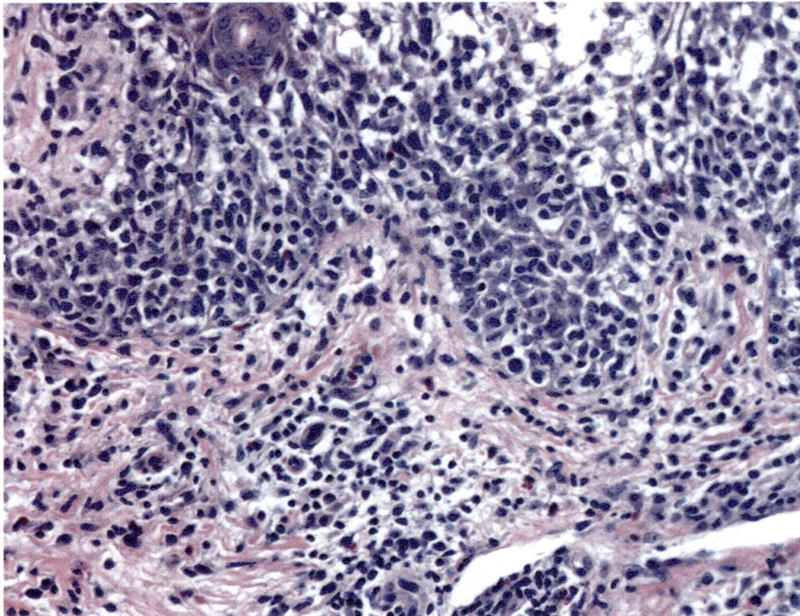

Fig. 24.3 Pagetoid reticulosis. Marked epidermotropism with pagetoid features

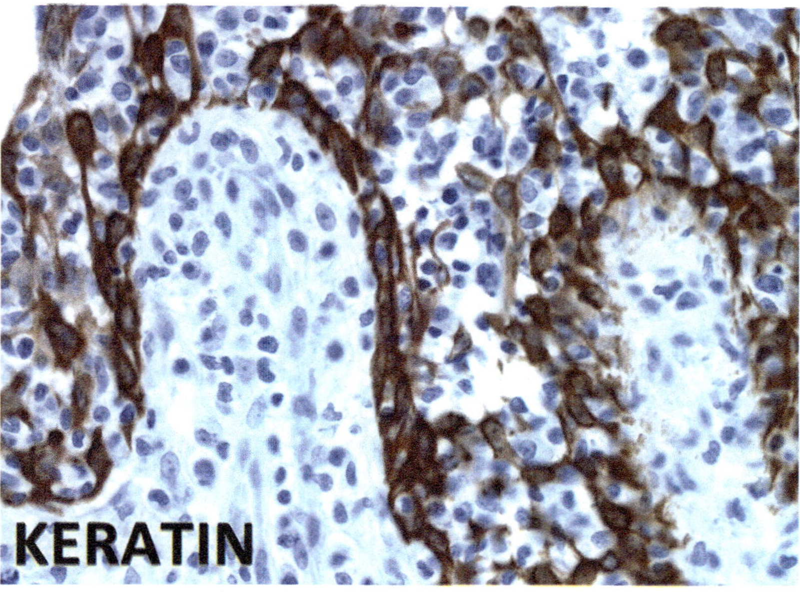

Fig. 24.4 Pagetoid reticulosis. The prominent epidermotropism is demonstrated by relatively minimal residual epidermal keratinocytes (highlighted by positive keratin staining, while lymphocytes are negative)

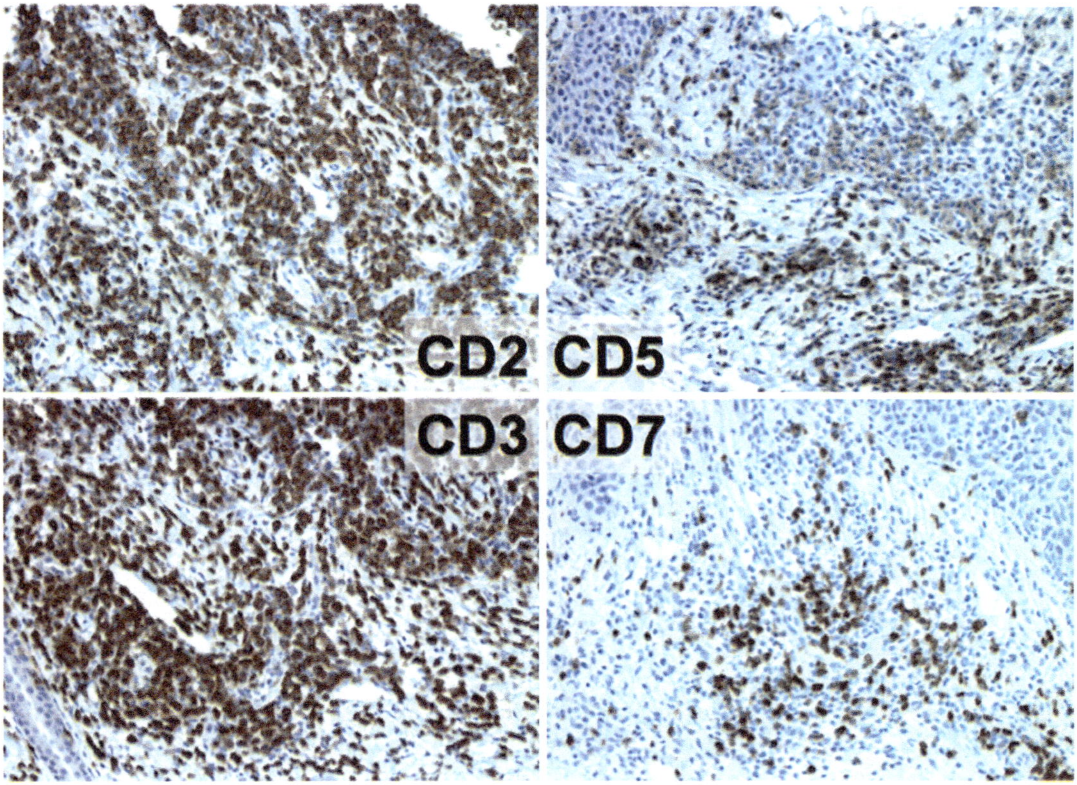

Fig. 24.5 Pagetoid reticulosis. Epidermotropic T cells are positive with CD2 and CD3 but show loss of CD5 and CD7

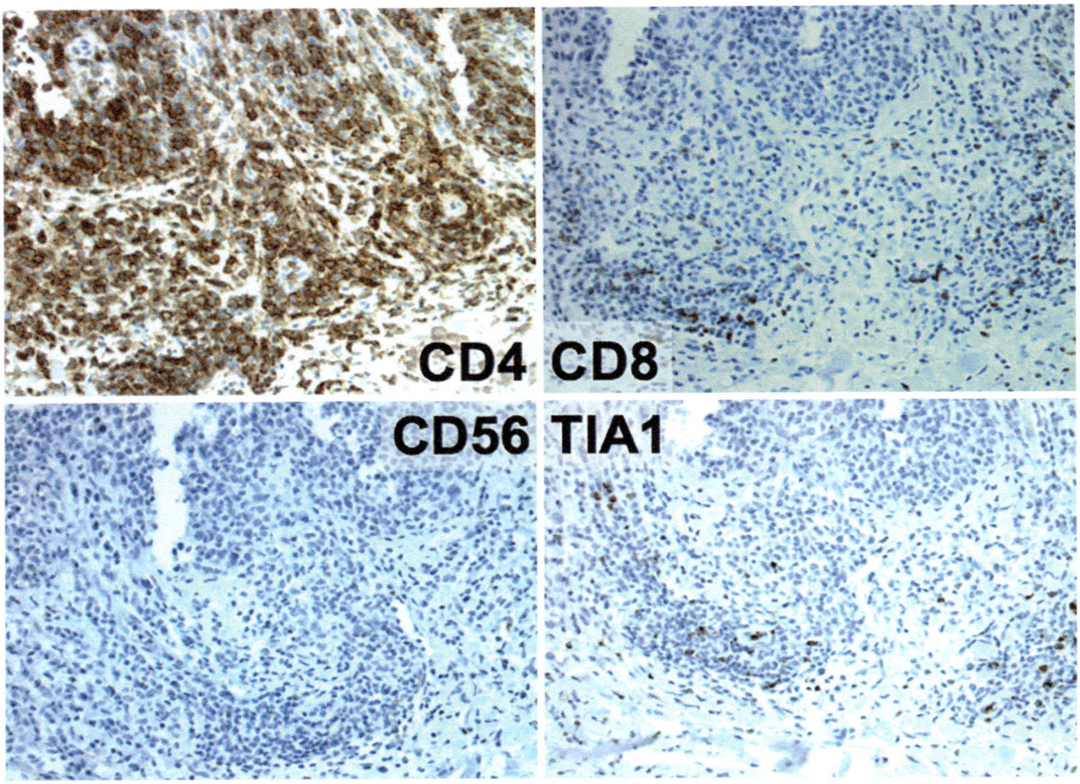

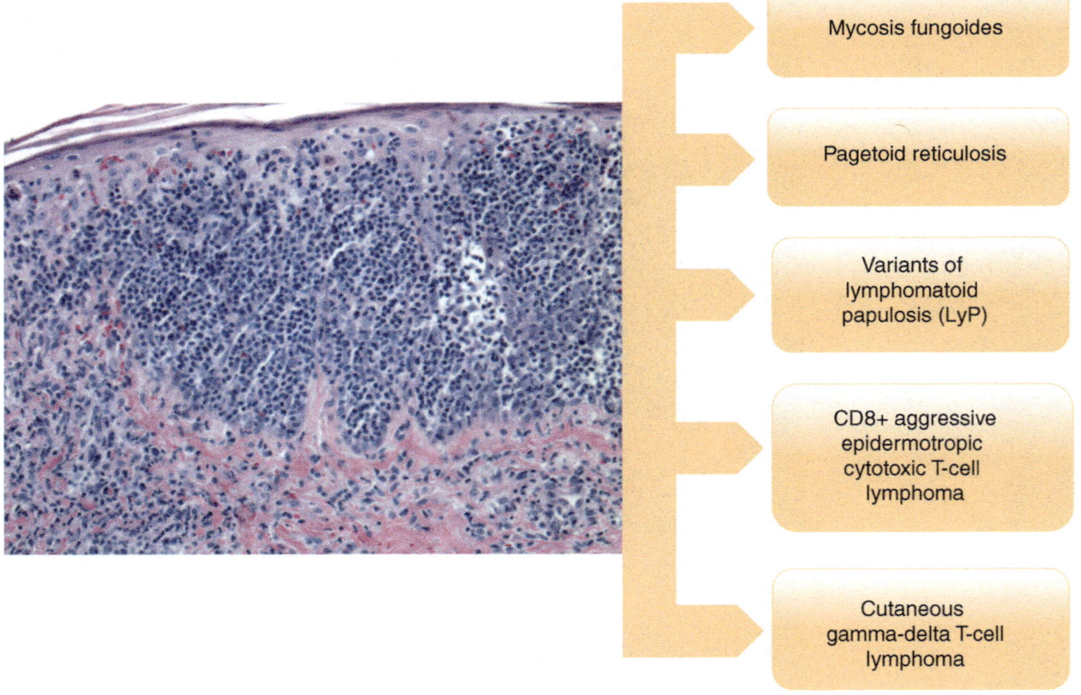

Fig. 24.6 Example of CD4+/CD8− pagetoid reticulosis (neoplastic T cells in pagetoid reticulosis may be CD4−/CD8+, CD4+/CD8− or CD4−/CD8−)

Fig. 24.7 Differential diagnosis of epidermotropism

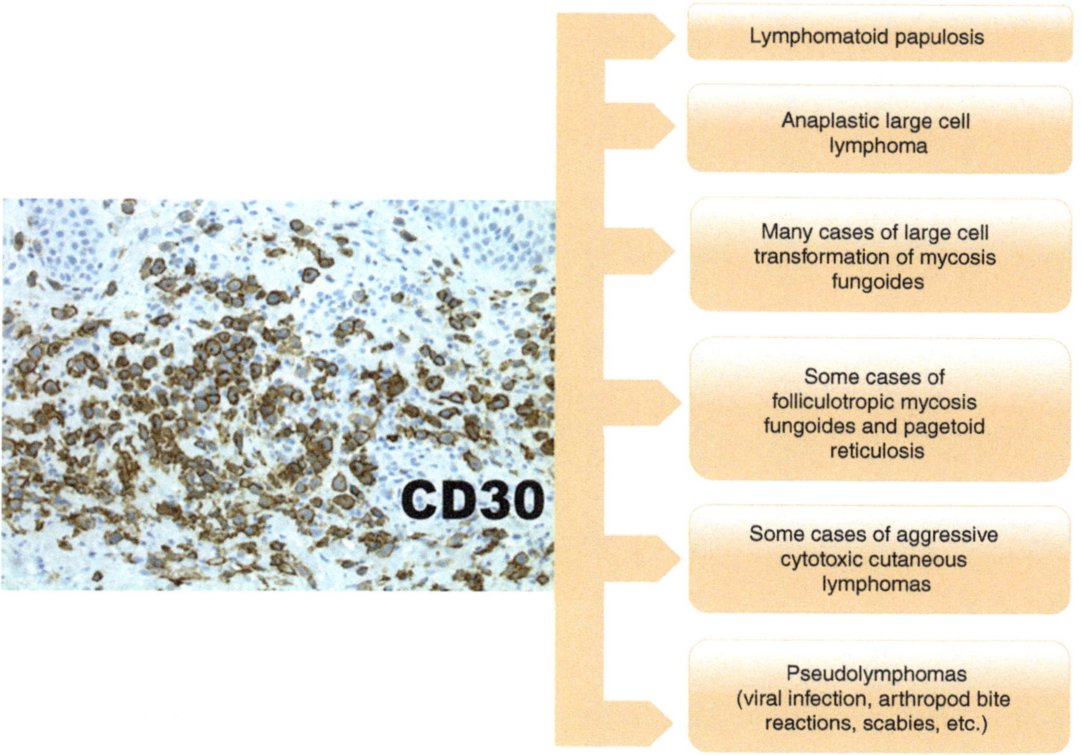

Fig. 24.8 Differential diagnosis of CD30 expression

Disease Definition

– Pagetoid reticulosis is a localized variant of mycosis fungoides characterized clinically by patches and/or plaques occurring mostly on acral sites and histologically by intraepidermal T cells (Table 24.1).

Epidemiology

– Rare disease
– May affect adults or children

Preferential Sites of Involvement

– Acral sites and distal extremities (hand, wrist, foot, ankle) (Fig. 24.1)

Clinical Features

– Solitary or localized, slow-growing patch(es) or plaque(s) on (or near) one acral site
– May be psoriasiform, verrucous (wartlike), erythematous, and/or scaly
– *Less common presentations*: may clinically resemble eczematous dermatitis

Histomorphology

– *Pattern*: prominent epidermotropism with numerous intraepidermal lymphocytes, often with a pagetoid pattern. Epidermal hyperplasia is common and may be prominent (Figs. 24.2 and 24.3).
– *Less common patterns*: in addition to the pagetoid epidermotropic component, there may be an associated band-like superficial dermal

lymphocytic component and/or focal adnexal extension of intraepithelial lymphocytes in eccrine ducts.

- *Neoplastic cells*: atypical hyperchromatic lymphocytes with convoluted nuclei (usually intermediate-sized but may be large).
- *Reactive cells*: relatively scant small reactive lymphocytes, mostly in the upper dermis.

Immunophenotype

- *Neoplastic cells*: the neoplastic CD3+ T cells may be CD4−/CD8+, CD4+/CD8−, or CD4−/CD8−. CD30 expression is common. Variable loss of pan-T-cell markers (Figs. 24.4, 24.5, and 24.6)
- *Reactive cells*: scant CD3+ T cells

Genetics

- Monoclonal rearrangement of T-cell receptor genes in majority of cases

Prognosis

- Indolent disease with excellent prognosis
- 5-year survival: 100%
- No reported cases of extracutaneous dissemination or disease-related deaths

Differential Diagnosis

- Cutaneous gamma-delta T-cell lymphoma and primary cutaneous CD8+ aggressive epidermotropic cytotoxic T-cell lymphoma may show marked epidermotropism with pagetoid features and may resemble localized pagetoid reticulosis. However, those cytotoxic lymphomas are aggressive, disseminated, and fast-growing, while pagetoid reticulosis is indolent, localized, and slow-growing. Clinical correlation and follow-up are essential for classification of epidermotropic infiltrates (Fig. 24.7).
- Epidermotropic variants of lymphomatoid papulosis (particularly CD8+ type D) may histologically resemble pagetoid reticulosis. In addition, both often show CD30 expression (Fig. 24.8). However, their clinical presentations are distinct (small self-regressing papules for lymphomatoid papulosis versus chronic slow-growing patch or plaque for pagetoid reticulosis).
- Cases of mycosis fungoides with simultaneous involvement of several acral sites (palms and soles) appear to be distinct from pagetoid reticulosis and may be better classified as "mycosis fungoides palmaris et plantaris."
- Spongiotic/eczematous dermatitis on acral skin may show a significant number of intraepidermal lymphocytes (in addition to spongiosis). However, the degree of epidermotropism in pagetoid reticulosis is extreme. If in doubt, it probably is not pagetoid reticulosis.

Pearls and Pitfalls
1. In general, mycosis fungoides (MF) variants do not look clinically like classic MF. In most cases of classic MF, the dermatologist suspects the possibility of MF in the clinical differential, while a histologic diagnosis of pagetoid reticulosis is usually unexpected. Pagetoid reticulosis is a rare MF variant and may be confused clinically with common hyperkeratotic lesions, such as verruca or squamous cell carcinoma.
2. Pagetoid reticulosis terminology should only be used for localized disease (Woringer-Kolopp type). The historic Ketron-Goodman type (disseminated disease) has been replaced by specific types of cytotoxic cutaneous lymphomas (cutaneous gamma-delta T-cell lymphoma, primary cutaneous CD8+ aggressive epidermotropic cytotoxic T-cell lymphoma, or extranodal NK/T-cell lymphoma, nasal type). Extended immunophenotyping (including determination of alpha-beta versus gamma-delta status) is necessary for classification of disseminated lymphomas with features resembling pagetoid reticulosis.

Suggested Reading

Elder DE, Massi D, Scolyer RA, Willemze R, editors. WHO classification of skin tumors. 4th ed. Lyon: IARC; 2018.

Haghighi B, Smoller BR, LeBoit PE, Warnke RA, Sander CA, Kohler S. Pagetoid reticulosis (Woringer-Kolopp disease): an immunophenotypic, molecular, and clinicopathologic study. Mod Pathol. 2000;13(5):502–10.

Martínez-Escala ME, González BR, Guitart J. Mycosis fungoides variants. Surg Pathol Clin. 2014;7(2):169–89.

Swerdlow SH, et al., editors. WHO Classification of tumors of hematopoietic and lymphoid tissues. Lyon: IARC; 2008.

Swerdlow SH, Campo E, Pileri SA, et al. The 2016 revision of the WHO classification of lymphoid neoplasms. Blood. 2016;127(20):2375–90.

Swerdlow SH, Campo E, Harris NL, Jaffe ES, Pileri SA, Stein H, Thiele J, editors. WHO classification of tumours of haematopoietic and lymphoid tissues (revised 4th ed). Lyon: IARC; 2017.

Willemze R, Jaffe ES, Burg G, et al. WHO-EORTC classification for cutaneous lymphomas. Blood. 2005;105(10):3768–85.

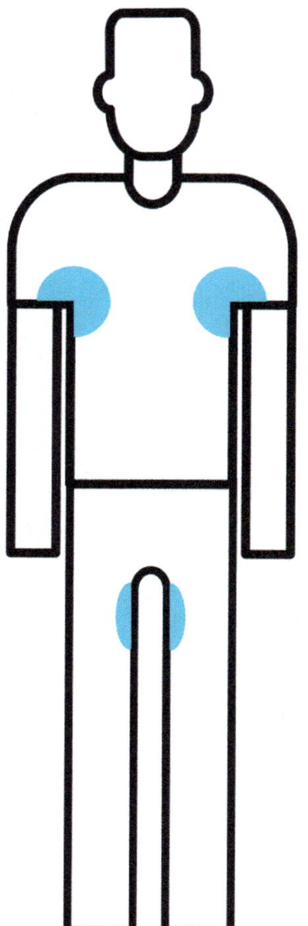

Fig. 25.1 Granulomatous slack skin classically involves flexural areas (axilla, groin)

Table 25.1 Key facts

Definition	
Granulomatous slack skin is a granulomatous variant of mycosis fungoides characterized by bulky, pendulous skin folds	
Prototypic clinical presentation	
Circumscribed area of bulky, pendulous, lax skin folds at a flexural site (axilla, groin)	
Histopathologic findings	
Dense diffuse dermal lymphohistiocytic infiltrate with pannicular extension. Abundant macrophages and large multinucleated giant cells with multiple nuclei and elastophagocytosis	
Most common immunophenotype: CD3+, CD4+, CD8−, variable loss of pan-T-cell markers	
Prognosis	
Excellent	

© Springer Nature Switzerland AG 2019

A. Subtil, *Diagnosis of Cutaneous Lymphoid Infiltrates*,

https://doi.org/10.1007/978-3-030-11654-5_25

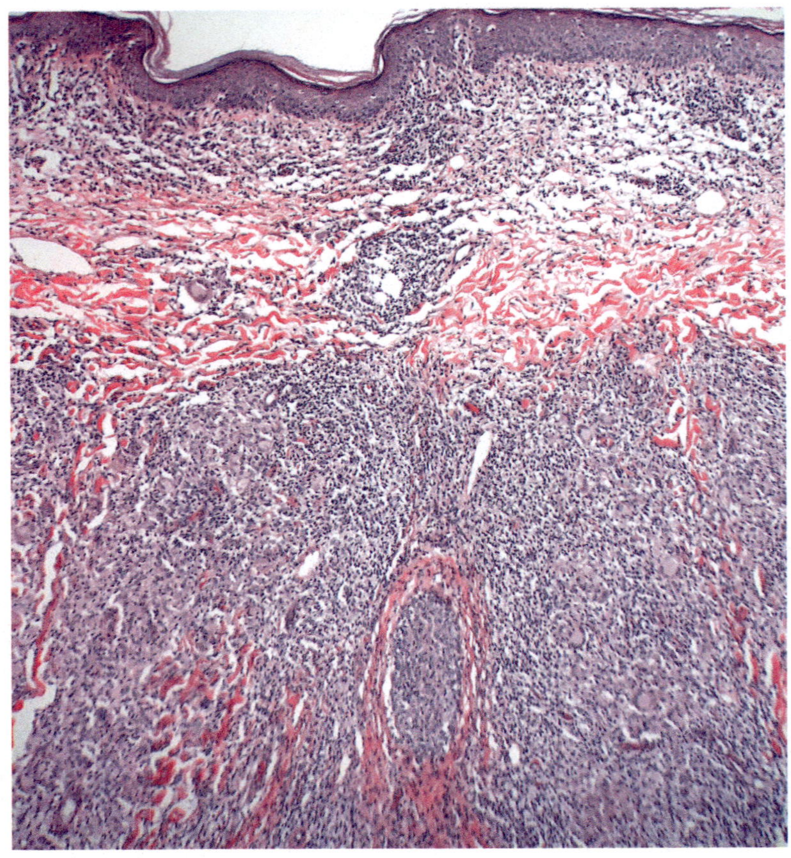

Fig. 25.2 Low-power magnification of granulomatous slack skin showing dense diffuse dermal infiltrate

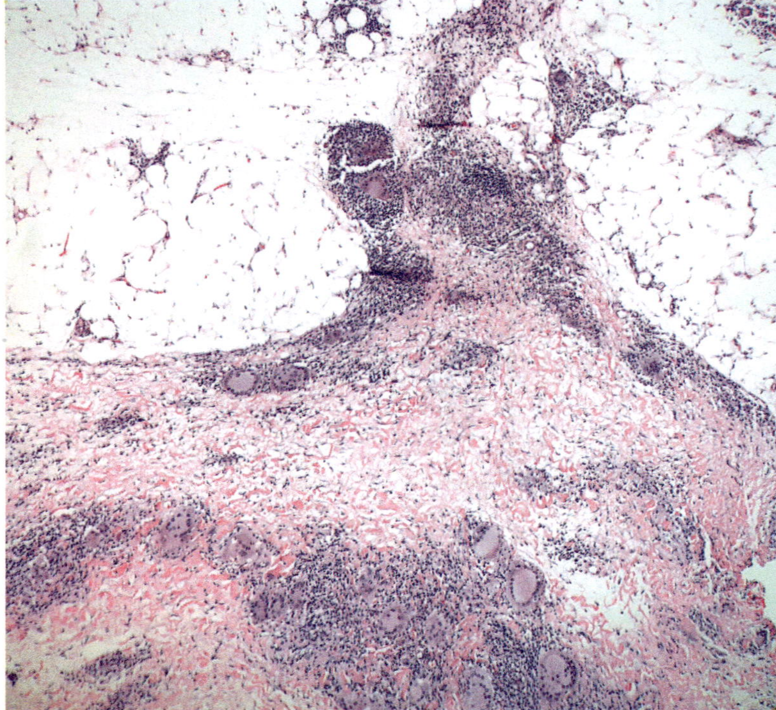

Fig. 25.3 Subcutaneous extension in granulomatous slack skin

Fig. 25.4
Granulomatous slack skin. Focal mild exocytosis of small lymphocytes in the epidermis

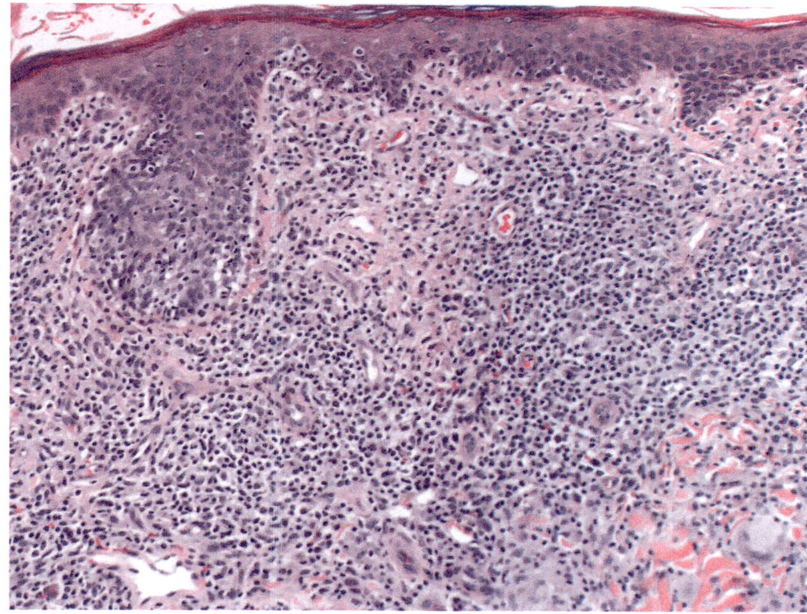

Fig. 25.5
Granulomatous slack skin. Dense diffuse dermal lymphohistiocytic infiltrate with exocytosis of lymphocytes in follicular epithelium

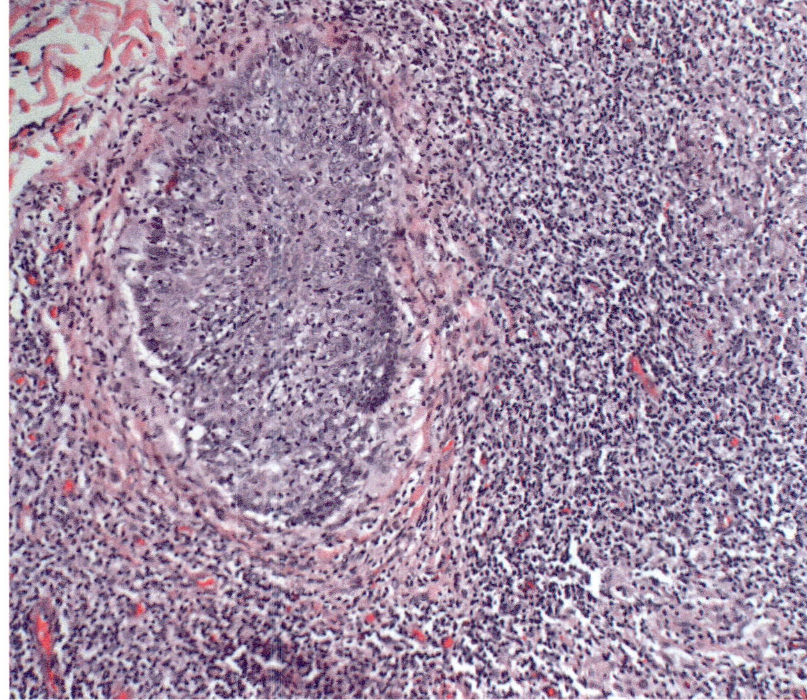

Fig. 25.6
Granulomatous slack skin. Dense diffuse dermal lymphocytic infiltrate with granuloma formation

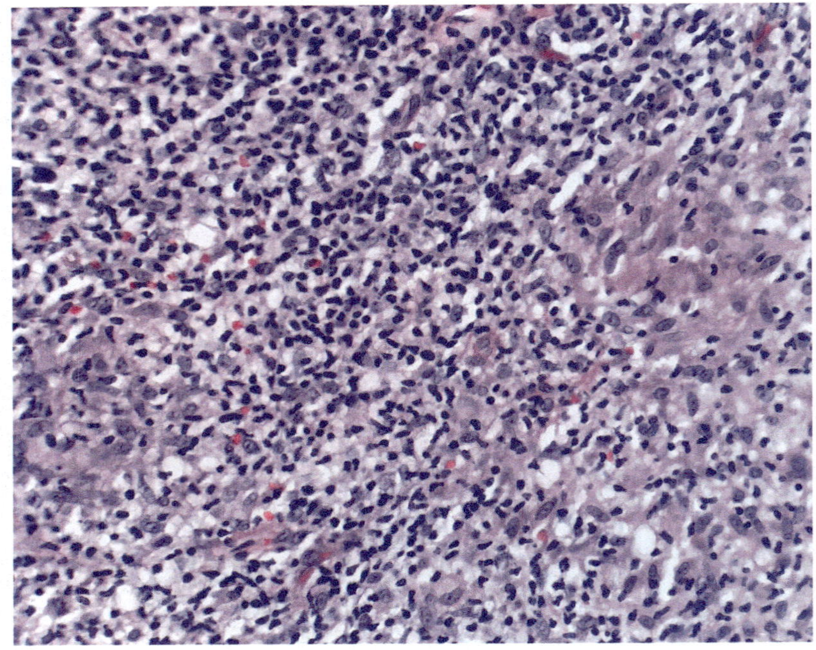

Fig. 25.7
Granulomatous slack skin. Large multinucleated giant cells with multiple nuclei

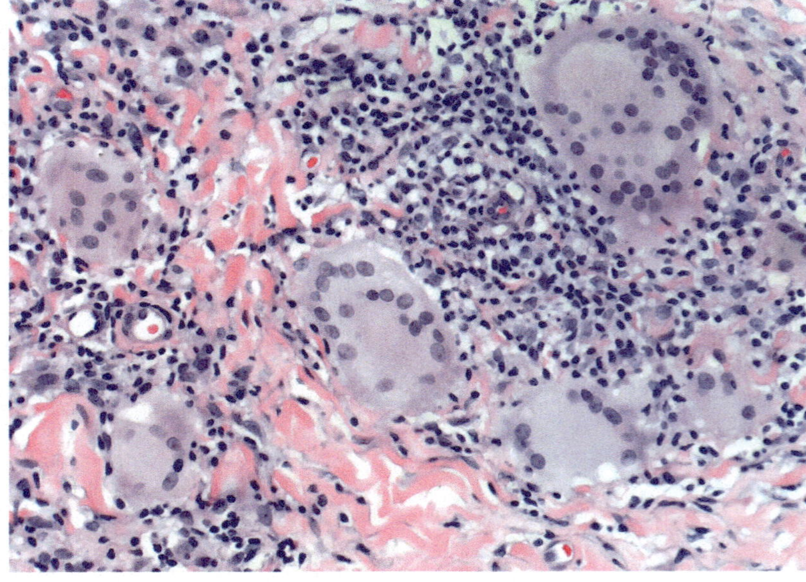

Fig. 25.8
Granulomatous slack
skin. Elastophagocytosis
(in brackets)

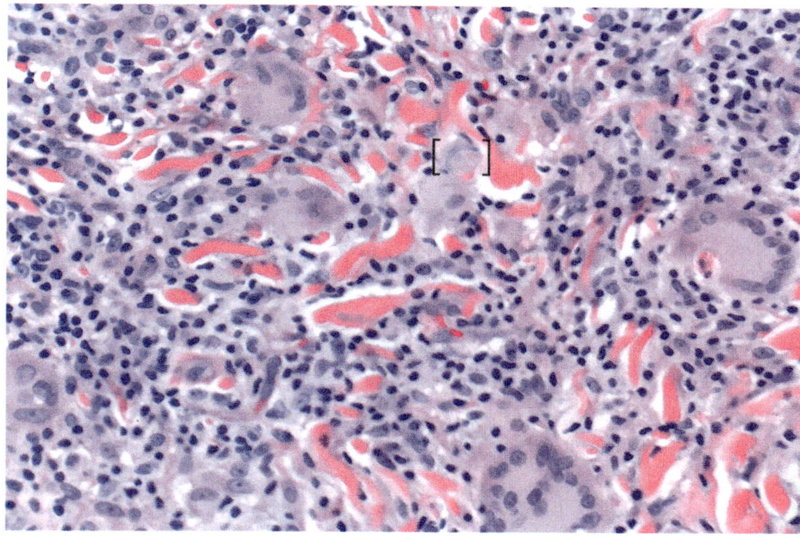

Disease Definition

- Granulomatous slack skin is a granulomatous variant of mycosis fungoides characterized by bulky, pendulous skin folds at flexural sites (Table 25.1).

Epidemiology

- Very rare
- Usually adults but onset may initiate in childhood
- May occasionally occur in association with Hodgkin lymphoma or classic mycosis fungoides

Preferential Sites of Involvement

- Flexural areas (axilla, groin) (Fig. 25.1)
- Generally limited to skin but regional lymph involvement may rarely occur

Clinical Features

- Clinically similar to classic mycosis fungoides in early stages, but eventually bulky, pendulous, lax skin folds develop at a flexural site.
- Overlying skin may be atrophic, wrinkled and/or erythematous.

Histomorphology

- *Pattern*: dense diffuse dermal lymphohistiocytic infiltrate with pannicular extension (Figs. 25.2 and 25.3)
- *Less common patterns*: variable epitheliotropism (usually limited) (Figs. 25.4 and 25.5)
- *Neoplastic cells*: small- to intermediate-sized lymphocytes with slightly indented to cerebriform nuclei and scant cytoplasm (Fig. 25.6)
- *Reactive cells*: abundant histiocytes and large multinucleated giant cells with multiple nuclei (Fig. 25.7). Elastophagocytosis and destruction of elastic fibers (Fig. 25.8)

Immunophenotype

- *Neoplastic cells*: CD3+, CD4+, CD8−, variable loss of pan-T-cell markers
- *Reactive cells*: CD68+ histiocytes

Genetics

- Monoclonal rearrangement of T-cell receptor genes in the majority of cases

Prognosis

- Indolent and slowly progressive. Better prognosis than classic mycosis fungoides
- 5-year survival: 100%

Differential Diagnosis

- Granulomatous cases of classic mycosis fungoides histologically resemble granulomatous slack skin, though pannicular extension is uncommon in the former. The distinction is made by the clinical presentation (conventional patches/plaques/tumors in granulomatous MF versus bulky, pendulous skin folds at flexural sites in GSS).
- Reactive granulomatous inflammatory infiltrates generally exhibit only a small component of lymphocytes, while histiocyte-rich T-cell lymphomas (such as granulomatous slack skin) contain abundant lymphocytes and epitheliotropism in addition to the prominent histiocytic component.

Suggested Reading

Elder DE, Massi D, Scolyer RA, Willemze R, editors. WHO classification of skin tumors. 4th ed. Lyon: IARC; 2018.

Martínez-Escala ME, González BR, Guitart J. Mycosis fungoides variants. Surg Pathol Clin. 2014;7(2):169–89.

Motta LMD, Soares CT, Nakandakari S, Silva GVD, Nigro MHMF, Brandão LSG. Granulomatous slack skin: a rare subtype of mycosis fungoides. An Bras Dermatol. 2017;92(5):694–7.

Swerdlow SH, et al., editors. WHO classification of tumors of hematopoietic and lymphoid tissues. Lyon: IARC; 2008.

Swerdlow SH, Campo E, Harris NL, Jaffe ES, Pileri SA, Stein H, Thiele J, editors. WHO classification of tumours of haematopoietic and lymphoid tissues (revised 4th ed). Lyon: IARC; 2017.

Willemze R, Jaffe ES, Burg G, et al. WHO-EORTC classification for cutaneous lymphomas. Blood. 2005;105(10):3768–85.

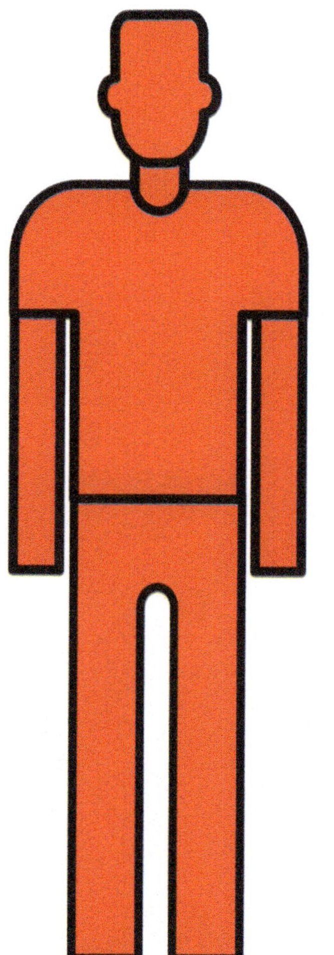

Fig. 26.1 Sézary syndrome is associated with erythroderma (>80% of total body erythema)

Table 26.1 Key facts

Definition

Sézary syndrome is the triad of erythroderma, generalized lymphadenopathy, and the presence of clonally related T cells in the skin, peripheral blood, and/or lymph nodes. At least one of the following additional criteria must also be present in the peripheral blood: absolute Sézary cell count ≥1000/μL, CD4/CD8 ratio ≥10, or loss of one or more T-cell antigens

Prototypic clinical presentation

Erythroderma (>80% of total body erythema) and generalized lymphadenopathy

Pruritus, alopecia, ectropion, and palmoplantar hyperkeratosis are common

Histopathologic findings

Often nonspecific histopathologic findings. Superficial dermal atypical lymphocytic infiltrate with variable epidermotropism

Most common immunophenotype: CD3+, CD4+, CD8−, PD1+, variable loss of pan-T-cell markers

Prognosis

Poor

© Springer Nature Switzerland AG 2019
A. Subtil, *Diagnosis of Cutaneous Lymphoid Infiltrates*,
https://doi.org/10.1007/978-3-030-11654-5_26

Fig. 26.2 Low-power magnification of a case of Sézary syndrome showing a mild superficial dermal lymphocytic infiltrate with epidermotropism. There are background changes of lichen simplex chronicus (epidermal hyperplasia and dermal fibrosis) due to prominent pruritus

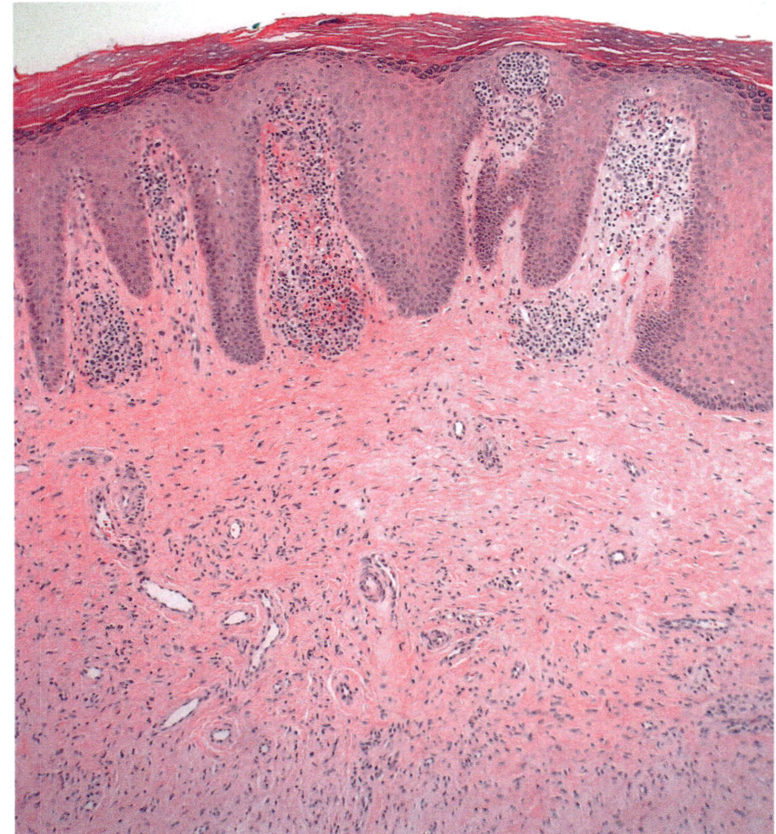

Fig. 26.3 High-power magnification of a case of Sézary syndrome showing a mild superficial dermal lymphocytic infiltrate with epidermotropism

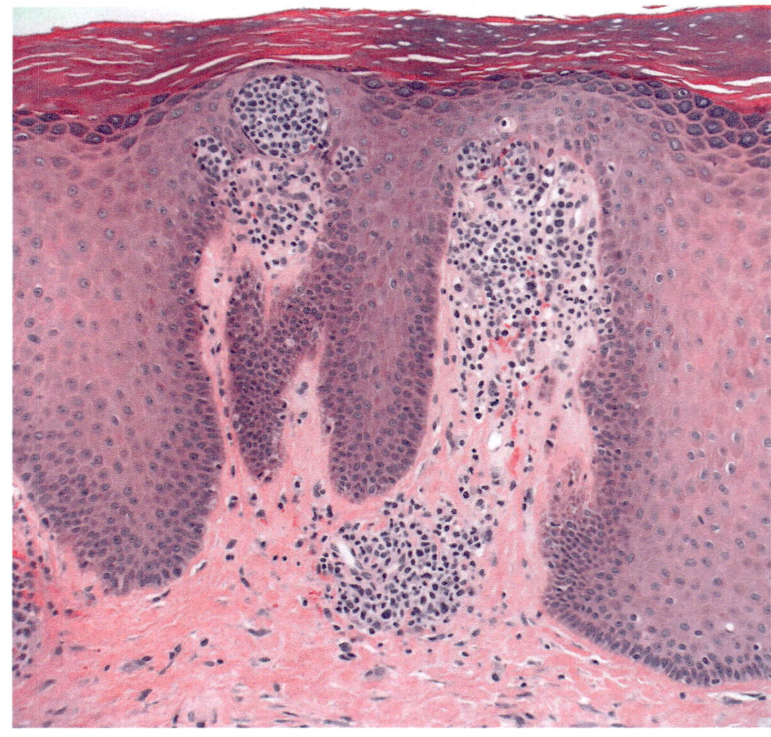

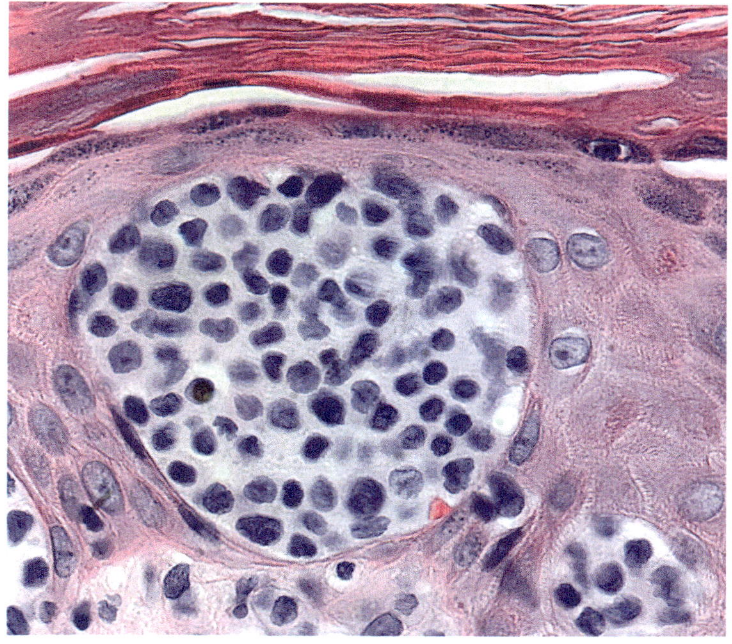

Fig. 26.4 High-power magnification of a case of Sézary syndrome showing Pautrier microabscesses. Atypical intraepidermal lymphocytes with cerebriform nuclei

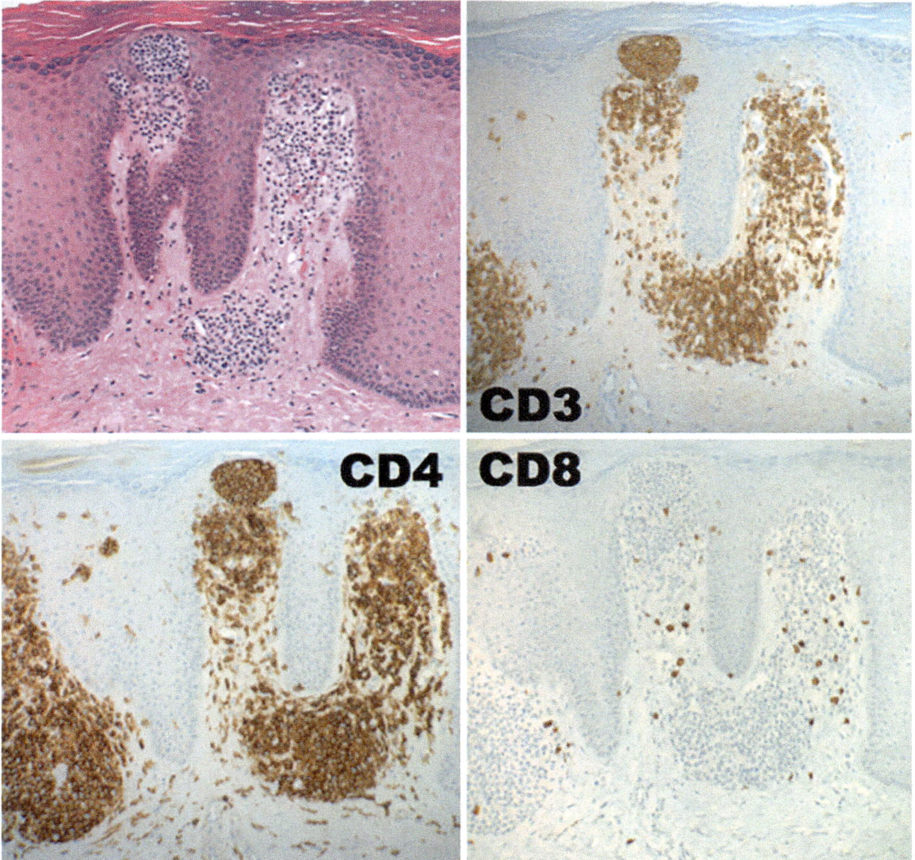

Fig. 26.5 Immunophenotype of Sézary syndrome. The neoplastic cells are CD3+/CD4+ T cells. Only rare reactive lymphocytes mark with CD8 stain

Fig. 26.6 Some cases of Sézary syndrome do not exhibit epidermotropism but may show atypical lymphocytes in the superficial dermis

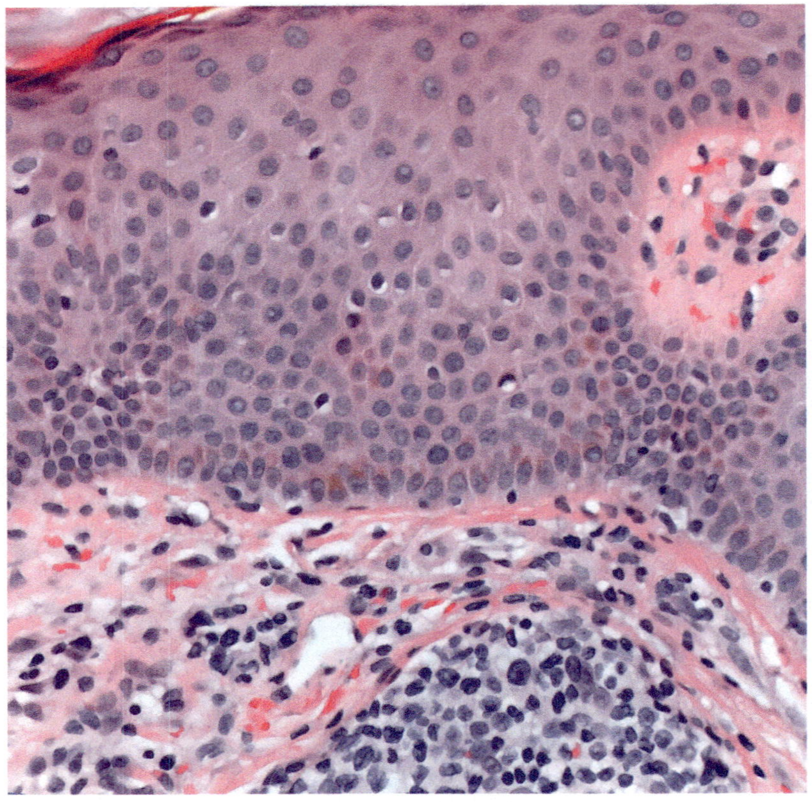

Disease Definition

- Sézary syndrome is the triad of erythroderma, generalized lymphadenopathy, and the presence of clonally related T cells in the skin, peripheral blood, and/or lymph nodes. At least one of the following additional criteria must also be present in the peripheral blood: absolute Sézary cell count ≥1000/μL, CD4/CD8 ratio ≥10, or loss of one or more T-cell antigens (usually CD7 or CD26) (Table 26.1).

Epidemiology

- Rare.
- Adults and elderly patients.
- Male predominance.

Preferential Sites of Involvement

- Generalized skin involvement with erythroderma (>80% of total body surface area with erythema) (Fig. 26.1).
- Generalized lymphadenopathy.
- Peripheral blood involvement (leukemic disease by definition).
- Bone marrow involvement may occur (but often sparse and interstitial infiltrates).
- Visceral involvement and cutaneous tumoral nodules may occur in advance disease.

Clinical Features

- Erythroderma ("red man syndrome"), occasionally with sparing of large skinfolds. Pruritus is common and may be severe.

- Palpable lymphadenopathy.
- Alopecia, ectropion, nail dystrophy, and palmoplantar hyperkeratosis.
- *Less common presentations*: presentation with only pruritus.

Histomorphology

- *Pattern*: In patients with Sézary syndrome, the majority of skin biopsies are histopathologically nondiagnostic with variable parakeratosis, mild spongiosis, and sparse inflammatory infiltrates (often overlapping with features of benign causes of erythroderma). Lichen simplex chronicus (hyperkeratosis, acanthosis, and superficial dermal fibrosis) may be seen due to chronic pruritus.
- *Less common patterns*: (a) Epidermotropic infiltrate of atypical lymphocytes, singly or in clusters (Pautrier microabscesses), similar to that seen in mycosis fungoides (Figs. 26.2 and 26.3). (b) Superficial dermal infiltrate of atypical lymphocytes without epidermotropism. (c) Rare cases may show folliculotropism with or without follicular mucinosis. (d) Large cell transformation may occur in a subset of patients.
- *Neoplastic cells*: Atypical small- to intermediate-sized pleomorphic lymphocytes with convoluted, cerebriform, hyperchromatic nuclei and scant cytoplasm (Fig. 26.4).
- *Reactive cells*: Sparse small lymphocytes.

Immunophenotype

- *Neoplastic cells*: CD3+, CD4+, CD8−, PD1+, variable loss of pan-T-cell markers (CD7, CD26, and/or CD2) (Fig. 26.5)
- *Reactive cells*: Sparse small CD8+ T cells

Genetics

- Monoclonal T-cell receptor gene rearrangement is required by definition, and the same clone should be demonstrated in the skin, peripheral blood, and/or lymph nodes.

Prognosis

- Poor. Median survival of 32–48 months.
- 5-year survival: 10–30%.
- Most common cause of death is infection (secondary to disease-related immunosuppression).

Differential Diagnosis

- Biopsies with epidermotropic infiltrates must be differentiated from other epidermotropic processes, largely on clinical grounds. In contrast to the erythroderma of Sézary syndrome, the other entities show distinct clinical findings: chronic patches/plaques in mycosis fungoides, self-regressing papules in lymphomatoid papulosis types B and D, and fast-progressing ulcerative disease in aggressive cytotoxic lymphomas.
- Sézary syndrome is a malignant cause of erythroderma but is a rare disease. Most patients with erythroderma will have benign causes (usually psoriasis, drug reaction, spongiotic/eczematous dermatitis, or pityriasis rubra pilaris). While this differential diagnosis is often difficult on clinical and histopathologic grounds, exclusion of Sézary syndrome would require hematologic and molecular studies.

Pearls and Pitfalls

1. While Sézary syndrome and mycosis fungoides are closely related, they are distinct entities. Sézary syndrome is associated with a significantly worse prognosis as well as marked immunosuppression.

2. A few patients with mycosis fungoides may progress from the conventional clinical picture of chronic patches/plaques into erythroderma during the course of their disease (erythrodermic mycosis fungoides). In contrast, Sézary syndrome starts with erythroderma.

3. In patients with Sézary syndrome, the skin biopsies are often histopathologically nondiagnostic, and the classic epidermotropic pattern is only seen in a minority of specimens. Some cases may show a superficial dermal infiltrate of atypical lymphocytes without epidermotropism (Fig. 26.6).

4. The diagnosis of Sézary syndrome is made clinically (erythroderma associated with generalized lymphadenopathy) and molecularly (presence of clonally related T cells in the skin, peripheral blood, and/or lymph node) and by examination of the peripheral blood (absolute Sézary cell count $\geq$1000/μL or flow cytometric identification of an expanded CD4+ T-cell population with CD4/CD8 ratio $\geq$10 and/or loss of one or more T-cell antigens). It is not a dermatopathologic diagnosis.

5. The skin histopathology is not part of the diagnostic criteria for Sézary syndrome (Table 26.1). In a patient with erythroderma and suspected Sézary syndrome, the main reason for the skin biopsy is to obtain tissue for T-cell receptor gene rearrangement and subsequent comparison of any T-cell clone with the peripheral blood.

6. Sézary cell counts in peripheral blood are often difficult to interpret and are not available in most medical centers. Flow cytometry has largely replaced their use.

7. Sézary patients are markedly immunocompromised and have an increased risk of infections and second malignancies.

Suggested Reading

Elder DE, Massi D, Scolyer RA, Willemze R, editors. WHO classification of skin tumors. 4th ed. Lyon: IARC; 2018.

Kubica AW, Pittelkow MR. Sézary syndrome. Surg Pathol Clin. 2014;7(2):191–202.

Kubica AW, Davis MD, Weaver AL, Killian JM, Pittelkow MR. Sézary syndrome: a study of 176 patients at Mayo Clinic. J Am Acad Dermatol. 2012;67(6):1189–99.

Swerdlow SH, et al., editors. WHO classification of tumors of hematopoietic and lymphoid tissues. Lyon: IARC; 2008.

Swerdlow SH, Campo E, Harris NL, Jaffe ES, Pileri SA, Stein H, Thiele J, editors. WHO classification of tumours of haematopoietic and lymphoid tissues (revised 4th ed). Lyon: IARC; 2017.

Willemze R, Jaffe ES, Burg G, et al. WHO-EORTC classification for cutaneous lymphomas. Blood. 2005;105(10):3768–85.

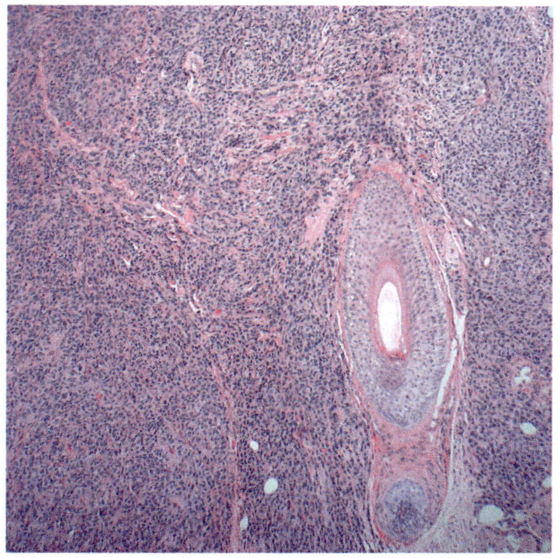

Fig. 27.1 Low-power magnification of primary cutaneous anaplastic large cell lymphoma showing a dense, vaguely nodular dermal lymphoid infiltrate

Table 27.1 Key facts

Definition
Primary cutaneous anaplastic large cell lymphoma is a skin lymphoma composed of large cells (anaplastic, pleomorphic, or immunoblastic morphology) with CD30 expression (>75%). There should be no clinical evidence or history of mycosis fungoides
Prototypic clinical presentation
Solitary or localized skin nodules or tumors. Ulceration and cutaneous relapses are common
Histopathologic findings
Dense, diffuse, or vaguely nodular dermal infiltrate of large atypical lymphoid cells in confluent sheets. Epidermotropism and/or pannicular extension may be seen. Ulceration is common
Most common immunophenotype: CD4+/CD8− phenotype with strong CD30 expression (>75% of neoplastic cells), variable loss of T-cell markers, and frequent expression of cytotoxic proteins (TIA-1, granzyme B, perforin). EMA and ALK are usually negative. PAX5 and EBV are negative
Prognosis
Indolent

© Springer Nature Switzerland AG 2019

A. Subtil, *Diagnosis of Cutaneous Lymphoid Infiltrates*,

https://doi.org/10.1007/978-3-030-11654-5_27

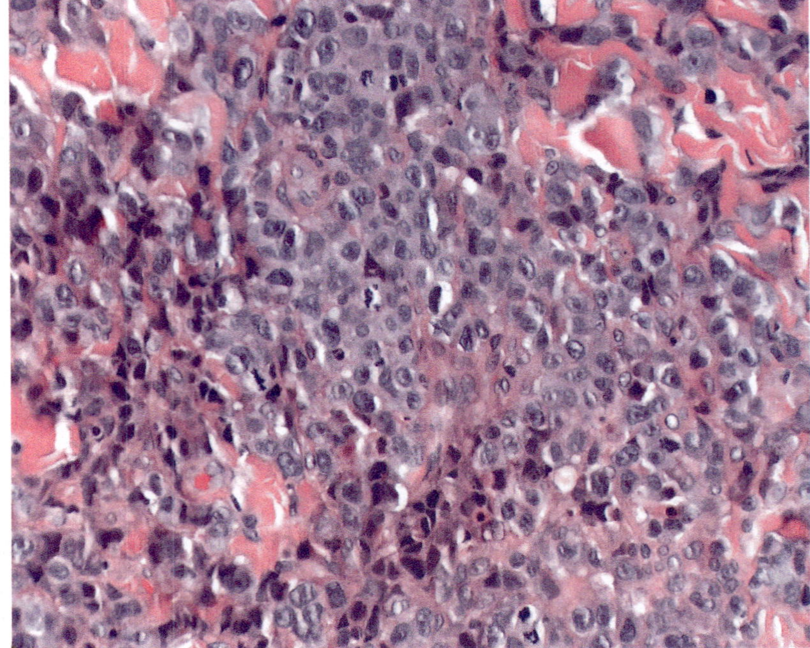

Fig. 27.2 High-power magnification of primary cutaneous anaplastic large cell lymphoma. Cohesive sheets of large atypical lymphoid cells in the dermis

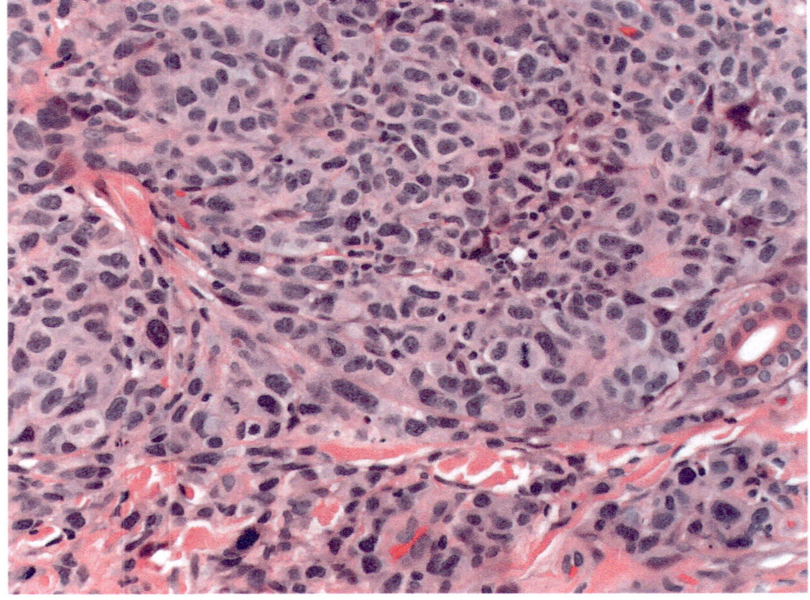

Fig. 27.3 High-power magnification of primary cutaneous anaplastic large cell lymphoma. Cohesive sheets of large atypical lymphoid cells with abundant cytoplasm and frequent mitotic figures

Fig. 27.4 High-power magnification of primary cutaneous anaplastic large cell lymphoma. Dense infiltrate of large atypical lymphoid cells with pleomorphic nuclei

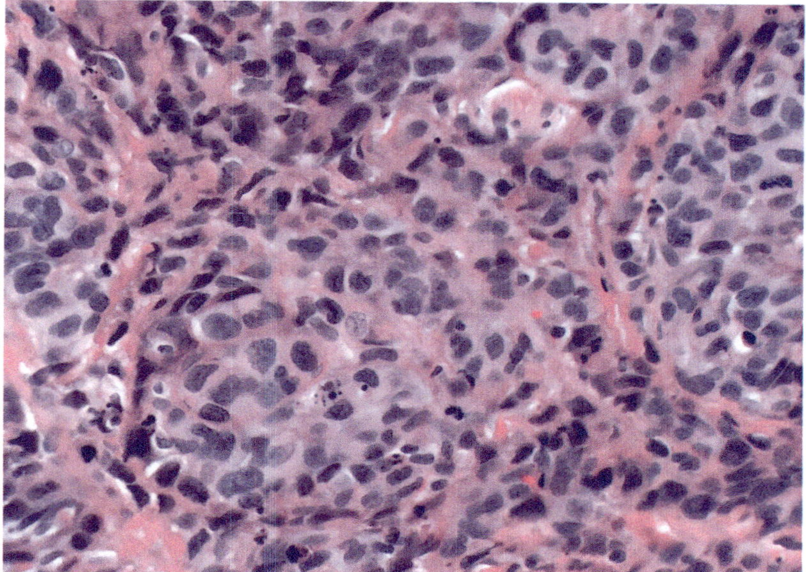

Fig. 27.5 Primary cutaneous anaplastic large cell lymphoma with epidermotropism

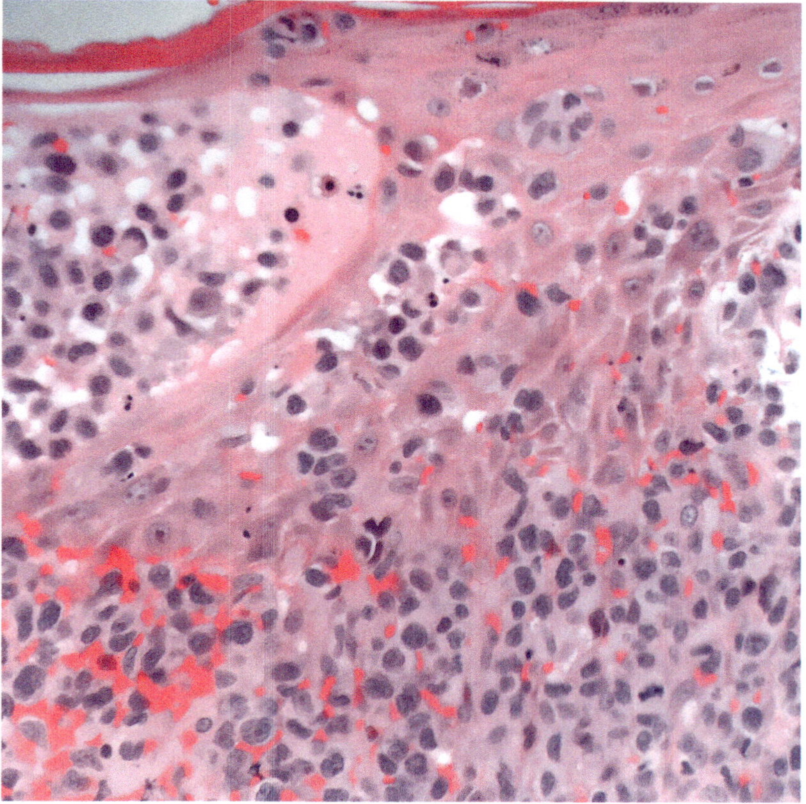

Fig. 27.6 Primary cutaneous anaplastic large cell lymphoma with myxoid stroma

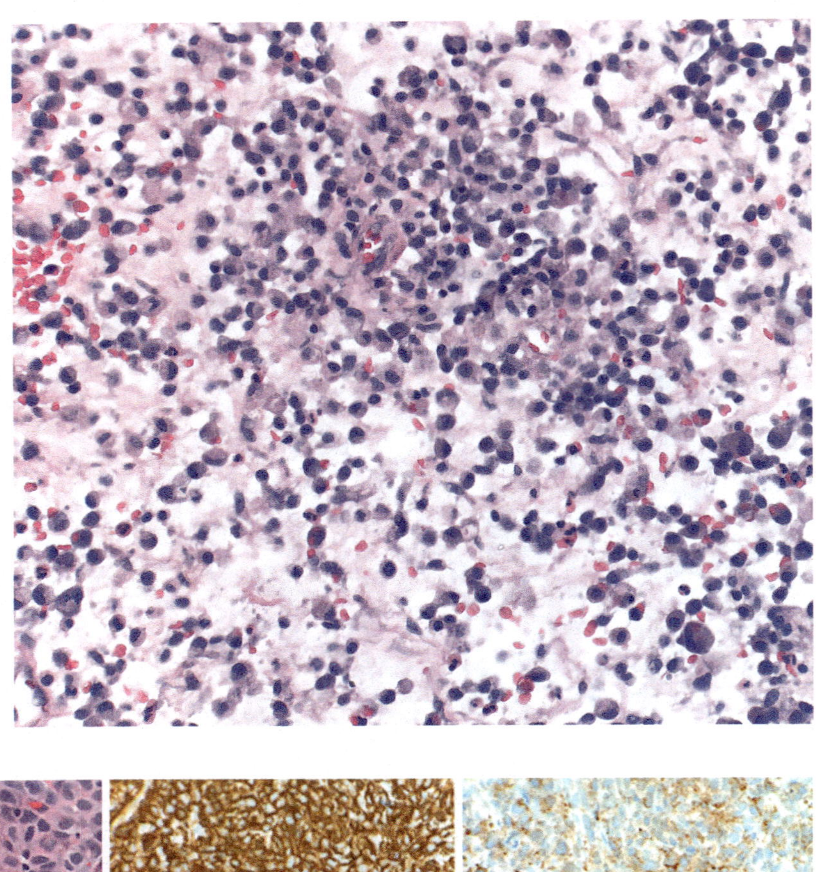

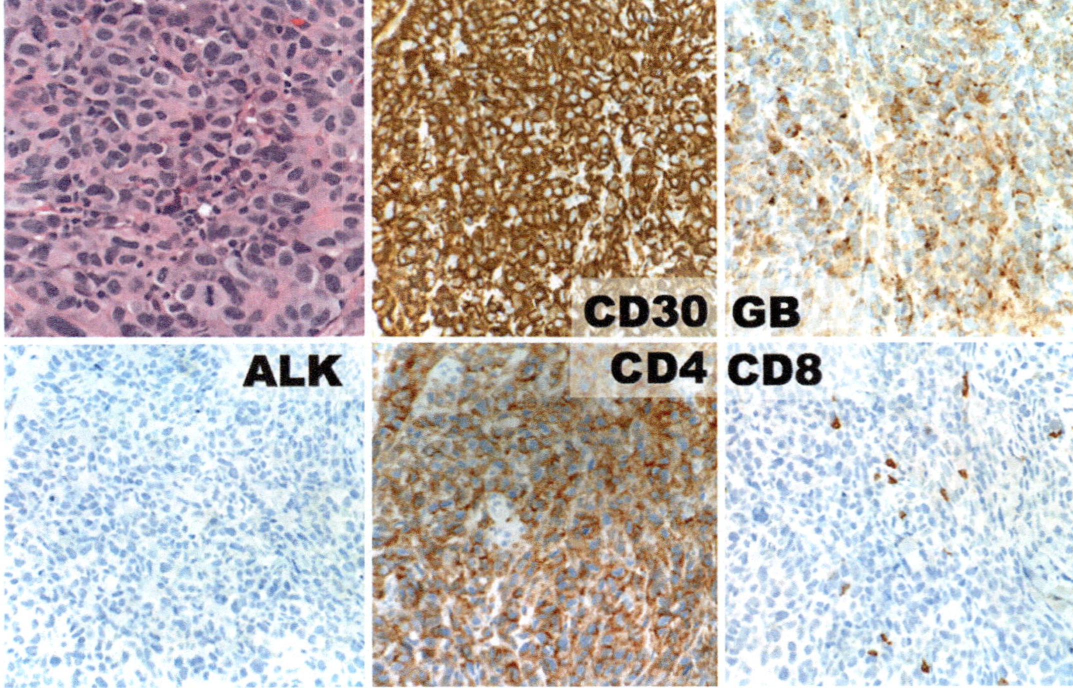

Fig. 27.7 Common immunophenotype of primary cutaneous anaplastic large cell lymphoma: CD30+ (>75% of atypical cells), CD4+, CD8−, ALK−, and granzyme B+

Fig. 27.8 Differential diagnosis of CD30 expression

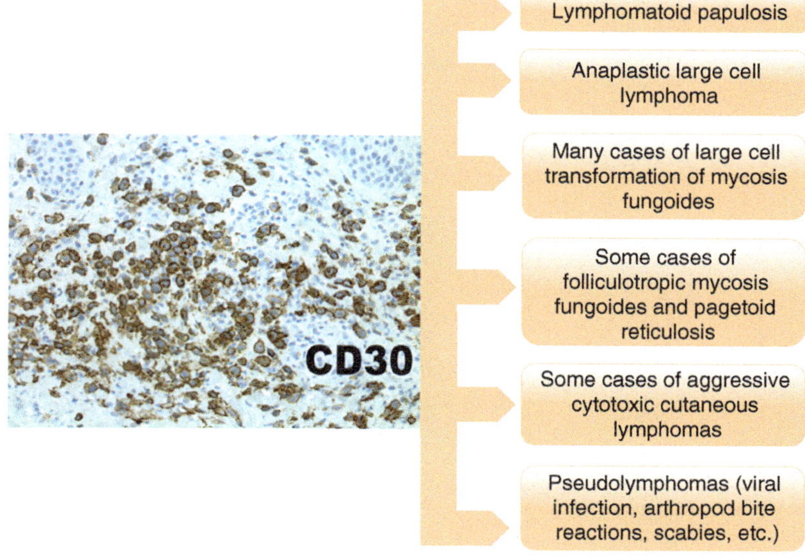

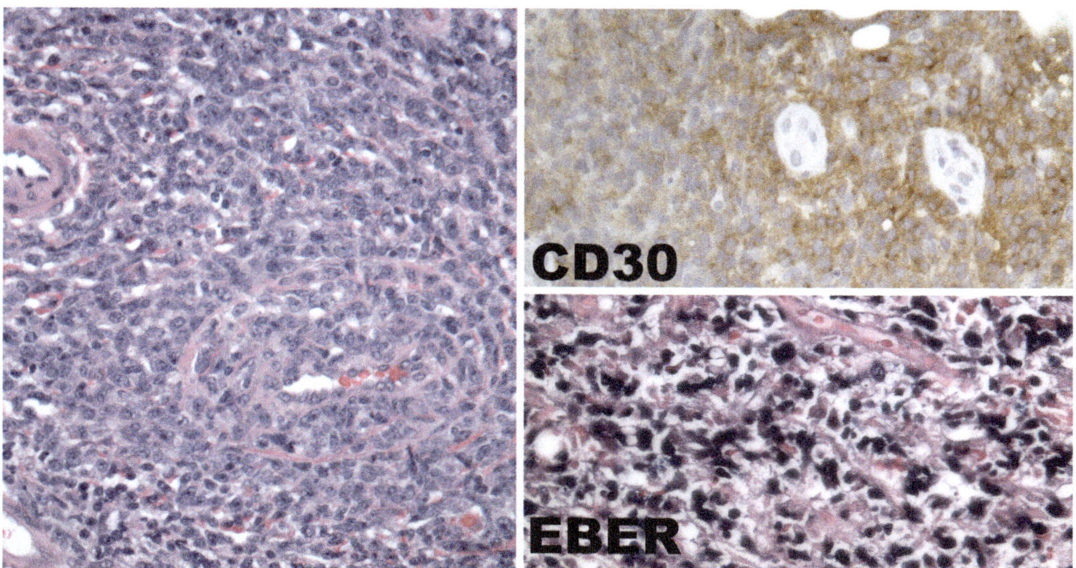

Fig. 27.9 Extranodal NK/T-cell lymphoma, nasal type mimicking cutaneous anaplastic large cell lymphoma. Some cases of aggressive cytotoxic lymphomas may exhibit large cell cytomorphology and variable CD30 expression. Subtle infiltration of the walls of a blood vessel (angiocentrism) is present in the lower half of the figure. Unlike anaplastic large cell lymphoma, EBV in situ hybridization (EBER) is positive

Fig. 27.10 Differential diagnosis of atypical large cell lymphoid infiltrate

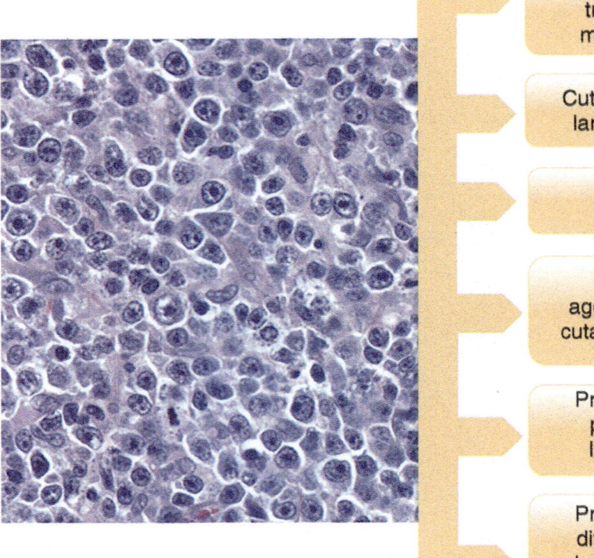

Fig. 27.11 Secondary skin involvement by systemic ALK-positive anaplastic large cell lymphoma

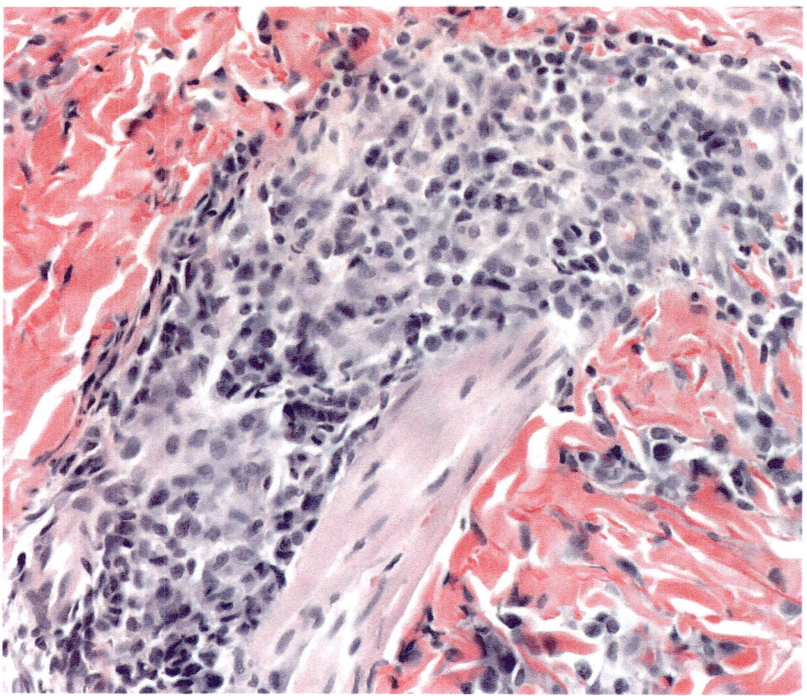

Lymphomatoid papulosis (LyP) and primary cutaneous anaplastic large cell lymphoma (C-ALCL) are part of the spectrum of cutaneous CD30-positive lymphoproliferative disorders, which also includes borderline lesions. Cutaneous anaplastic large cell lymphoma generally presents with skin tumors, while LyP exhibits small self-regressing papules.

Disease Definition

- Primary cutaneous anaplastic large cell lymphoma is a skin lymphoma composed of large cells (anaplastic, pleomorphic or immunoblastic cytomorphology) with CD30 expression (>75%). There should be no clinical evidence or history of mycosis fungoides (Table 27.1).

Epidemiology

- Usually adults and elderly patients
- May occur during childhood
- Male predominance
- Second most common form of primary cutaneous T-cell lymphoma

Preferential Sites of Involvement

- Trunk, face, and/or extremities
- Generally limited to the skin but extracutaneous dissemination may occur in 10% of cases (usually regional lymph nodes)

Clinical Features

- Solitary or localized, reddish-brown nodules or tumors.
- Ulceration and cutaneous relapses are common.
- Partial (and occasionally complete) self-regression may occur.
- *Less common presentations*: small satellite papules at the periphery of tumors, multifocal skin lesions, extensive limb disease.

Histomorphology

- *Pattern*: dense, diffuse, or vaguely nodular dermal infiltrate of large atypical lymphoid cells (in confluent sheets) with variable pannicular extension (Figs. 27.1, 27.2, 27.3, and 27.4). Ulceration is common.
- *Less common patterns*: epidermotropism in the overlying epidermis may also be seen (Fig. 27.5). Pleomorphic, immunoblastic, or signet ring cytomorphology. Pseudocarcinomatous epidermal hyperplasia. Neutrophil-rich variant. Eosinophil-rich variant. Intravascular variant. Myxoid stroma (Fig. 27.6).
- *Neoplastic cells*: usually anaplastic cytomorphology with round, oval, or irregular nuclei, prominent eosinophilic nucleoli, and abundant cytoplasm. Multinucleation may be seen.
- *Reactive cells*: usually sparse (predominantly small lymphocytes). If ulceration is present, neutrophils and histiocytes may be prominent.

Immunophenotype

- *Neoplastic cells*: most cases show a CD4+/CD8− phenotype with strong CD30 expression (>75% of neoplastic cells), variable loss of T-cell markers (CD3, CD2, CD5, and/or CD7), and frequent expression of cytotoxic proteins (TIA-1, granzyme B, perforin). EMA and ALK are usually negative (Fig. 27.7). PAX5 and EBV are negative. CD15 expression may be seen. CD56 expression is rare. Occasional cases are CD4−/CD8+, CD4+/CD8+, or CD4−/CD8−.
- *Reactive cells*: usually sparse small CD8+ T cells.

Genetics

- Monoclonal rearrangement of T-cell receptor genes in the majority of cases.
- DUSP22-IRF4 rearrangement in a minority of cases of primary cutaneous ALCL (20–25%). Epidermotropism is often marked in these

cases. This rearrangement may also be found in <5% of LyP and in 30% of systemic ALK-negative ALCL.

– Most cases do not have ALK translocations.

Prognosis

– Indolent
– 5-year survival: 95%
– Adverse risk factors: immunodeficiency, extensive leg involvement

Differential Diagnosis

– In the absence of adequate clinical information, distinction between LyP type C and C-ALCL is generally not possible (Table 27.2). In addition, ulcerated cases of C-ALCL show neutrophils and histiocytes in the infiltrate and may closely mimic LyP type A in a partial biopsy. In such cases, the diagnosis should be "cutaneous CD30+ lymphoproliferative disorder," and the final classification should be made by the clinician.
– Borderline cases of primary cutaneous CD30+ lymphoproliferative disorders. Some lesions are difficult to differentiate between lymphomatoid papulosis and anaplastic large cell lymphoma at presentation. However, the diagnosis is usually revealed by careful clinical examination during close follow-up (complete regression versus persistence/progression of each individual lesion).
– Some variants of mycosis fungoides may show variable CD30 expression, particularly folliculotropic mycosis fungoides and pagetoid reticulosis (Fig. 27.8). Large cell transformation of mycosis fungoides (LCT-MF) requires at least 25% of large atypical cells in the infiltrate or the formation of microscopic nodules of large cells. Once the histomorphologic criteria have been met, some cases express CD30, while other cases do not. It is important to emphasize that the definition of LCT-MF is based on H&E findings (not on the level of CD30 expression). LyP in association with MF must be excluded on clinical grounds for the CD30-positive cases. However, ALCL is not an option in this setting since the absence of MF is part of the diagnostic criteria for cutaneous ALCL.
– Some cases of aggressive cytotoxic cutaneous lymphomas (such as extranodal NK/T-cell lymphoma, nasal type; Fig. 27.9) may demonstrate large cell infiltrates in the initial biopsy. It is important to include them in the differential diagnosis of large T-cell infiltrates (Fig. 27.10). Since variable CD30 expression may occur in cytotoxic lymphomas, these aggressive cases may be misdiagnosed as anaplastic large cell lymphoma (an indolent process).
– The differential diagnosis for primary cutaneous ALCL includes secondary skin involvement by systemic ALCL (ALK-positive or ALK-negative) (Fig. 27.11). Staging is usually the best method to rule out this possibility, since there have been rare reports of ALK-positive ALCL apparently limited to the skin.
– Reactive inflammatory and infectious skin diseases. CD30 is an activation marker and is often positive in various reactive infiltrates, including viral conditions (inflamed molluscum contagiosum, herpes folliculitis, orf, milker's nodule, EBV-positive mucocutaneous ulcer), drug reactions, and arthropod bite reactions (including scabies). CD30 expression by itself is not enough for a diagnosis of anaplastic large cell lymphoma. Careful clinical correlation and proactively searching for histopathologic features of other conditions (e.g., viral cytopathic effect, scabietic organisms) may help prevent misdiagnosis.

Table 27.2 Comparison of cutaneous CD30-positive lymphoproliferative disorders

	Lymphomatoid papulosis (LyP)	Cutaneous anaplastic large cell lymphoma (C-ALCL)
Clinical findings	Solitary or multiple, recurrent, small self-healing papules	Solitary or localized large skin lesions (nodules or tumors)
Histologic findings	Variable findings depending of the histologic subtype, resembling different types of lymphoma (type C resembles ALCL)	Dense diffuse dermal infiltrate of large atypical CD30+ lymphoid cells Usually scant inflammation
Differential diagnoses	C-ALCL and other lymphomas Reactive inflammatory infiltrates with activated CD30+ lymphocytes (reactions to drugs, arthropod bites, and viral infections)	LyP Secondary cutaneous involvement by systemic/nodal CD30+ ALCL Large cell transformation of mycosis fungoides with CD30 expression

Pearls and Pitfalls

1. CD30 is an activation marker that is characteristically expressed by cutaneous CD30-positive lymphoproliferative disorders (lymphomatoid papulosis and anaplastic large cell lymphoma). However, CD30 is not specific for these entities and may show significant expression in a variety of benign and malignant cutaneous lymphoid infiltrates (Fig. 27.8). The identification of CD30 expression by itself is not enough to make a diagnosis. Additional immunophenotyping and clinical correlation are necessary for proper classification.
2. The threshold of positivity is variable for different CD markers. For example, for anaplastic large cell lymphoma, CD30 must be positive in at least 75% of atypical cells (i.e., even if 60% of an infiltrate marks with CD30, that level of staining is not sufficient for ALCL, and other entities should be considered in the differential diagnosis).

Suggested Reading

Elder DE, Massi D, Scolyer RA, Willemze R, editors. WHO classification of skin tumors. 4th ed. Lyon: IARC; 2018.

Feldman AL, Law M, Remstein ED, Macon WR, Erickson LA, Grogg KL, Kurtin PJ, Dogan A. Recurrent translocations involving the IRF4 oncogene locus in peripheral T-cell lymphomas. Leukemia. 2009;23(3):574–80.

Kempf W. Cutaneous CD30-positive lymphoproliferative disorders. Surg Pathol Clin. 2014;7(2):203–28.

Swerdlow SH, et al., editors. WHO classification of tumors of hematopoietic and lymphoid tissues. Lyon: IARC; 2008.

Swerdlow SH, Campo E, Harris NL, Jaffe ES, Pileri SA, Stein H, Thiele J, editors. WHO classification of tumours of haematopoietic and lymphoid tissues (revised 4th ed). Lyon: IARC; 2017.

Werner B, Massone C, Kerl H, et al. Large CD30-positive cells in benign, atypical lymphoid infiltrates of the skin. J Cutan Pathol. 2008;35(12):1100–7.

Willemze R, Jaffe ES, Burg G, et al. WHO-EORTC classification for cutaneous lymphomas. Blood. 2005;105(10):3768–85.

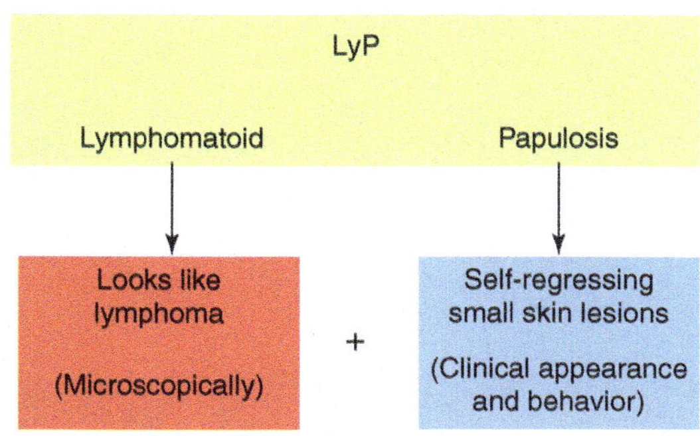

Fig. 28.1 Basic equation for the diagnosis of lymphomatoid papulosis

Table 28.1 Key facts

Definition
Lymphomatoid papulosis is a chronic, recurrent, self-healing skin disease that combines an indolent clinical course with histopathologic features of different types of cutaneous T-cell lymphomas
Prototypic clinical presentation
Self-regressing papules or small nodules, with or without ulceration
Histopathologic findings
Highly variable depending on subtype (see text) Most common immunophenotype: CD3+, CD4+, CD8−, CD30+, ALK− in types A (most common), B, and C. Usually CD4−,CD8+ in the other subtypes
Prognosis
Excellent

© Springer Nature Switzerland AG 2019

A. Subtil, *Diagnosis of Cutaneous Lymphoid Infiltrates*,

https://doi.org/10.1007/978-3-030-11654-5_28

Fig. 28.2 Low-power magnification of a case of lymphomatoid papulosis type A showing a wedge-shaped dermal infiltrate (upside-down triangle)

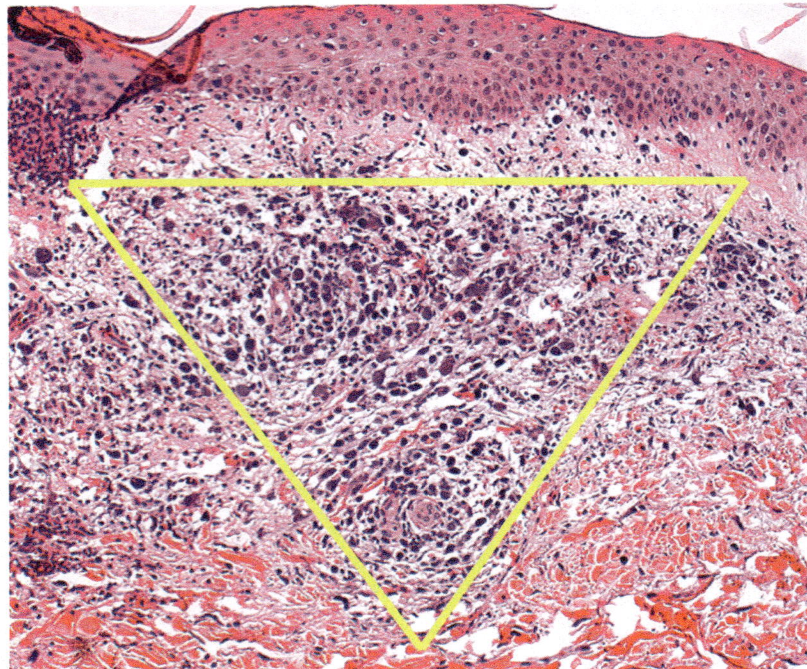

Fig. 28.3 High-power magnification of a case of lymphomatoid papulosis type A showing large atypical lymphoid cells admixed with a dermal infiltrate of neutrophils, eosinophils, histiocytes, and small lymphocytes

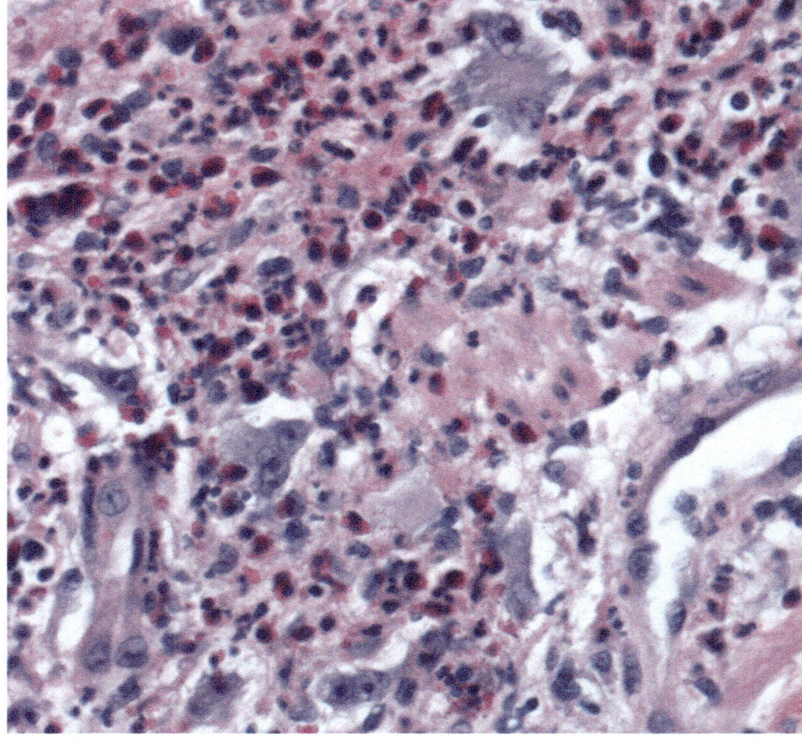

Fig. 28.4 CD30 expression in a case of lymphomatoid papulosis type A

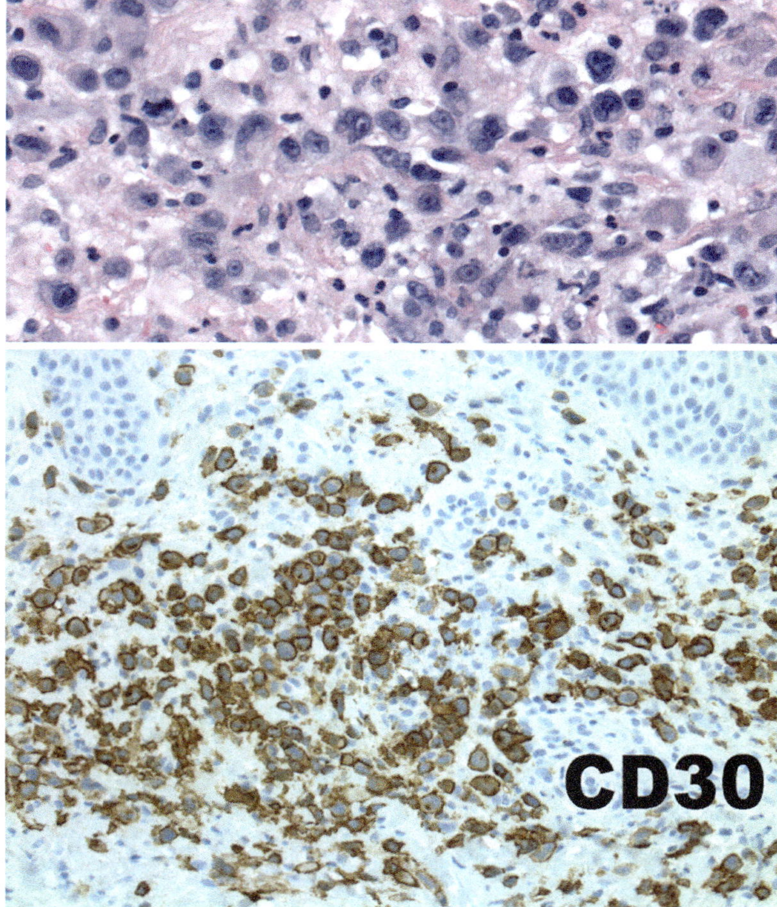

Fig. 28.5 High-power magnification of a case of lymphomatoid papulosis type B showing an atypical intraepidermal lymphocytic infiltrate resembling mycosis fungoides

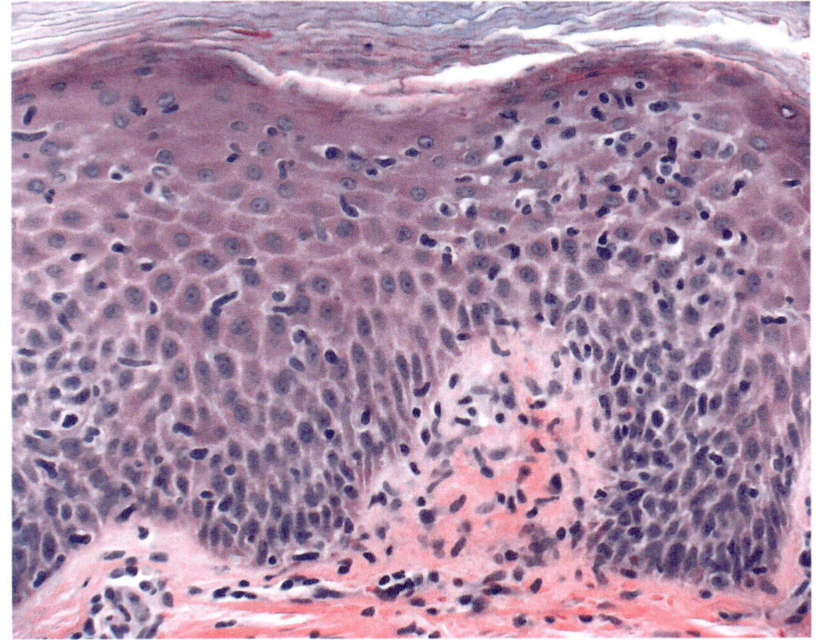

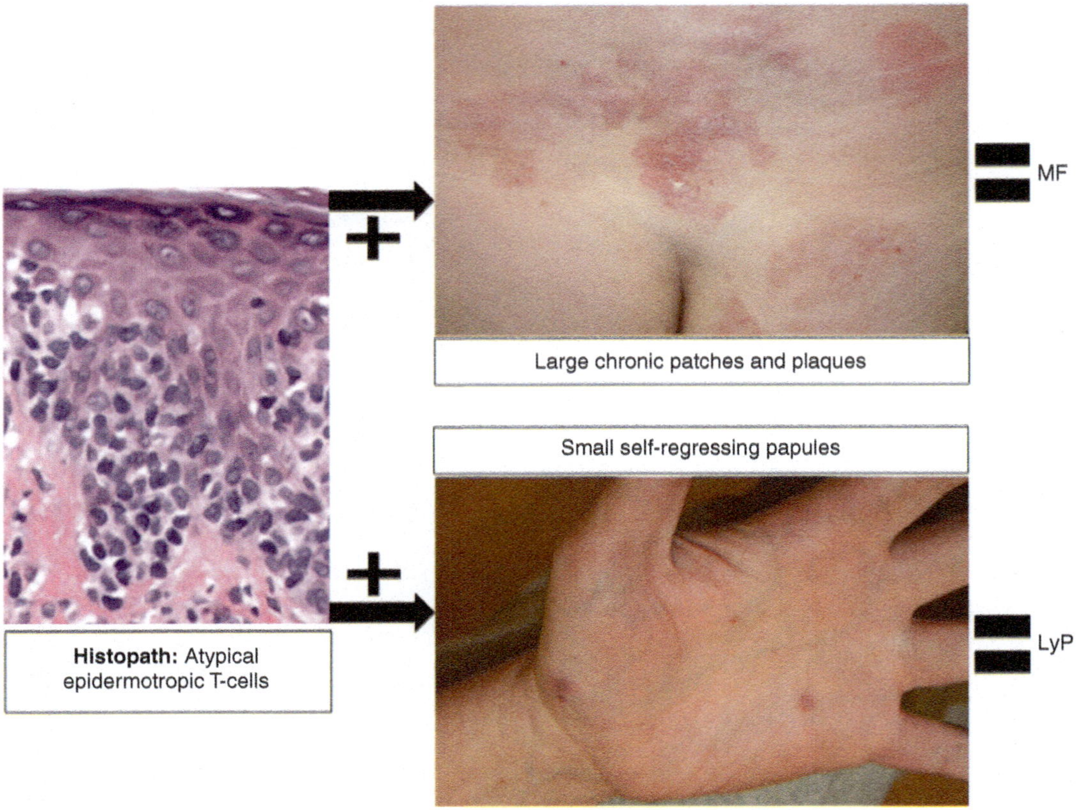

Fig. 28.6 Clinical pathologic correlation is essential to correctly classify cutaneous lymphoid infiltrates. The same histopathologic pattern of epidermotropism would result in different diagnoses depending on the clinical picture: classic mycosis fungoides (large, chronic patches and/or plaques on sun-protected skin) vs. lymphomatoid papulosis type B (small, self-regressing papules)

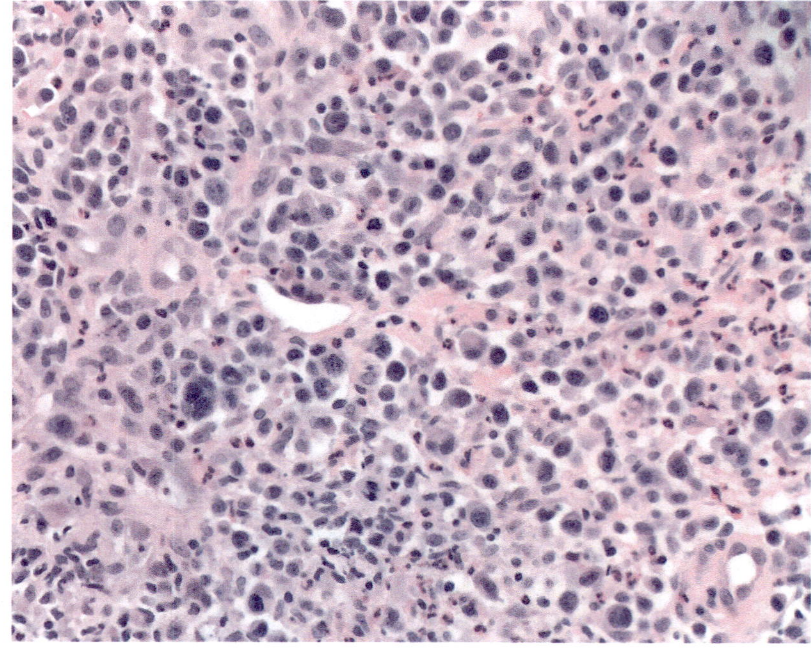

Fig. 28.7 High-power magnification of a case of lymphomatoid papulosis type C showing a dense diffuse dermal infiltrate of large atypical lymphoid cells resembling anaplastic large cell lymphoma

Fig. 28.8 High-power magnification of a case of lymphomatoid papulosis type D showing ulceration and an atypical intraepidermal lymphocytic infiltrate resembling an aggressive cytotoxic lymphoma

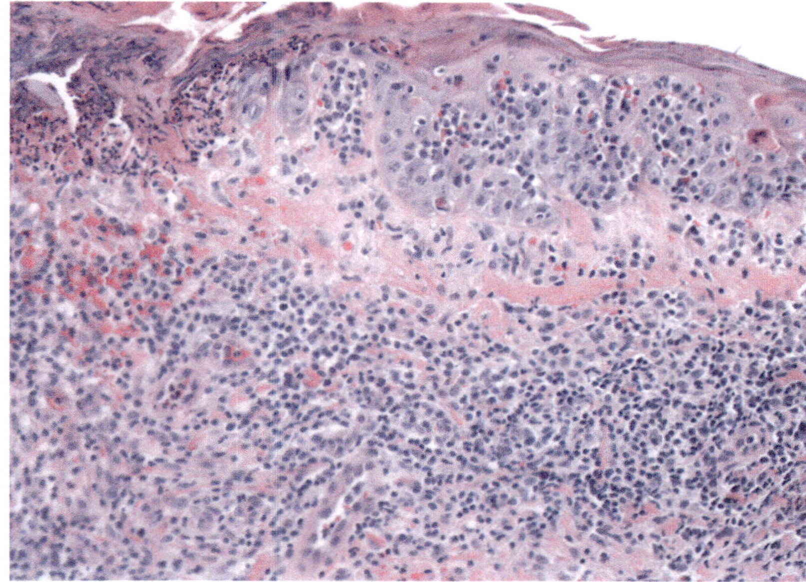

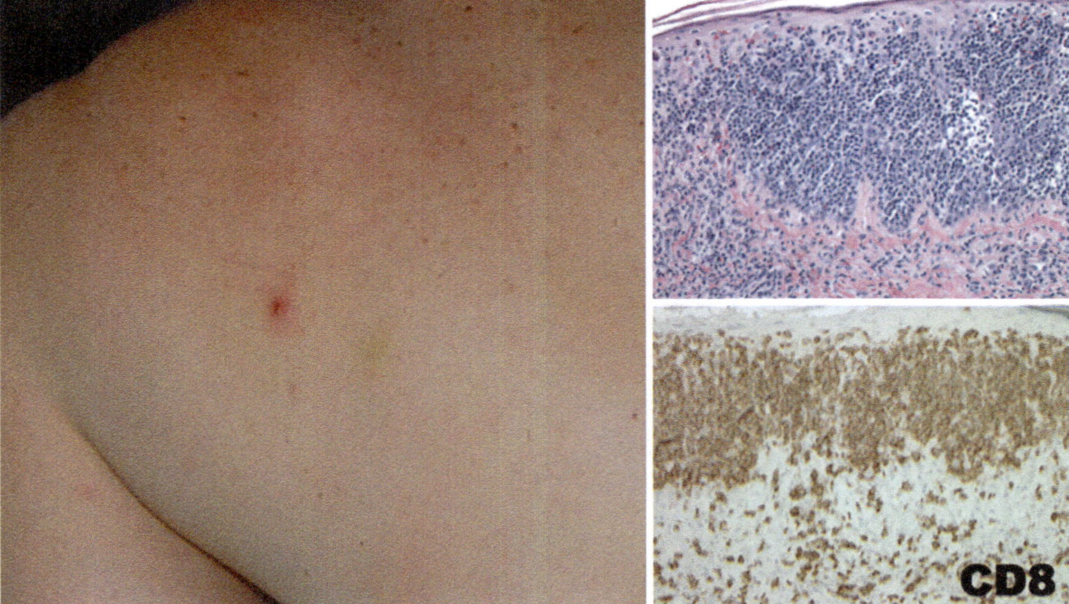

Fig. 28.9 Clinical pathologic correlation is essential to correctly classify cutaneous lymphoid infiltrates. While lymphomatoid papulosis type D histopathologically resembles primary cutaneous CD8+ aggressive epidermo-tropic cytotoxic T-cell lymphoma, the clinical appearance and behavior are distinct (small, self-regressing papules vs. progressive ulcerative disease)

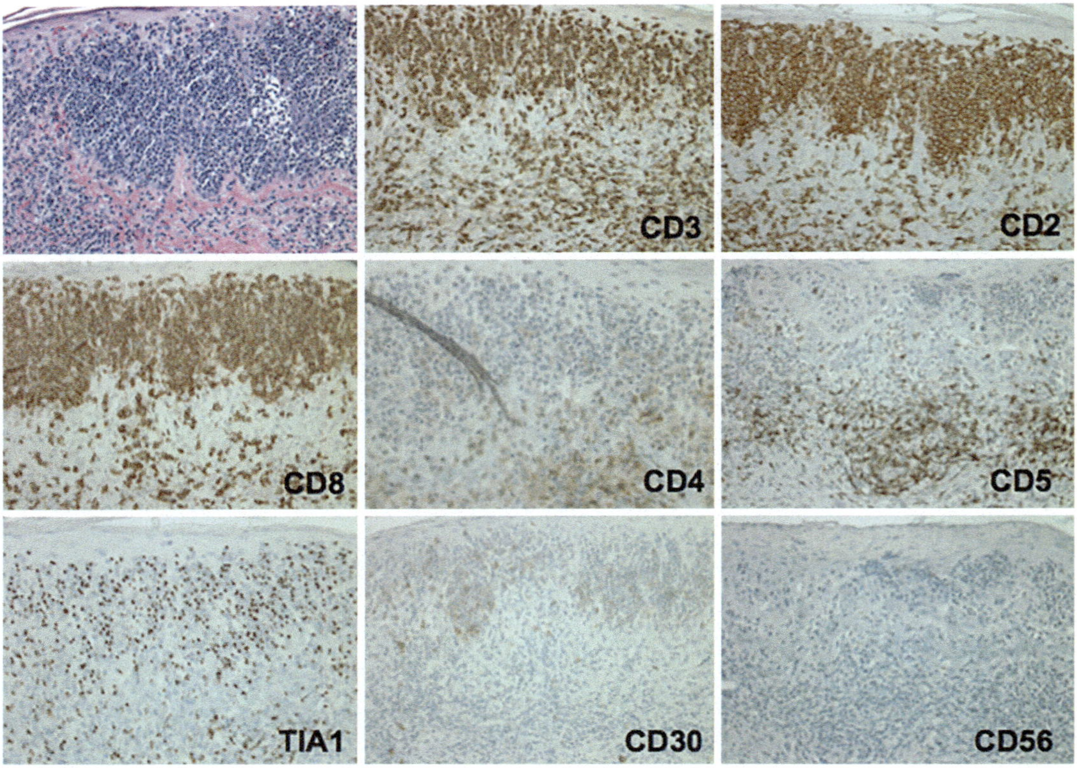

Fig. 28.10 Immunophenotype of a case of lymphomatoid papulosis type D

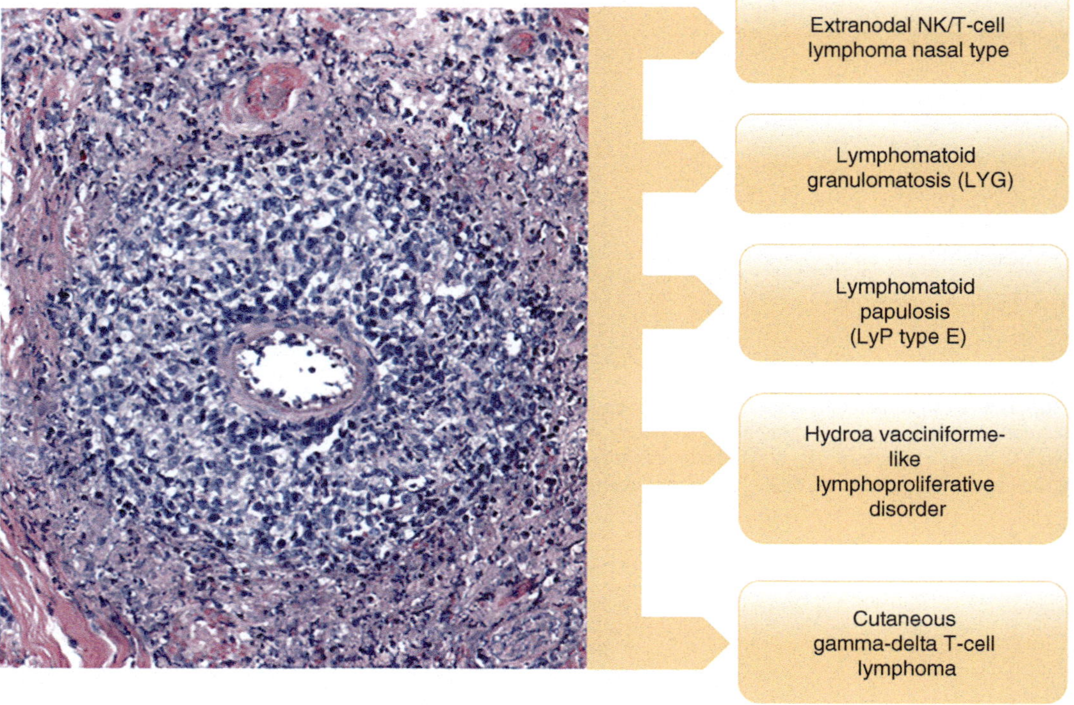

Fig. 28.11 Differential diagnosis of atypical lymphoid infiltrate with angiocentrism

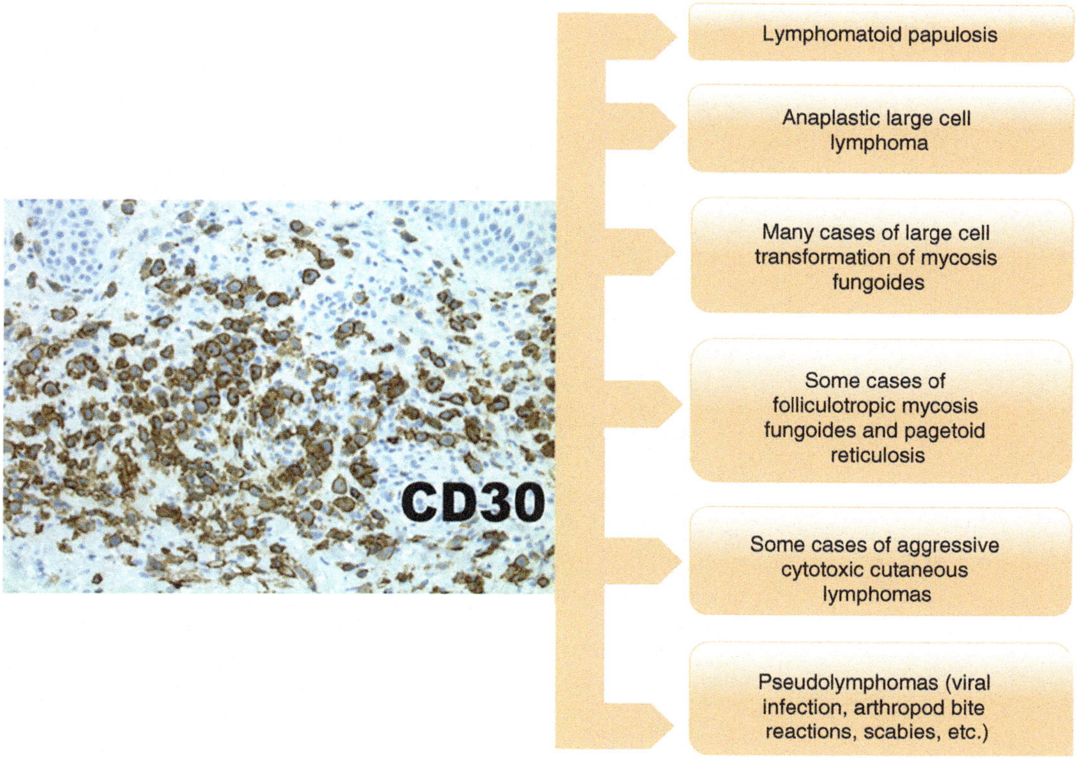

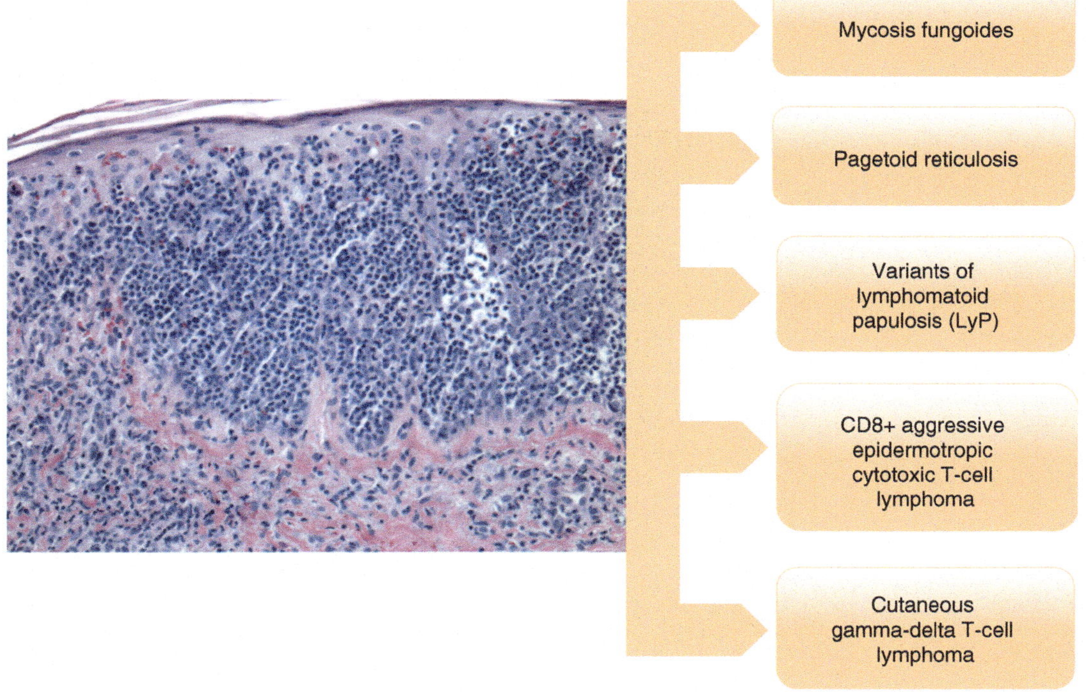

Fig. 28.12 Differential diagnosis of CD30 expression

Fig. 28.13 Differential diagnosis of atypical lymphocytic infiltrate with epidermotropism

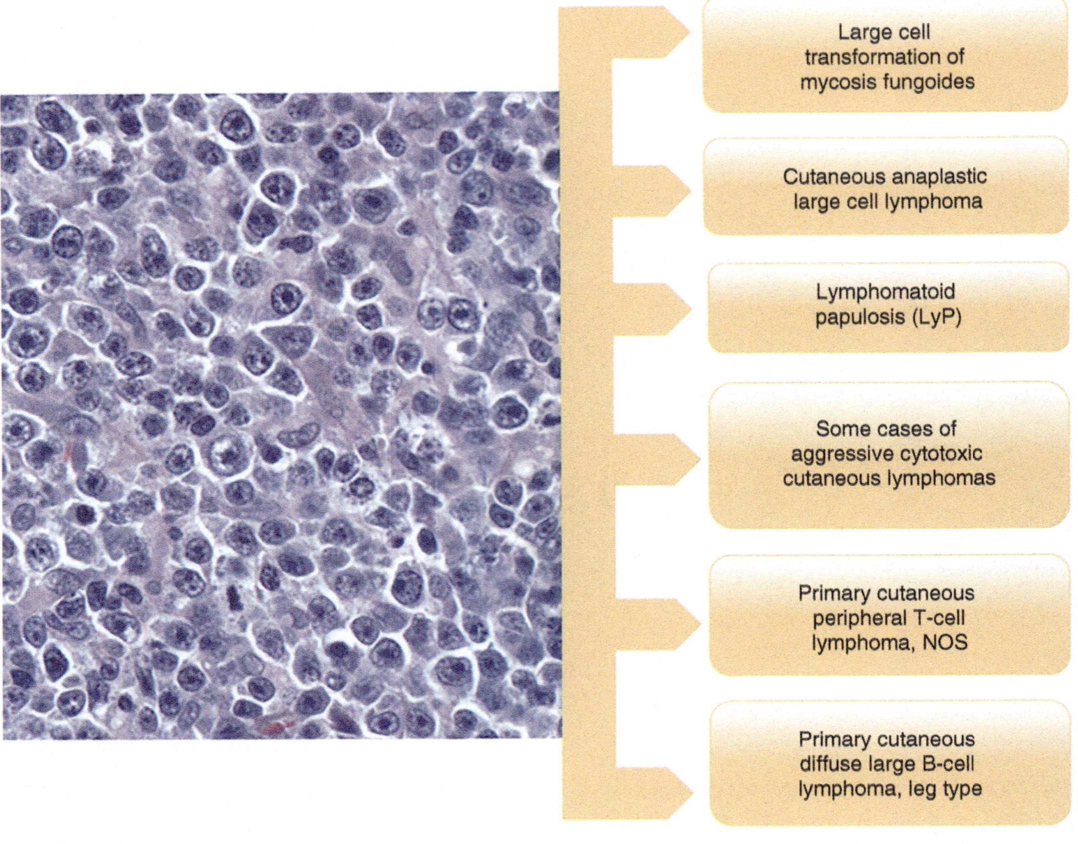

Fig. 28.14 Differential diagnosis of atypical large cell lymphoid infiltrate

Lymphomatoid papulosis (LyP) and cutaneous anaplastic large cell lymphoma (C-ALCL) are part of the spectrum of cutaneous CD30-positive lymphoproliferative disorders, which also includes borderline lesions. LyP presents with solitary or multiple, small, self-healing papules. While the histopathology is atypical and resembles that of a lymphoma ("lymphomatoid"), the clinical course is benign ("papulosis") (Fig. 28.1). There are several histopathologic variants, which mimic different lymphomas.

Disease Definition

– Lymphomatoid papulosis (LyP) is a chronic, recurrent, self-regressing skin disease that combines an indolent clinical course with his-topathologic features of different types of cutaneous T-cell lymphomas (Table 28.1).

Epidemiology

– Usually adults.
– May also occur in childhood.
– Male predominance.

Preferential Sites of Involvement

– Usually trunk and/or extremities.
– Acral skin may be involved.
– Limited to the skin but may occasionally involve oral mucosa.

Clinical Features

- Papules or small nodules, with or without ulceration (usually less than 2 cm).
- Lesions may be scattered or grouped (regional/agminated).
- By definition, each individual lesion must self-regress (within 12 weeks), leaving behind a superficial scar. However, new lesions may develop, while others are involuting, and lesions in various stages of evolution and involution often coexist.
- Highly variable number of lesions (from rare to over a 100).
- *Less common presentations*: necrotic eschar-like skin lesions in LyP type E due to angiodestruction; confluent papules associated with post-inflammatory hyperpigmentation.

Histomorphology

- *Pattern*: several histopathologic subtypes, which may mimic different lymphomas. Pattern may vary in different lesions or in different stages of the same lesion. Some lesions may show a combination of subtypes. LyP type A (most common): wedge-shaped dermal infiltrate of large atypical lymphoid cells with variable cytoplasm (scattered or in small clusters), admixed with a significant background inflammatory infiltrate of neutrophils, eosinophils, histiocytes, and small lymphocytes (Figs. 28.2, 28.3, and 28.4). Atypical cells may be multinucleated and may resemble Reed-Sternberg cells. Ulceration is common (Table 28.2). LyP type B (mimics early mycosis fungoides): epidermotropic infiltrate of small atypical lymphocytes with convoluted, hyperchromatic nuclei and scant cytoplasm (Figs. 28.5 and 28.6). A band-like superficial dermal component may also be seen. LyP type C (mimics cutaneous anaplastic large cell lymphoma): dense diffuse monotonous dermal infiltrate of large atypical lymphoid cells with relatively few admixed inflammatory cells (Fig. 28.7). Ulceration is common. LyP type D (mimics primary cutaneous CD8+ aggressive epidermotropic cytotoxic T-cell lymphoma): markedly epidermotropic infiltrate of small to intermediate-sized atypical lymphocytes with hyperchromatic nuclei and scant cytoplasm. Epidermal hyperplasia (reminiscent of pagetoid reticulosis) may be seen. Ulceration is common (Table 28.3 and Figs. 28.8, 28.9, and 28.10). LyP type E (mimics extranodal NK/T-cell lymphoma nasal type): angiocentric and angiodestructive infiltrate of variably sized atypical lymphocytes (Fig. 28.11 and Table 28.4). Prominent necrosis, hemorrhage, fibrin, and ulceration are common. LyP with DUSP22-IRF4 rearrangement (mimics advanced mycosis fungoides with large cell transformation) is genetically defined (DUSP22-IRF4 rearrangement at 6p25.3) but generally shows a biphasic histopathologic pattern: epidermotropic component of small- to intermediate-sized atypical lymphocytes with convoluted nuclei and dermal component of large atypical lymphoid cells.
- *Less common patterns*: some cases may be associated with hyperplasia of Langerhans cells, granulomatous inflammation, subepidermal edema, epidermal hyperplasia, or adnexal involvement (hair follicles/"type F" or sweat glands).
- *Neoplastic cells*: variable depending on subtype. Usually small- and intermediate-sized within the epidermis and large atypical cells in the dermis.
- *Reactive cells*: variable depending on subtype (scant to prominent mixed infiltrates of neutrophils, eosinophils, histiocytes, and/or small lymphocytes).

Immunophenotype

- *Neoplastic cells*: usually CD3+, CD4+, and CD8− in types A (most common), B, and C. Types D and E are generally CD3+, CD4−, and CD8+. LyP with DUSP22-IRF4 rearrangement may be CD4− and CD8+ or CD4− and CD8−. Usually prominent CD30 expression; however, intraepidermal cells may show weak to negative CD30 (subtypes B and D and the intraepidermal component of LyP with DUSP22-IRF4 rearrangement) (Fig. 28.10). Usually betaF1+, but rare cases may show a gamma-delta T-cell phenotype. CD56 may occasionally be expressed. ALK is negative. EBV (EBER in situ hybridization) is negative.

- *Reactive cells*: variable depending on subtype.

Genetics

- Monoclonal rearrangement of T-cell receptor genes in 40–60% of cases. Cases of LyP with an associated lymphoma generally show the same rearrangement.

Prognosis

- Excellent.
- 5-year survival: 100%. By definition, LyP shows a benign clinical course.
- Adverse risk factors: development of a lymphoma. In approximately 20% of patients, LyP may be preceded by, concomitant with, or followed by lymphoma (usually mycosis fungoides, cutaneous anaplastic large cell lymphoma, or Hodgkin lymphoma). Therefore, follow-up is recommended for LyP patients.

Differential Diagnosis (Figs. 28.12, 28.13, and 28.14)

- In the absence of adequate clinical information, distinction between LyP and ALCL is generally not possible (Table 28.5). In such cases, the diagnosis should be "cutaneous CD30+ lymphoproliferative disorder," and subsequently the final classification should be made by the clinician.

- Borderline cases of primary cutaneous CD30+ lymphoproliferative disorders. Some lesions are difficult to differentiate between lymphomatoid papulosis and anaplastic large cell lymphoma at presentation. However, the diagnosis is usually revealed by careful clinical examination during close follow-up (regression versus persistence/progression of each individual lesion).

- By definition, LyP is lymphomatoid and mimics different types of lymphoma. LyP subtype A may resemble Hodgkin lymphoma, which is extremely rare in the skin (and usually only seen in patients with nodal Hodgkin lymphoma). In addition, Hodgkin is generally negative with T-cell markers and shows expression of CD15 and PAX-5.

- Other LyP variants resemble different types of lymphoma: patch-stage mycosis fungoides (type B), anaplastic large cell lymphoma (type C), aggressive epidermotropic CD8-positive cytotoxic T-cell lymphoma (type D), extranodal NK/T-cell lymphoma (type E), and tumor-stage mycosis fungoides with large cell transformation (LyP with DUSP22-IRF4 rearrangement). While there may be histopathologic clues for LyP (e.g., CD30 expression in most cases of LyP; lack of dermal fibrosis in LyP B; negative EBV in LyP E), the best way to differentiate among these possibilities is correlation with clinical findings (small self-regressing skin lesions).

- Reactive inflammatory and infectious skin diseases. CD30 is an activation marker and is often positive in various reactive infiltrates, including viral conditions (inflamed molluscum contagiosum, herpes folliculitis, orf, milker's nodule, EBV-positive mucocutaneous ulcer), drug reactions, and arthropod bite reactions (including scabies). CD30 expression by itself is not enough for a diagnosis of LyP; significant cytologic atypia or epidermotropism should also be present. Careful clinical correlation and proactively searching for histopathologic features of other conditions (e.g., viral cytopathic effect, scabietic organisms) may help prevent misdiagnosis.

Table 28.2 Differential diagnosis of ulceration

Lymphomas/lymphoproliferative disorders	Benign dermatoses/pseudolymphomas
Tumor-stage mycosis fungoides	Pityriasis lichenoides et varioliformis acuta (PLEVA)
CD30-positive lymphoproliferative disorders: lymphomatoid papulosis, cutaneous anaplastic large cell lymphoma	Inflamed molluscum contagiosum
Primary cutaneous aggressive epidermotropic CD8-positive cytotoxic T-cell lymphoma	Herpesvirus infection
Cutaneous gamma-delta T-cell lymphoma	Primary syphilis
Extranodal NK/T-cell lymphoma, nasal type	Leishmania infection

Table 28.3 Differential diagnosis of CD8-positive cutaneous lymphoid infiltrate

Some cases of otherwise classical or hypopigmented mycosis fungoides
Many cases of localized pagetoid reticulosis
Lymphomatoid papulosis (LyP), type D
Some cases of anaplastic large cell lymphoma (ALCL)
Primary cutaneous CD8+ aggressive epidermotropic cytotoxic T-cell lymphoma
Many cases of cutaneous gamma-delta T-cell lymphoma
Subcutaneous panniculitis-like T-cell lymphoma
Indolent CD8+ lymphoid proliferation of the ear (primary cutaneous acral CD8+ T-cell lymphoma)
Cutaneous pseudolymphoma: CD8-positive infiltrates in the setting of advanced AIDS, many cases of pityriasis lichenoides

Table 28.4 Differential diagnosis of an atypical angiocentric lymphoid infiltrate in relation to Epstein-Barr virus (EBV) and immunophenotype

EBV	Angiocentric process	Immunophenotype
Positive (+)	Extranodal NK/T-cell lymphoma nasal type	T cell or NK cell
	Hydroa vacciniforme-like lymphoproliferative disorder	T cell or NK cell
	Lymphomatoid granulomatosis (LYG)	B cell
Negative (−)	Cutaneous gamma-delta T-cell lymphoma	Gamma-delta T cell
	Lymphomatoid papulosis (LyP type E)	CD30-positive T cell

Table 28.5 Comparison of cutaneous CD30-positive lymphoproliferative disorders

	Lymphomatoid papulosis (LyP)	Cutaneous anaplastic large cell lymphoma (C-ALCL)
Clinical findings	Solitary or multiple, recurrent, self-regressing papules	Solitary or localized nodules or tumors
Histologic findings	Variable findings depending of the histologic subtype, resembling different types of lymphoma	Dense diffuse dermal infiltrate of large atypical CD30+ lymphoid cells Usually scant inflammation
Differential diagnoses	C-ALCL and other lymphomas Reactive inflammatory infiltrates with activated CD30+ lymphocytes (reactions to drugs, arthropod bites, and viral infections)	LyP Secondary cutaneous involvement by systemic/nodal CD30+ ALCL Large cell transformation of MF with CD30 expression

Pearls and Pitfalls

1. The epidermotropic variants of LyP (B and D) may lack prominent CD30 expression.
2. The main reason for histologic subtype classification in LyP is to avoid misdiagnosis of various (often-aggressive) lymphomas. Prognostic differences have not been demonstrated.
3. While the inflammatory background in LyP type A is quite mixed (neutrophils, eosinophils, histiocytes, and small lymphocytes), certain inflammatory components would be unusual (e.g., plasma cells, lymphoid follicles). If either of the latter is found in a mixed infiltrate with CD30 expression, other conditions should be entertained in the differential diagnosis.

Suggested Reading

Karai LJ, Kadin ME, Hsi ED, Sluzevich JC, Ketterling RP, Knudson RA, Feldman AL. Chromosomal rearrangements of 6p25.3 define a new subtype of lymphomatoid papulosis. Am J Surg Pathol. 2013;37(8):1173–81.

Kempf W. Cutaneous CD30-positive lymphoproliferative disorders. Surg Pathol Clin. 2014;7(2):203–28.

Swerdlow SH, et al., editors. WHO classification of tumors of hematopoietic and lymphoid tissues. Lyon: IARC; 2008.

Swerdlow SH, Campo E, Pileri SA, et al. The 2016 revision of the WHO classification of lymphoid neoplasms. Blood. 2016;127(20):2375–90.

Swerdlow SH, et al., editors. WHO classification of tumors of hematopoietic and lymphoid tissues (revised 4th ed). Lyon: IARC; 2017.

Willemze R, Jaffe ES, Burg G, et al. WHO-EORTC classification for cutaneous lymphomas. Blood. 2005;105(10):3768–85.

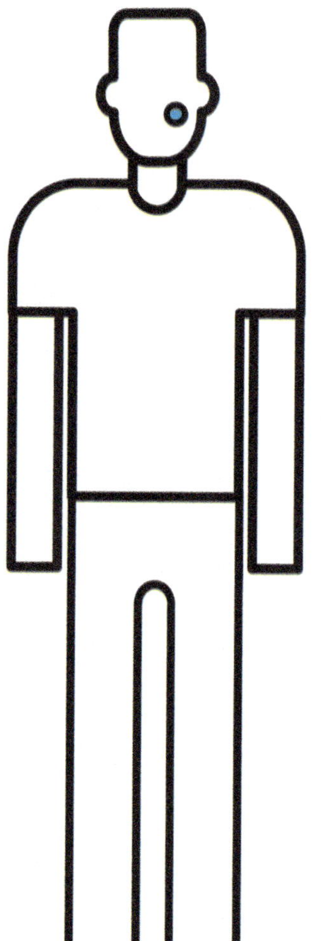

Fig. 29.1 Primary cutaneous CD4+ small/medium T-cell lymphoproliferative disorder is an indolent lymphoproliferative disorder characterized clinically by a solitary skin lesion, often on the face

Table 29.1 Key facts

Definition
Primary cutaneous CD4+ small/medium T-cell lymphoproliferative disorder is an indolent lymphoproliferative disorder characterized clinically by a solitary skin lesion (without patches/plaques typical of mycosis fungoides) and histopathologically by a cutaneous infiltrate of small- and medium-sized pleomorphic CD4-positive T cells
Prototypic clinical presentation
Solitary plaque or tumor on the head/neck region (face) or upper trunk
Histopathologic findings
Dense, diffuse and/or nodular, superficial and deep dermal infiltrate of small- and medium-sized pleomorphic lymphocytes (<30% large cells) Most common immunophenotype: CD3+, CD4+, CD8−, CD30−, CD56−, PD1+, CD2+, CD5+/−, CD7−/+, TIA1−, betaF1+, and low Ki-67
Prognosis
Excellent

© Springer Nature Switzerland AG 2019

A. Subtil, *Diagnosis of Cutaneous Lymphoid Infiltrates*,

https://doi.org/10.1007/978-3-030-11654-5_29

Fig. 29.2 Primary cutaneous CD4+ small/medium T-cell lymphoproliferative disorder is composed of a dense, dermal-based lymphoid infiltrate with a diffuse and/or nodular pattern

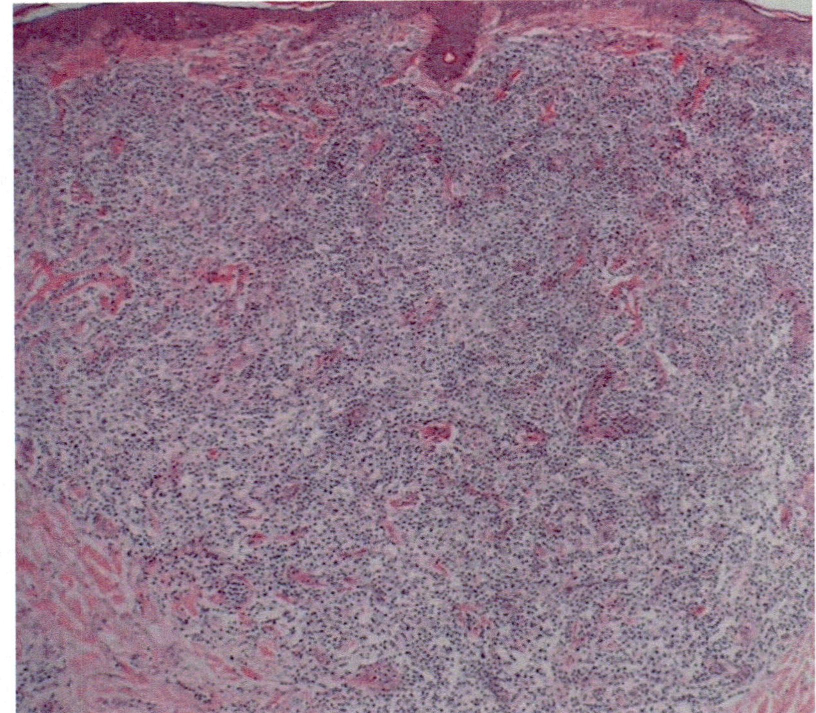

Fig. 29.3 Epitheliotropism is generally not prominent in primary cutaneous CD4+ small/medium T-cell lymphoproliferative disorder. However, focal exocytosis of lymphocytes may be observed in the overlying epidermis

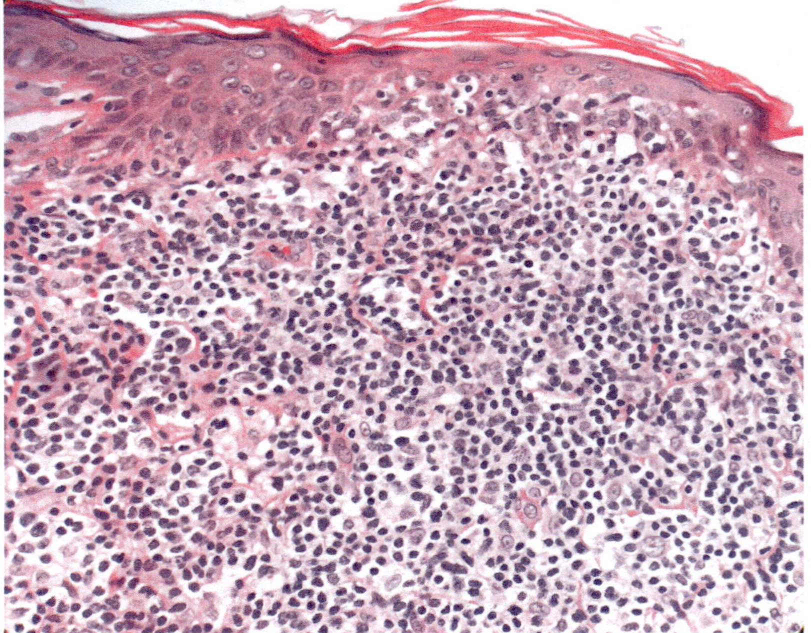

Fig. 29.4 Focal exocytosis of lymphocytes into the epithelium of hair follicles is frequently observed in primary cutaneous CD4+ small/medium T-cell lymphoproliferative disorder

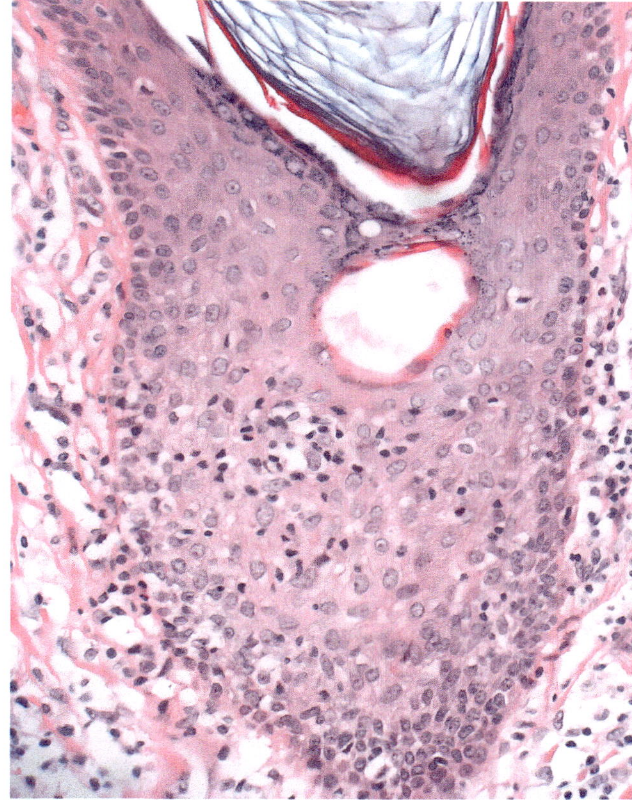

Fig. 29.5 As its name implies, primary cutaneous CD4+ small/medium T-cell lymphoproliferative disorder is composed of small- and intermediate-sized lymphocytes. While small lymphocytes predominate, a significant component of irregular, hyperchromatic (pleomorphic) medium-sized lymphocytes should be present (arrows)

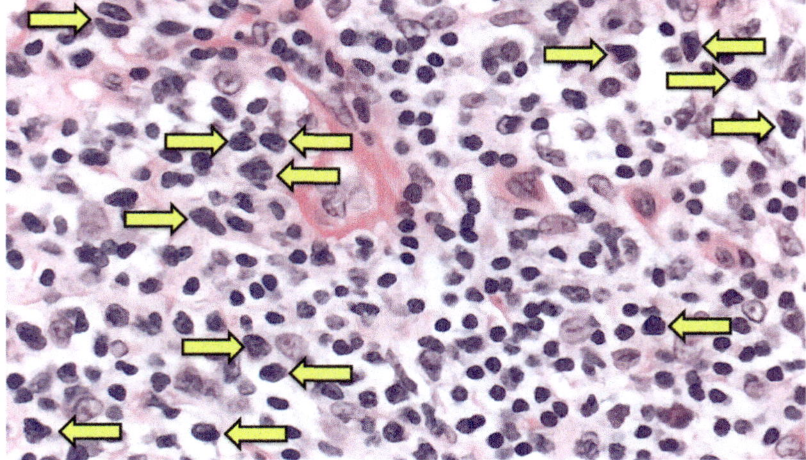

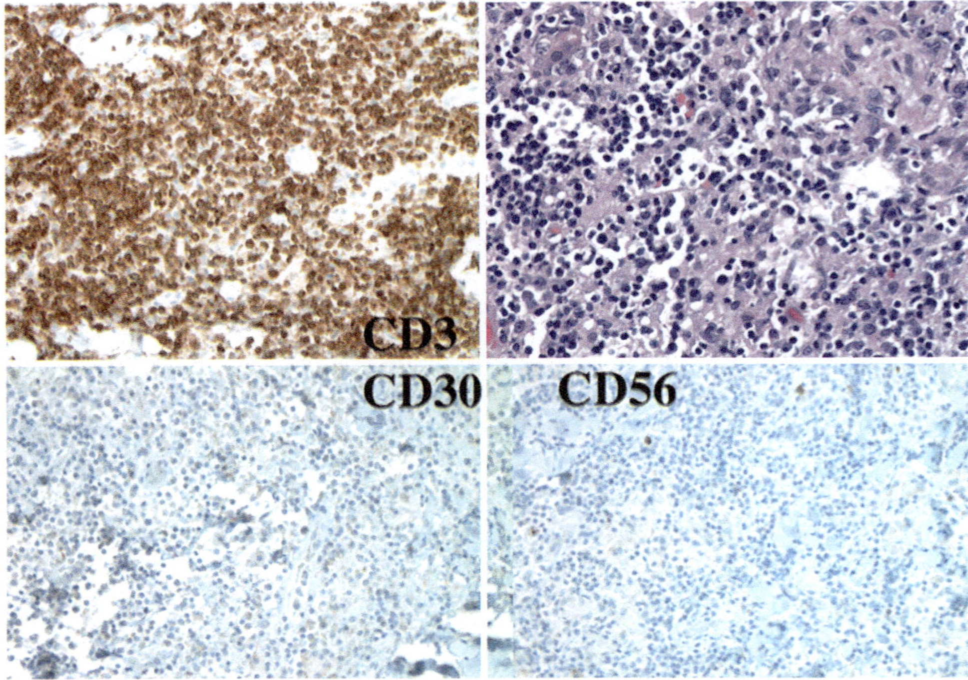

Fig. 29.6 Primary cutaneous CD4+ small/medium T-cell lymphoproliferative disorder. The infiltrate consists predominantly of CD3-positive T cells without significant expression of CD30 or CD56

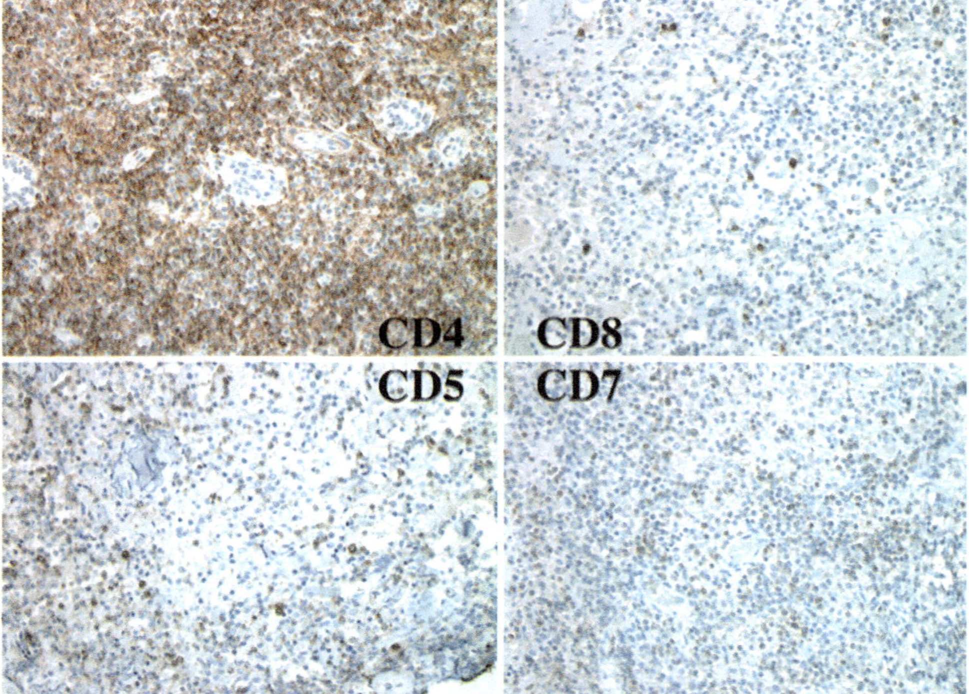

Fig. 29.7 As its name implies, primary cutaneous CD4+ small/medium T-cell lymphoproliferative disorder is composed predominantly of CD4-positive T cells, while only a small subset of predominantly small reactive CD8-positive T cells is present. Loss of pan-T-cell markers may be seen (usually CD7, rarely CD5)

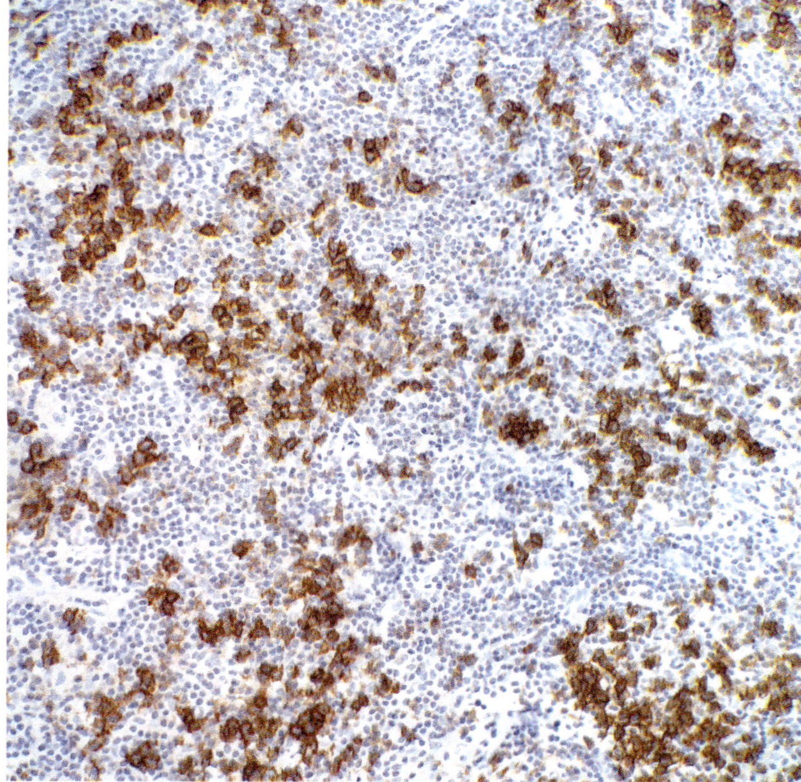

Fig. 29.8 Primary cutaneous CD4+ small/medium T-cell lymphoproliferative disorder. Frequent expression of PD1 by atypical lymphocytes, often arranged in clusters

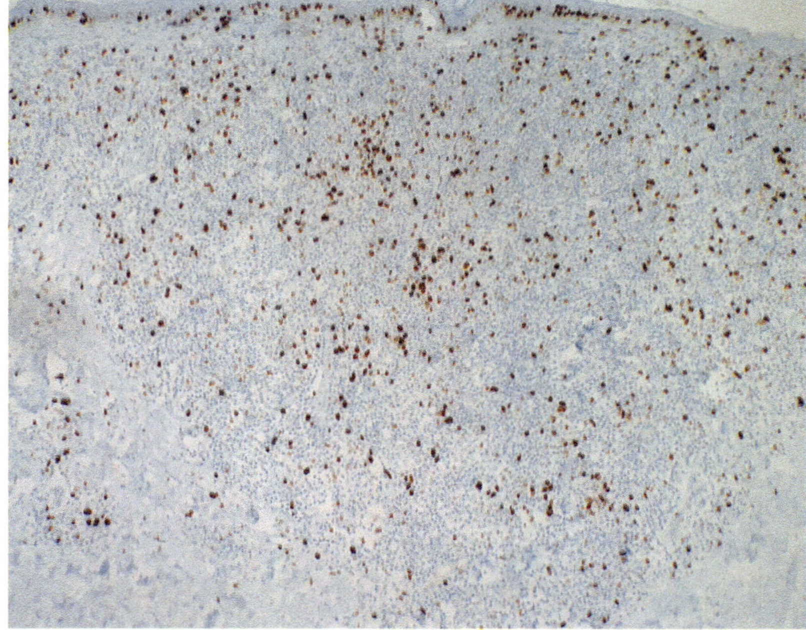

Fig. 29.9 The Ki-67 proliferation index is generally low in primary cutaneous CD4+ small/medium T-cell lymphoproliferative disorder

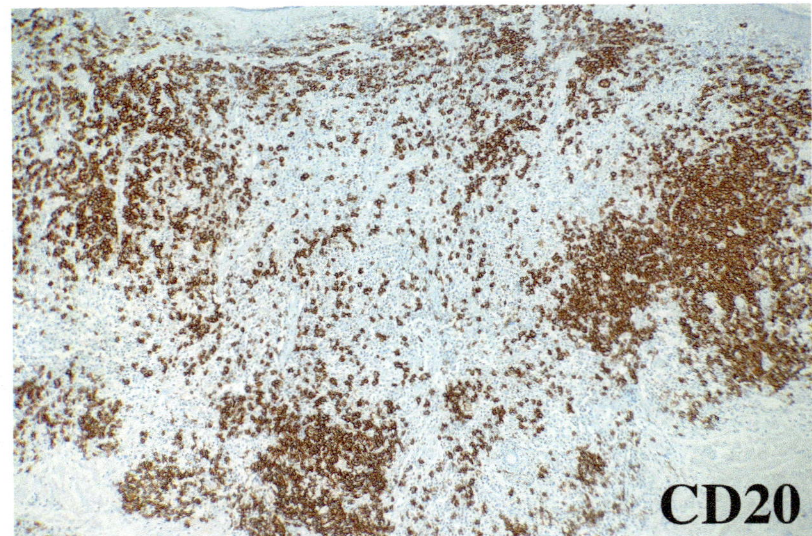

Fig. 29.10 While T cells predominate in primary cutaneous CD4+ small/medium T-cell lymphoproliferative disorder, a sizable component of CD20-positive B cells is generally present and may cause diagnostic confusion with pseudolymphoma and low-grade cutaneous B-cell lymphoma

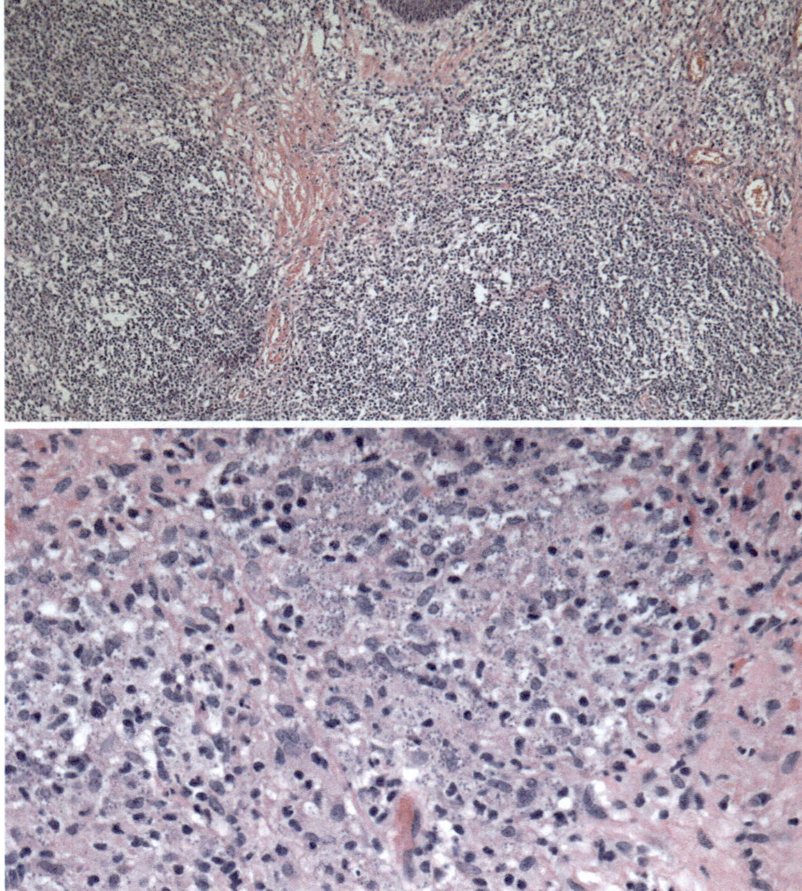

Fig. 29.11 Cutaneous Leishmaniasis may mimic primary cutaneous CD4+ small/medium T-cell lymphoproliferative disorder since both may present with a solitary lesion on exposed skin lasting several months and cutaneous infiltrates with prominent lymphocytes and histiocytes. However, ulceration and Leishmania organisms are absent in primary cutaneous CD4-positive small/medium T-cell lymphoproliferative disorder

Disease Definition

- Primary cutaneous CD4+ small/medium T-cell lymphoproliferative disorder is an indolent lymphoproliferative disorder characterized clinically by a solitary skin lesion (without patches/plaques typical of mycosis fungoides) and histopathologically by a cutaneous infiltrate of small- and medium-sized pleomorphic CD4-positive T cells (Table 29.1).

Epidemiology

- Usually adult and elderly patients, but pediatric cases may occasionally occur.

Preferential Sites of Involvement

- Face (central face, forehead).
- Neck.
- Upper trunk.
- Ear.

Clinical Features

- Solitary plaque or nodule/tumor (Fig. 29.1).
- Erythematous or purplish surface without ulceration. Slow growing.
- Absence of patches and/or plaques typical of mycosis fungoides (must be excluded clinically).
- *Less common presentations*: more than one lesion but in a localized area. If multiple widespread lesions occur, consider another diagnosis.

Histomorphology

- *Pattern*: dense, diffuse and/or nodular, superficial and deep dermal infiltrate (Fig. 29.2). Epitheliotropism is usually not prominent; however, focal exocytosis of lymphocytes may be observed in the epidermis and hair follicles (Figs. 29.3 and 29.4). Ulceration, prominent necrosis, or angiodestruction is not seen.
- *Less common patterns*: plaque-like superficial and mid-dermal infiltrate. Variable extension into superficial panniculus.
- *Neoplastic cells*: small- and medium-sized lymphocytes. While small lymphocytes predominate, a significant component of irregular, hyperchromatic (pleomorphic) medium-sized lymphocytes should be present (Fig. 29.5). Large lymphoid cells with vesicular chromatin and prominent nucleolus should be rare and scattered (<30% of the infiltrate).
- *Reactive cells*: histiocytes can be quite prominent (Fig. 29.6). Occasional plasma cells and multinucleated giant cells.

Immunophenotype

- *Neoplastic cells*: the infiltrate consists predominantly of CD3-positive alpha-beta T cells without significant expression of CD30 or CD56 (Fig. 29.6). There is a significant predominance of CD4 expression. Loss of pan-T-cell markers may occur (usually CD7, rarely CD5) (Fig. 29.7). Because of the T follicular helper (TFH) phenotype, there is frequent expression of PD1 (CD279) by atypical lymphocytes, often arranged in clusters (Fig. 29.8). Other TFH markers may be expressed (BCL6, CXCL13, ICOS, rarely CD10). The Ki-67 proliferation index is low (below 50%) (Fig. 29.9).
- *Reactive cells*: small subset of predominantly small reactive CD8-positive T cells. While T cells predominate, a significant component of reactive CD20-positive B cells is generally present (Fig. 29.10). Variable component of CD68-positive histiocytes. Occasional polytypic plasma cells. CD21 is generally negative since lymphoid follicle formation is uncommon.

Genetics

- Monoclonal rearrangement of T-cell receptor genes in majority of cases.
- EBV (EBER in situ hybridization) is negative.

Prognosis

- Excellent. Rare local recurrence.
- Because of its indolent behavior, "lymphoproliferative disorder" is the currently preferred term rather than "lymphoma."
- 5-year survival: close to 100%. The initially reported 5-year survival of 75% has not been observed in subsequent series; it appears that the initial series may have been contaminated by systemic lymphomas presenting in the skin.
- Adverse risk factors: cases incorrectly classified; recurrence/progression after initial treatment.

Differential Diagnosis

- Pseudolymphoma. Primary cutaneous CD4-positive small/medium T-cell lymphoproliferative disorder has similar features and benign behavior analogous to cutaneous T-cell pseudolymphoma with nodular growth pattern. It is conceivable that it may represent a clonal variant of the latter.
- Cutaneous Leishmaniasis may cause diagnostic confusion since it often presents with a solitary lesion on exposed skin that lasts several months and often demonstrates cutaneous infiltrates with prominent lymphocytes and histiocytes (Fig. 29.11). However, the infiltrate is generally more granulomatous and more plasmacytic than in primary cutaneous CD4-positive small/medium T-cell lymphoproliferative disorder. In addition, ulceration and Leishmania organisms would be absent in primary cutaneous CD4-positive small/medium T-cell lymphoproliferative disorder. Careful examination of superficial dermal histiocytes at high-magnification is recommended.
- Primary cutaneous marginal zone B-cell lymphoma may have features similar to primary cutaneous CD4-positive small/medium T-cell lymphoproliferative disorder: indolent behavior, frequently solitary nodular skin lesion, presence of mixed dermal infiltrates with prominent T-cell and B-cell populations, and frequent PD1 expression (Figs. 29.8 and 29.10). However, marginal zone lymphoma lacks a significant component of hyperchromatic pleomorphic medium-sized cells and is generally associated with lymphoid follicles and monotypic plasma cells. In contrast, prominent lymphoid follicles would be an unusual finding in primary cutaneous CD4-positive small/medium T-cell lymphoproliferative disorder. Plasma cells are uncommon and polytypic in primary cutaneous CD4-positive small/medium T-cell lymphoproliferative disorder.
- Cutaneous presentation of systemic T-cell lymphoma. Systemic T-cell lymphomas (which may have T follicular helper phenotype) may occasionally present in the skin and may closely mimic primary cutaneous CD4-positive small/medium T-cell lymphoproliferative disorder. Therefore, adequate staging at initial diagnosis and/or close follow-up would be judicious to exclude this possibility. This differential is important because of the significantly worse prognosis of systemic T-cell lymphoma.
- Mycosis fungoides. As part of the definition of primary cutaneous CD4-positive small/medium T-cell lymphoproliferative disorder, mycosis fungoides must be excluded clinically by the absence of patches and/or plaques. This distinction is critical because of the significantly worse prognosis of tumor-stage mycosis fungoides. By definition, a patient with mycosis fungoides can never be subsequently diagnosed with primary cutaneous CD4-positive small/medium T-cell lymphoproliferative disorder (if a similar lesion develops in a patient with known mycosis fungoides, the diagnosis is tumor-stage mycosis fungoides).
- Primary cutaneous peripheral T-cell lymphoma NOS. The diagnostic criteria for primary cutaneous CD4-positive small/medium T-cell lymphoproliferative disorder should be carefully followed. Cases presenting with multiple/widespread/generalized skin lesions, rapidly growing large tumors, >30% large

lymphocytes, and/or high proliferative index should be classified as peripheral T-cell lymphoma NOS (which may be primary cutaneous or systemic). This distinction is imperative because of the significantly worse prognosis of peripheral T-cell lymphoma NOS.

Pearls and Pitfalls

1. Some have considered primary cutaneous acral CD8-positive T-cell lymphoma (indolent CD8-positive lymphoid proliferation of the ear/face) as a phenotypic variant of primary cutaneous CD4-positive small/medium T-cell lymphoproliferative disorder, since both are indolent conditions and generally present with solitary lesions (often on the head and neck region). However, the cytomorphology is distinct (monomorphic/blastoid versus pleomorphic/hyperchromatic, respectively), and some epitheliotropism and PD1 expression are generally present in the CD4-positive cases (as opposed to grenz zone in CD8-positive cases).

Suggested Reading

Beltraminelli H, Leinweber B, Kerl H, Cerroni L. Primary cutaneous CD4+ small-/medium-sized pleomorphic T-cell lymphoma: a cutaneous nodular proliferation of pleomorphic T lymphocytes of undetermined significance? a study of 136 cases. Am J Dermatopathol. 2009;31(4):317–22.

Elder DE, Massi D, Scolyer RA, Willemze R, editors. WHO classification of skin tumors. 4th ed. Lyon: IARC; 2018.

James E, Sokhn JG, Gibson JF, Carlson K, Subtil A, Girardi M, Wilson LD, Foss F. CD4 + primary cutaneous small/medium-sized pleomorphic T-cell lymphoma: a retrospective case series and review of literature. Leuk Lymphoma. 2015;56(4):951–7.

Swerdlow SH, et al., editors. WHO classification of tumors of hematopoietic and lymphoid tissues. Lyon: IARC; 2008.

Swerdlow SH, Campo E, Pileri SA, et al. The 2016 revision of the WHO classification of lymphoid neoplasms. Blood. 2016;127(20):2375–90.

Swerdlow SH, Campo E, Harris NL, Jaffe ES, Pileri SA, Stein H, Thiele J, editors. WHO classification of tumours of haematopoietic and lymphoid tissues (revised 4th ed). Lyon: IARC; 2017.

Willemze R, Jaffe ES, Burg G, et al. WHO-EORTC classification for cutaneous lymphomas. Blood. 2005;105(10):3768–85.

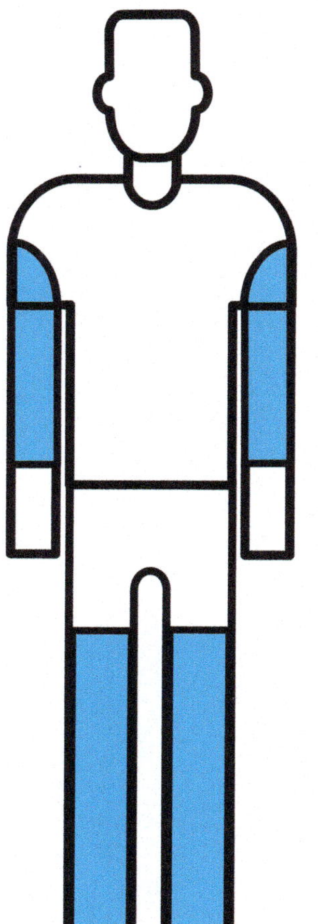

Fig. 30.1 Subcutaneous panniculitis-like T-cell lymphoma is an indolent lymphoma composed of subcutaneous infiltrates of alpha-beta CD8-positive T cells. The extremities are common sites of involvement

Table 30.1 Key facts

Definition
Subcutaneous panniculitis-like T-cell lymphoma (SPTCL) is a cytotoxic alpha-beta T-cell lymphoma that preferentially infiltrates the subcutaneous tissue
Prototypic clinical presentation
Multiple subcutaneous nodules on extremities without ulceration or lymphadenopathy
Histopathologic findings
Atypical lymphocytic infiltrate confined to the panniculus (lobular pattern) without involvement of the overlying dermis or epidermis. Rimming of atypical lymphocytes surrounding individual adipocytes
Most common immunophenotype: CD3+, CD4−, CD8+, CD30−, CD56−, TIA1+, TCRbetaF1+, EBV−. High proliferation rate with Ki-67
Prognosis
Indolent (5-year survival >80%)

© Springer Nature Switzerland AG 2019
A. Subtil, *Diagnosis of Cutaneous Lymphoid Infiltrates*,
https://doi.org/10.1007/978-3-030-11654-5_30

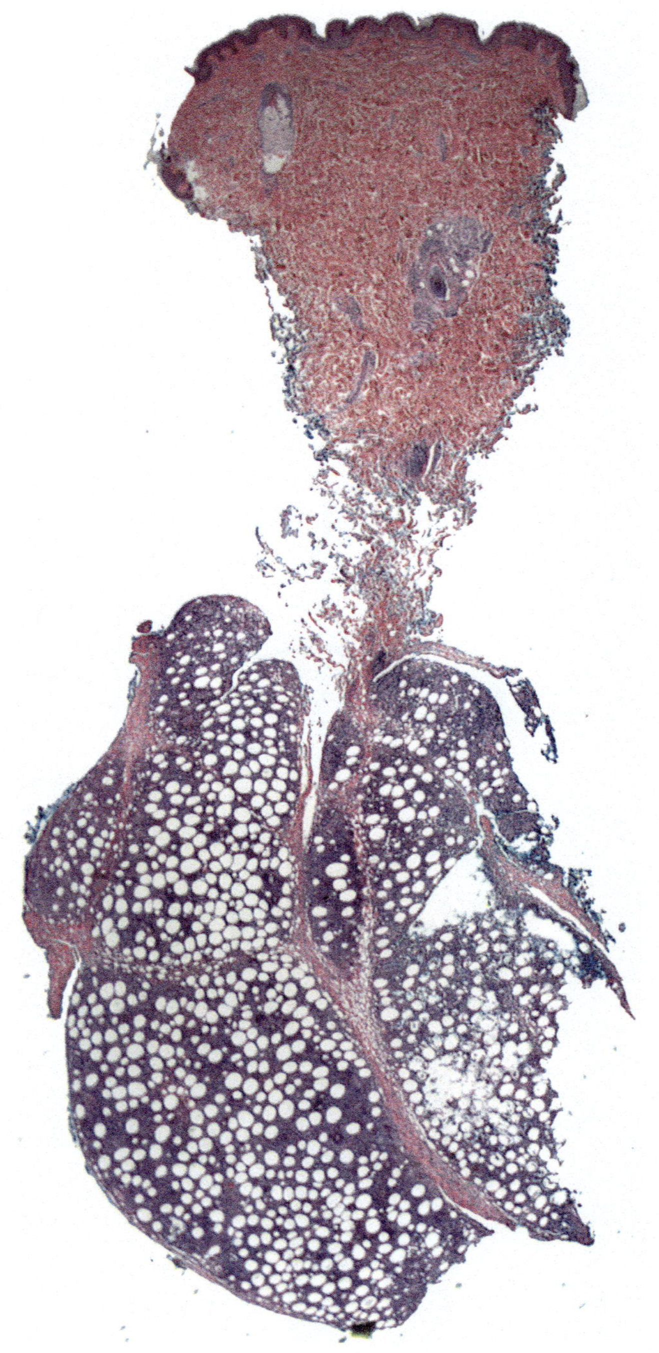

Fig. 30.2 Subcutaneous panniculitis-like T-cell lymphoma shows preferential involvement of the panniculus. A deep biopsy is necessary to adequately sample the infiltrate

Fig. 30.3
Unremarkable epidermis and dermis overlying subcutaneous panniculitis-like T-cell lymphoma. Ulceration, epidermotropism, interface change, or diffuse reticular dermal infiltrates are not identified

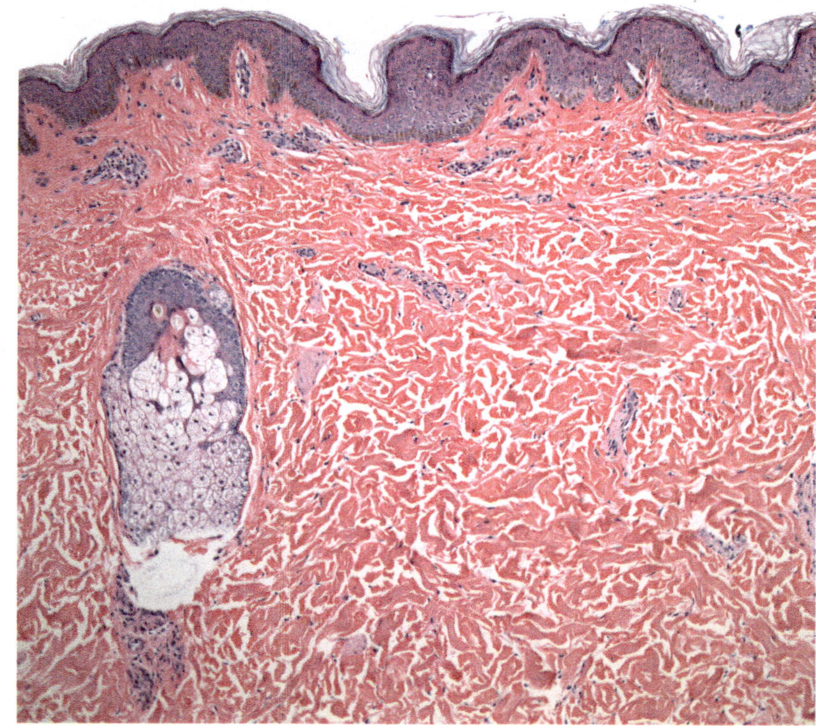

Fig. 30.4 Subcutaneous panniculitis-like T-cell lymphoma (SPTCL) with focal involvement of periadnexal adipose tissue. Dermal periadnexal fat is continuous with underlying subcutaneous tissue and may be involved by SPTCL. Dense diffuse dermal infiltrates are not identified

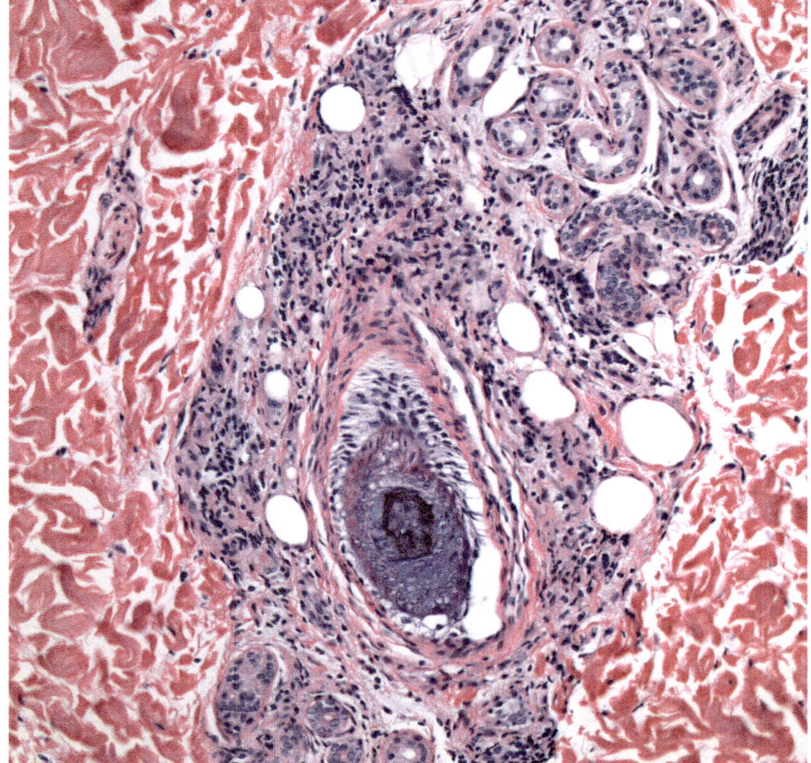

Fig. 30.5 Subcutaneous panniculitis-like T-cell lymphoma. Dense lobular pannicular lymphocytic infiltrate

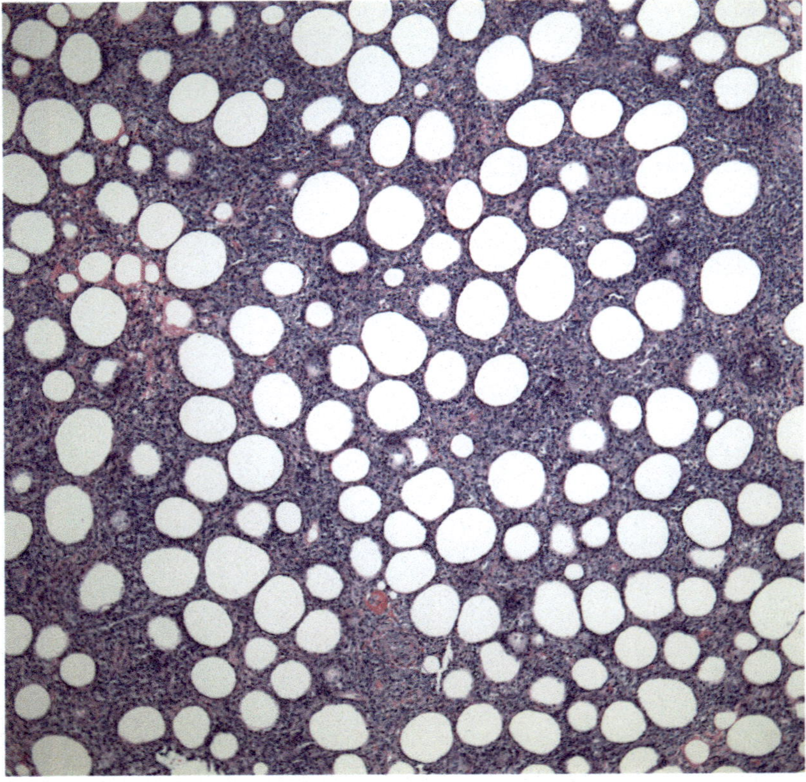

Fig. 30.6 Subcutaneous panniculitis-like T-cell lymphoma. Pannicular-based infiltrate of atypical lymphocytes with rimming of adipocytes

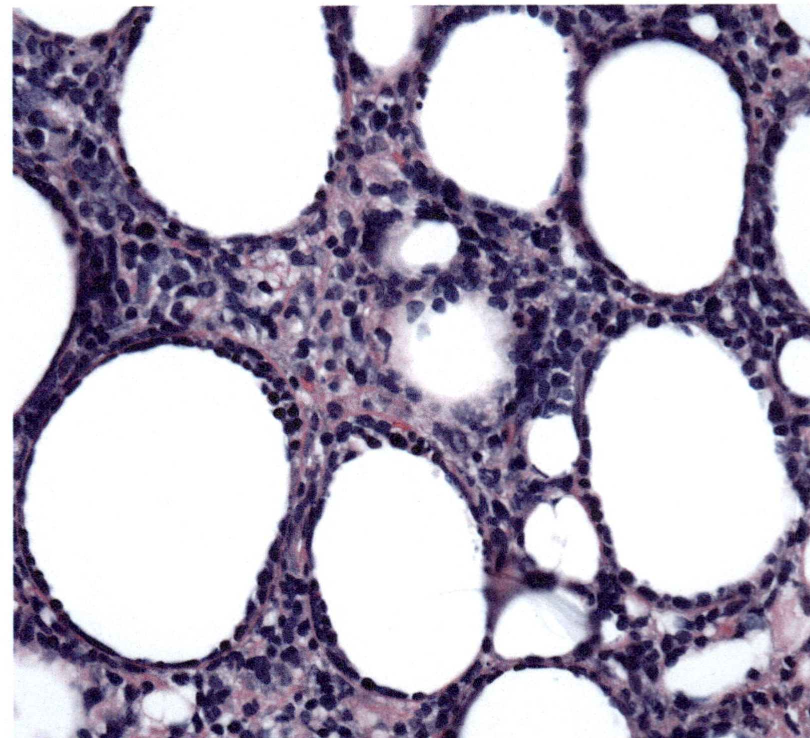

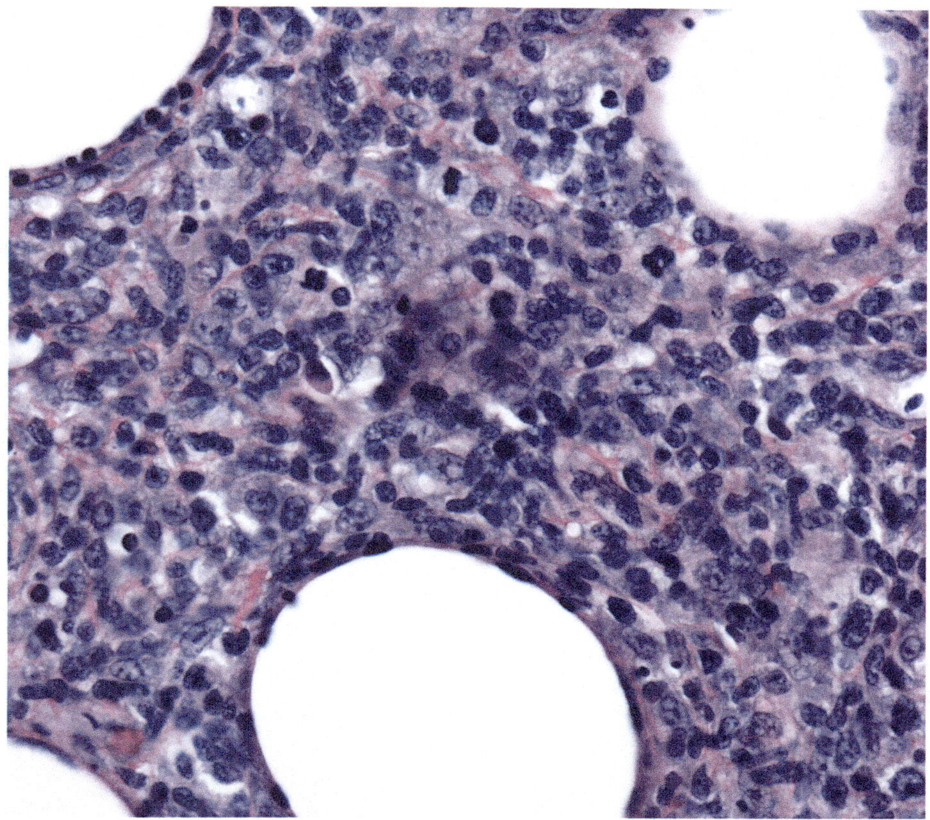

Fig. 30.7 Subcutaneous panniculitis-like T-cell lymphoma. Cytologic atypia, mitotic figures, and apoptosis are common

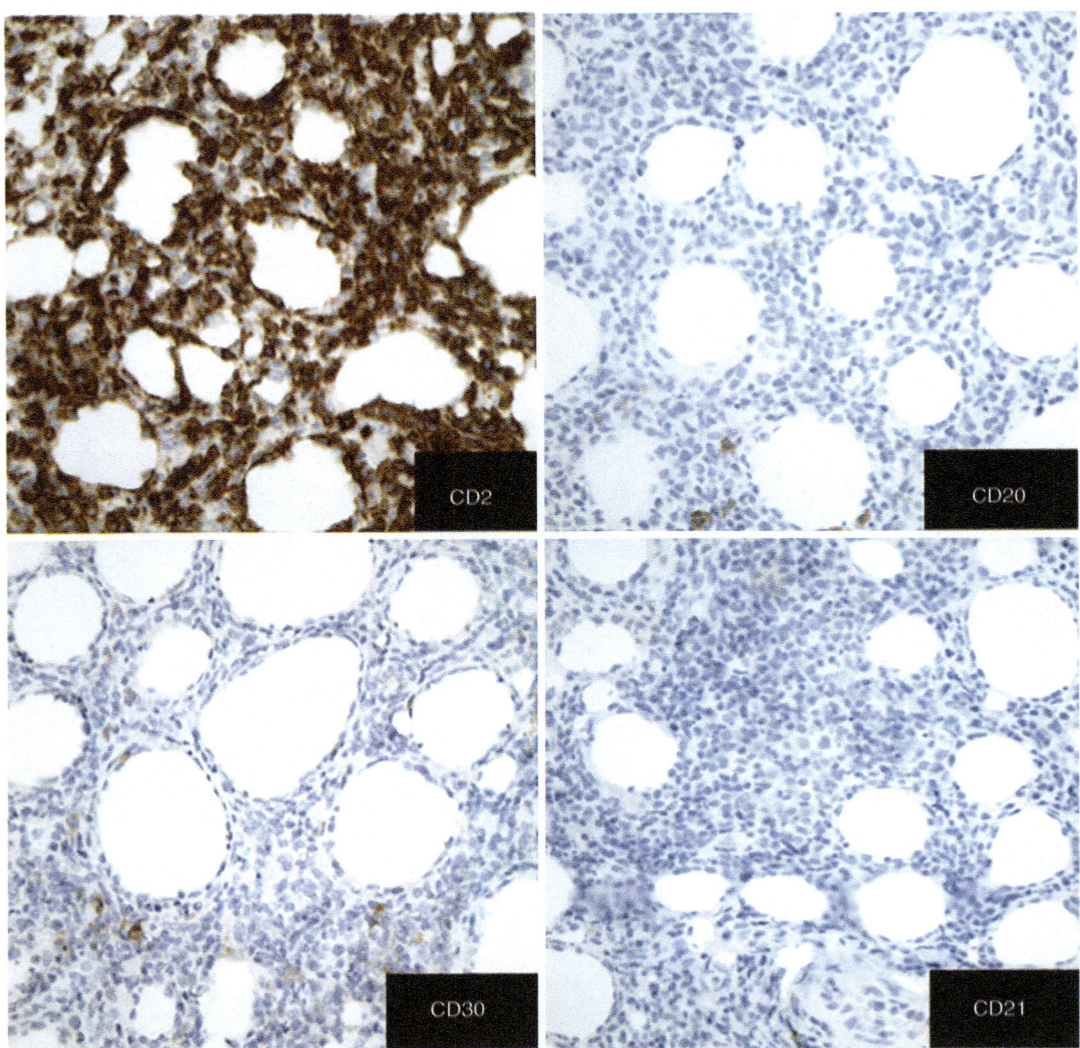

Fig. 30.8 Subcutaneous panniculitis-like T-cell lymphoma. The infiltrate is composed of CD2-positive T cells. A prominent component of B cells is not identified with CD20 stain. Significant CD30 expression is not present. A component of follicular dendritic cells is not identified with CD21 stain

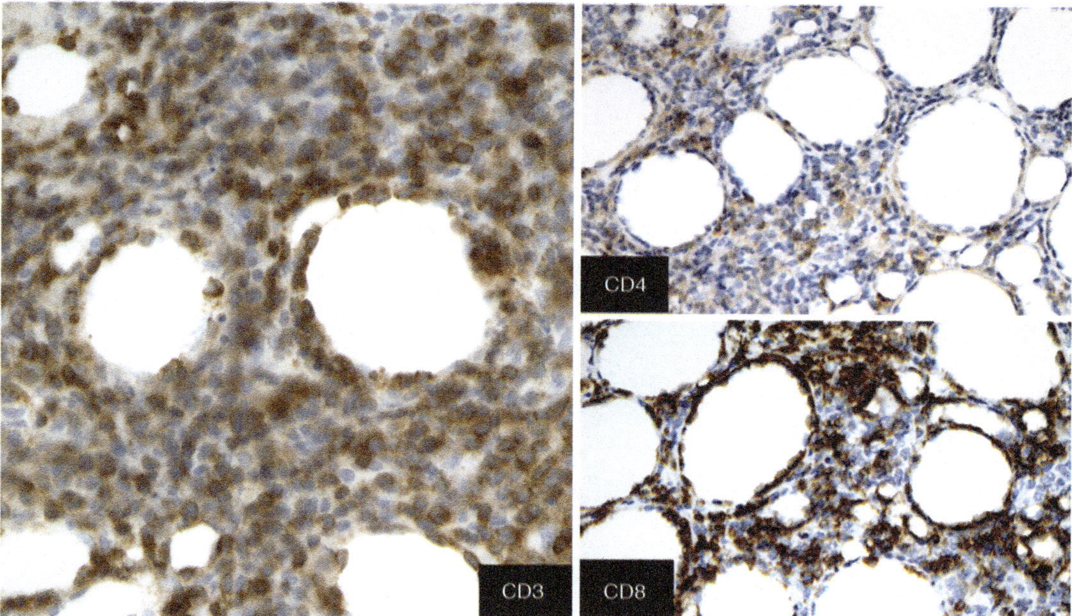

Fig. 30.9 Subcutaneous panniculitis-like T-cell lymphoma. The infiltrate is composed of CD3-positive/CD8-positive cytotoxic T cells. CD4 stain highlights a small subset of scattered, reactive T cells and histiocytes

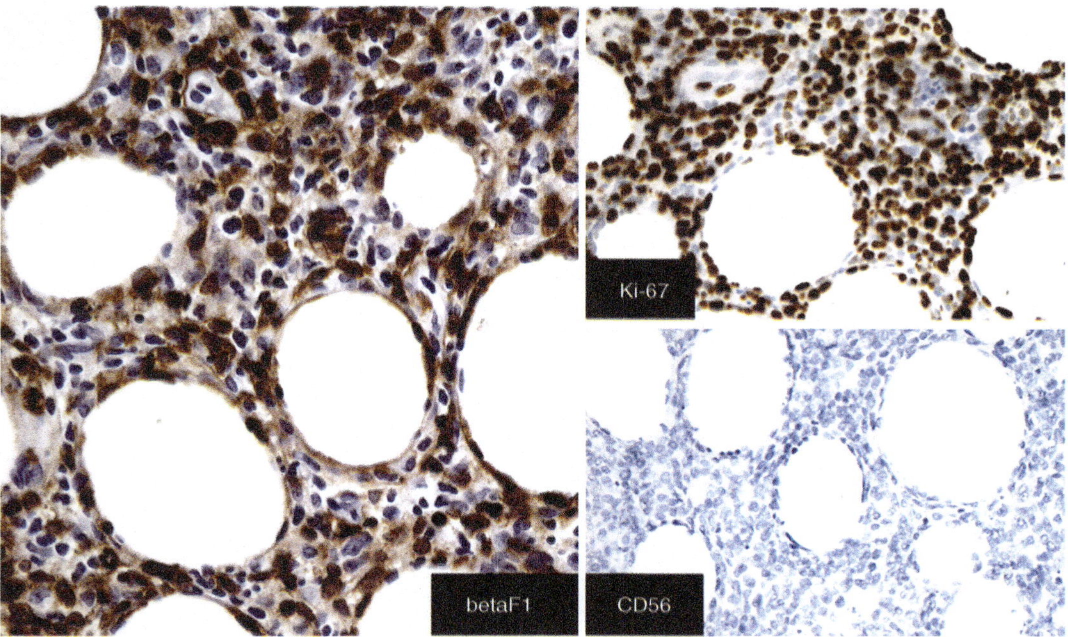

Fig. 30.10 Subcutaneous panniculitis-like T-cell lymphoma (SPTCL). Unlike gamma-delta T-cell lymphoma, SPTCL is composed of alpha-beta T cells (positive staining with TCRbetaF1) without significant CD56 expression. A high proliferation rate with Ki-67 stain can be helpful in the differential diagnosis with lupus erythematosus panniculitis

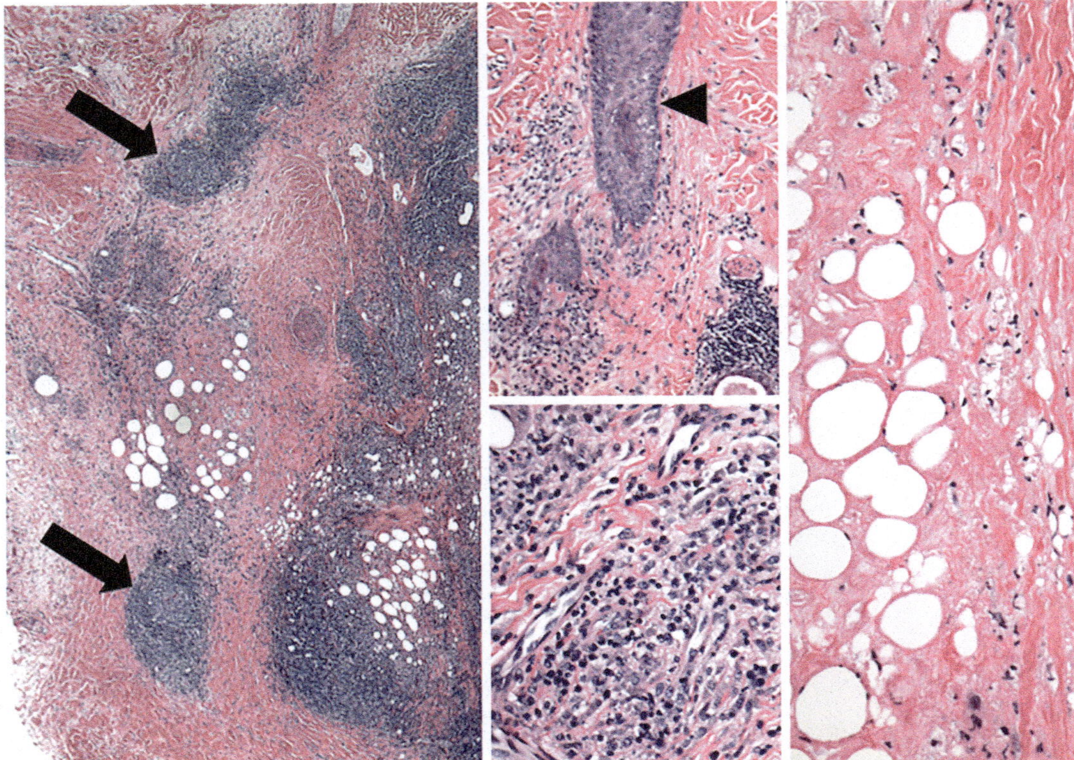

Fig. 30.11 Lupus erythematosus panniculitis. Lobular panniculitis composed predominantly of lymphocytes and plasma cells. Lymphoid follicles (arrows) and hyaline fat necrosis (right panel) are present. The overlying skin shows changes of discoid lupus erythematosus, including perifollicular (arrowhead) and perieccrine inflammation

Disease Definition

- Subcutaneous panniculitis-like T-cell lymphoma (SPTCL) is a cytotoxic alpha-beta T-cell lymphoma that preferentially infiltrates the subcutaneous tissue (Table 30.1). Pannicular lymphomas composed of gamma-delta T cells are now reclassified as cutaneous gamma-delta T-cell lymphoma.

Epidemiology

- <1% of all lymphomas.
- Slight female predominance.
- Variable age range, often occurring in young patients.
- A subset of patients has a history of autoimmune disease, particularly lupus erythematosus and occasionally lupus panniculitis.

Preferential Sites of Involvement

- Extremities (particularly lower extremities) and sometimes the trunk (Fig. 30.1).

Clinical Features

- Usually multiple subcutaneous nodules without ulceration or lymphadenopathy. Variable size.
- Some patients may have a history of panniculitis.
- *Less common presentations*: involvement of head and neck area. Solitary lesion. B symptoms (e.g., fever, weight loss). Cytopenias and abnormal liver function tests. Hemophagocytic syndrome (may occur in up to 20% of patients and is associated with significant mortality risk).

Histomorphology

- *Pattern*: Atypical lymphocytic infiltrate confined to the panniculus (lobular pattern) without involvement of the overlying dermis or epidermis (Figs. 30.2 and 30.3). The density of the infiltrate may be variable and patchy. Rimming of atypical lymphocytes surrounding individual adipocytes is characteristic (though rimming may also be seen when other lymphomas involve the panniculus). Necrosis is common. Mitotic figures are easily identified.
- *Less common patterns*: Periadnexal adipocytes in the dermis are contiguous with subcutaneous tissue, and the pannicular lymphocytic infiltrate may extend into the adipose tissue around eccrine sweat glands and hair follicles (however, reticular dermal collagen is not significantly involved) (Fig. 30.4). Vascular invasion may occasionally be seen. Interface dermatitis may rarely be seen and would raise the possibilities of SPTCL in association with autoimmune disease and of gamma-delta T-cell lymphoma.
- *Neoplastic cells*: Variable nuclear size (small, medium, or large). Irregular, pleomorphic, hyperchromatic nuclei with usually inconspicuous nucleoli and variable, often pale cytoplasm. Karyorrhexis and rimming are common (Figs. 30.5, 30.6, and 30.7).
- *Reactive cells*: Usually abundant histiocytes with vacuolated cytoplasm and apoptotic debris. Plasma cells are usually infrequent.

Immunophenotype

- *Neoplastic cells*: Alpha-beta T cells (positive staining with TCRbetaF1) with expression of cytotoxic proteins (TIA-1, granzyme B, and/or perforin). CD3+, CD4−, CD8+, CD30−, and CD56− (Figs. 30.8, 30.9, and 30.10). High proliferation rate with Ki-67 stain. Epstein-Barr virus (EBV) is absent.
- *Reactive cells*: CD68-positive histiocytes (which also stain with CD4). A prominent B-cell or plasma cell component is generally not seen (limited to absent staining with CD20, CD79a, CD138, kappa, or lambda). CD21 stain is usually negative (absent follicular dendritic cell meshworks of lymphoid follicles). Prominent CD123 staining is usually not identified.

Genetics

- Monoclonal rearrangement of T-cell receptor genes in majority of cases.

Prognosis

- Indolent (in contrast to gamma-delta T-cell lymphoma). Lymph node or visceral involvement is rare.
- 5-year survival: >80%.
- Adverse risk factors: Cases that develop hemophagocytic syndrome have a significantly worse survival.

Differential Diagnosis

- Lupus erythematosus panniculitis (LEP) and subcutaneous panniculitis-like T-cell lymphoma (SPTCL) may demonstrate significant clinical and histopathologic overlap. In addition, a significant subset of patients with SPTCL has a history of autoimmune disease, particularly lupus. While the differential diagnosis for a pannicular lymphocytic infiltrate includes LEP and SPTCL, a few patients may have both entities. A prominent component of CD20-positive B cells (often forming CD21+ lymphoid follicles), plasma cells (CD79a+, CD138+), and plasmacytoid dendritic cells (CD123+) as well as hyaline fat necrosis would favor a diagnosis of LEP (Fig. 30.11). Lymphocytic atypia, adipocyte rimming by cytotoxic alpha-beta T cells (betaF1+, CD3+, CD4−, CD8+, CD56−, TIA1+), an increased proliferation rate (overall Ki-67 index >20% and/or "hotspots" of lymphocytic aggregates with Ki-67 > 30%), and positive clonal T-cell receptor gene rearrangement would favor SPTCL.

– Besides LEP, other benign conditions and indolent lymphoproliferative disorders may also demonstrate pannicular infiltrates including lymphocytes. The differential diagnosis would also include necrobiosis lipoidica, morphea, cold panniculitis, and Rosai-Dorfman disease. Careful evaluation of clinical and histopathologic findings is essential for accurate diagnosis.

– CD8 expression may be seen in other lymphomas (Table 30.2).

– Gamma-delta T-cell lymphoma (GDTCL) is an important differential diagnosis in this setting. Because GDTCL may be CD8-positive and involve the panniculus, it is important to perform TCRbetaF1 immunostain. While SPTCL is an indolent lymphoma of alpha-beta T cells involving the panniculus, GDTCL is an aggressive lymphoma of gamma-delta T cells (TCRbetaF1–, CD3+, CD5–, CD4–, CD8–/+, CD56+, TIA1+) that may involve any combination of panniculus, dermis, and epidermis. Ulceration and significant angiocentrism may also occur in GDTCL.

– Extranodal NK/T-cell lymphoma nasal type is EBV-positive.

– Other lymphomas that may show variable involvement of the subcutaneous adipose tissue include tumor-stage mycosis fungoides and diffuse large B-cell lymphoma, leg type (Table 30.3). Comprehensive immunophenotyping and correlation with clinical findings must be obtained.

Table 30.2 Differential diagnosis of CD8-positive cutaneous lymphoid infiltrates

Some cases of otherwise classical or hypopigmented mycosis fungoides
Many cases of localized pagetoid reticulosis
Lymphomatoid papulosis (LyP), type D
Some cases of anaplastic large cell lymphoma (ALCL)
Primary cutaneous CD8+ aggressive epidermotropic cytotoxic T-cell lymphoma
Many cases of cutaneous gamma-delta T-cell lymphoma
Subcutaneous panniculitis-like T-cell lymphoma
Indolent CD8+ lymphoid proliferation of the ear (primary cutaneous acral CD8+ T-cell lymphoma)
Cutaneous pseudolymphoma: CD8-positive infiltrates in the setting of advanced AIDS, many cases of pityriasis lichenoides

Table 30.3 Differential diagnosis of lymphocytic infiltrates with pannicular involvement

Lymphomas	Benign conditions/indolent lymphoproliferative disorders
Subcutaneous panniculitis-like T-cell lymphoma	Lupus erythematosus panniculitis
Gamma-delta T-cell lymphoma	Rosai-Dorfman disease
Tumor-stage mycosis fungoides	Cold panniculitis
Diffuse large B-cell lymphoma, leg type	Morphea
	Necrobiosis lipoidica

Pearls and Pitfalls

1. Subcutaneous lymphomas often demonstrate patchy distribution in the panniculus. Therefore, a large and deep specimen is generally necessary for diagnosis.

2. Manuscripts published prior to the 2005 WHO-EORTC classification include gamma-delta T-cell lymphomas in the subcutaneous panniculitis-like T-cell lymphoma category (beware of marked differences in prognosis as well as different diagnostic criteria in older literature). Historically, these lymphomas were often labeled histiocytic cytophagic panniculitis and Weber-Christian panniculitis in the past.

3. Histiocytes are generally abundant in SPCTL. Since histiocytes generally mark with CD4, interpretation of CD4 staining must be careful. At low-power magnification, it may appear that the infiltrate has a predominance of CD4 expression (due to staining of histiocytes). To avoid misinterpreting a CD8-positive T-cell infiltrate as CD4-positive, it is often easier to look at the CD8 stain first (while comparing it to CD3) and then look at the CD4 stain.

Suggested Reading

LeBlanc RE, Tavallaee M, Kim YH, et al. Useful parameters for distinguishing subcutaneous panniculitis-like T-cell lymphoma from lupus erythematosus panniculitis. Am J Surg Pathol. 2016;40(6):745–54.

Pincus LB, Leboit PE, McCalmont TH, et al. Subcutaneous panniculitis-like T-cell lymphoma with overlapping clinicopathologic features of lupus erythematosus: coexistence of 2 entities? Am J Dermatopathol. 2009;31:520–6.

Swerdlow SH, et al., editors. WHO classification of tumors of hematopoietic and lymphoid tissues. Lyon: IARC; 2008.

Swerdlow SH, Campo E, Pileri SA, et al. The 2016 revision of the WHO classification of lymphoid neoplasms. Blood. 2016;127(20):2375–90.

Willemze R, Jaffe ES, Burg G, et al. WHO-EORTC classification for cutaneous lymphomas. Blood. 2005;105(10):3768–85.

Wu X, Subtil A, Craiglow B, et al. The coexistence of lupus erythematosus panniculitis and subcutaneous panniculitis-like T-cell lymphoma in the same patient. JAAD Case Rep. 2018;4(2):179–84.

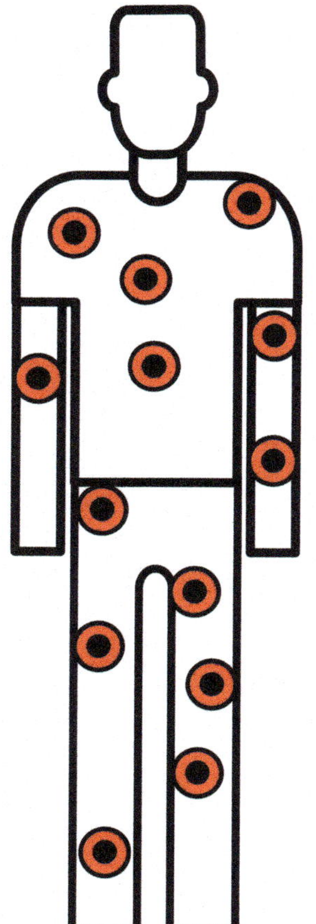

Fig. 31.1 Primary cutaneous gamma-delta T-cell lymphoma is an aggressive cytotoxic lymphoma. Ulceration and disseminated disease are common

Table 31.1 Key facts

Definition
Primary cutaneous gamma-delta T-cell lymphoma is an aggressive skin lymphoma composed of mature gamma-delta T cells with a cytotoxic phenotype
Prototypic clinical presentation
Variable clinical presentation, but the disease is rapidly growing and eventually becomes generalized. Some cases may be predominantly epidermotropic and present with patches/plaques, which are often red-brown and may exhibit superficial erosions. Other cases may present with deep dermal/subcutaneous tumors. Ulceration is common. Mucosal involvement may also occur
Histopathologic findings
Any (or all) of the layers of the skin may be involved. Any of the three patterns (epidermotropic, dermal, and subcutaneous) may be combined or present in isolation in the same specimen or in different biopsies of the same patient. Keratinocyte necrosis, interface change, and ulceration are common. Variable cell size. Angioinvasion may occur
Most common immunophenotype: CD3+, CD2+, CD5−, CD7+/−, CD4−, CD8−/+, CD30−, CD56+, TIA1+, betaF1−, TCR gamma+, and EBV−
Prognosis
Poor. 5-year survival: 0–11%

© Springer Nature Switzerland AG 2019
A. Subtil, *Diagnosis of Cutaneous Lymphoid Infiltrates*,
https://doi.org/10.1007/978-3-030-11654-5_31

Fig. 31.2 Primary cutaneous gamma-delta T-cell lymphoma showing epidermotropism. The epidermis shows intraepithelial atypical lymphocytes and necrotic keratinocytes. The atypical lymphocytes are immunoreactive with TCR gamma and negative with TCRbetaF1 (positive internal control in reactive alpha-beta T cells in the dermis)

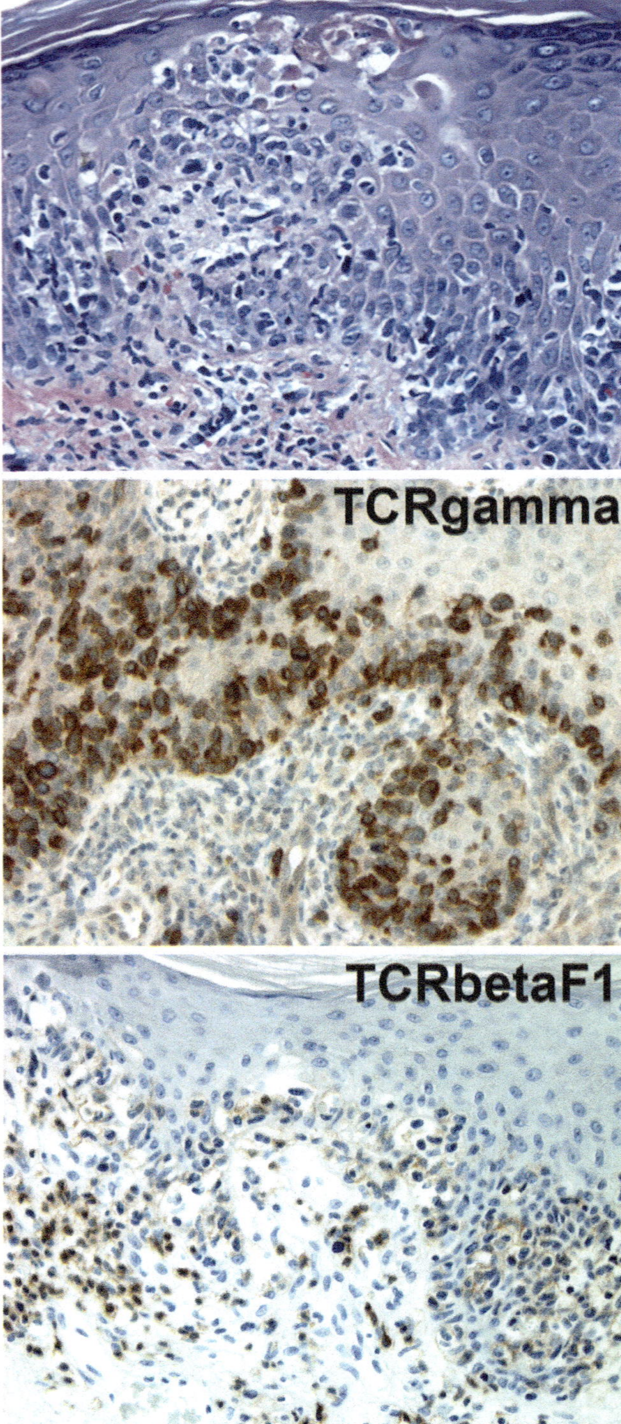

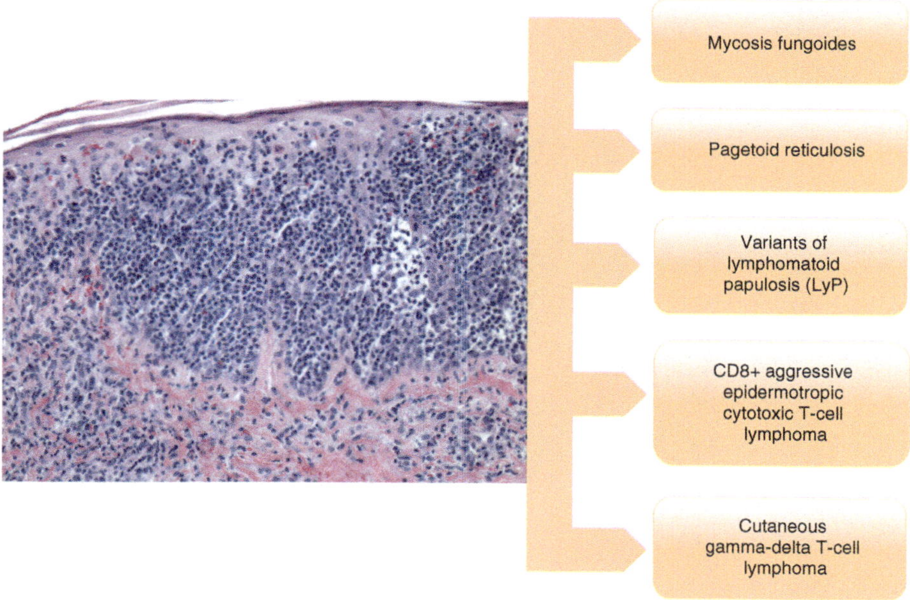

Fig. 31.3 Differential diagnosis of atypical lymphoid infiltrate with epidermotropism

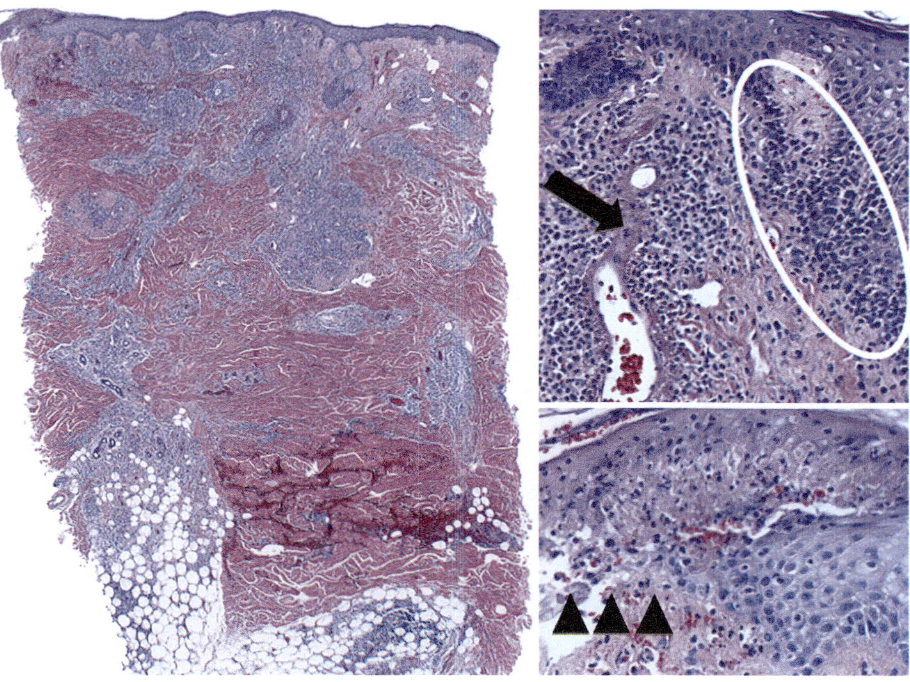

Fig. 31.4 Primary cutaneous gamma-delta T-cell lymphoma involving all layers of the skin (epidermis, dermis, and panniculus). The epidermis shows intraepithelial atypical lymphocytes (circle) and ulceration (arrowheads). Vasculitic changes with fibrin deposition are present (arrow)

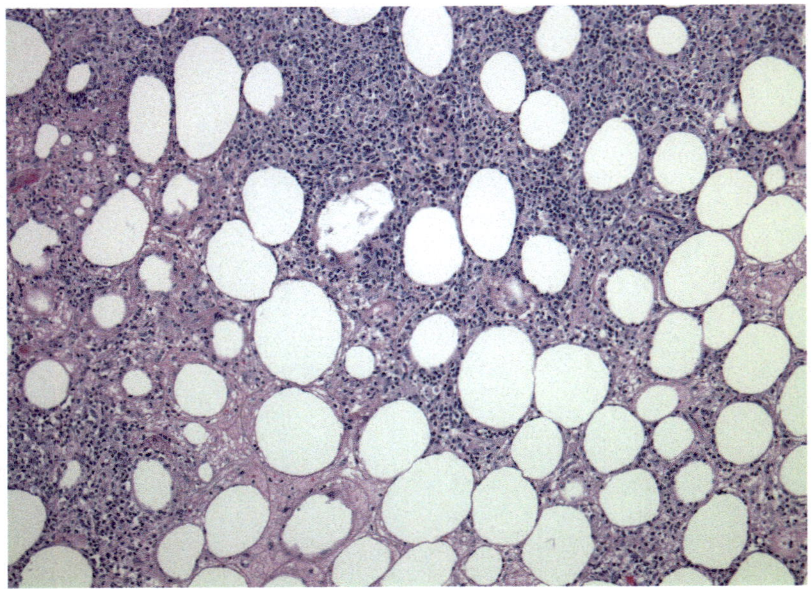

Fig. 31.5 Primary cutaneous gamma-delta T-cell lymphoma involving the panniculus

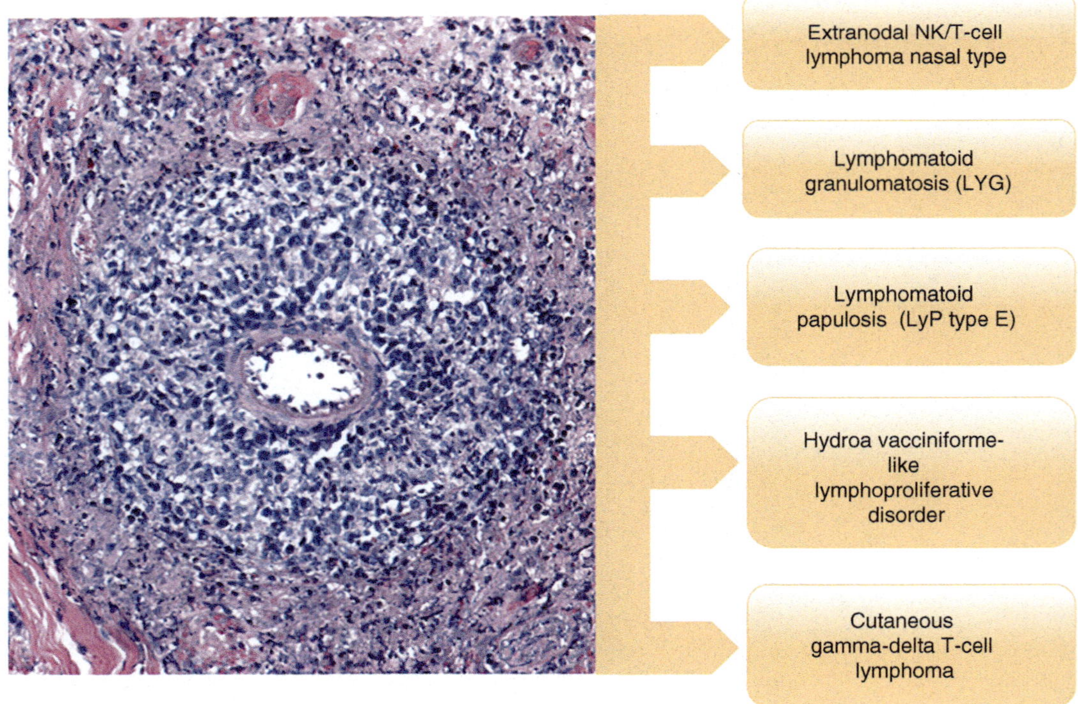

Fig. 31.6 Differential diagnosis of atypical lymphoid infiltrate with angiocentrism

Disease Definition

- *Primary cutaneous gamma-delta T-cell lymphoma* is an aggressive skin lymphoma composed of mature gamma-delta T cells with a cytotoxic phenotype (Table 31.1). Since the 2005 WHO-EORTC classification, this category includes cases previously known as subcutaneous panniculitis-like T-cell lymphoma with gamma-delta phenotype.

Epidemiology

- Rare (1% of all cutaneous T-cell lymphomas)
- Usually adults but may occur in children
- No gender predilection

Preferential Sites of Involvement

- Usually presents with generalized skin lesions (Fig. 31.1).
- Extremities are commonly affected, but other sites may be involved.
- Dissemination to mucosal and extranodal sites is frequent. CNS involvement may occur.
- Involvement of lymph nodes, bone marrow, or spleen is uncommon.

Clinical Features

- Variable clinical presentation.
- Some cases may be predominantly epidermotropic and present with patches/plaques, which are often red-brown and may exhibit superficial erosions. Other cases may present with deep dermal/ subcutaneous tumors with variable ulceration. Mucosal involvement may also occur. In general, the disease is rapidly growing and eventually becomes generalized.
- Hemophagocytic syndrome may occur, particularly in patients with subcutaneous tumors.
- B symptoms (fever, night sweats, and unintended weight loss) and elevated LDH (lactate dehydrogenase) are common.

- *Less common presentations*: solitary or localized lesion(s) on the lower extremities.

Histomorphology

- *Pattern*: Any (or all) of the layers of the skin may be involved. Any of the three patterns (epidermotropic, dermal, and subcutaneous) may be combined or present in isolation in the same specimen or in different biopsies of the same patient.
- The degree of epidermal involvement is variable (from absent to mild epidermotropism to marked epidermotropism resembling pagetoid reticulosis; Figs. 31.2 and 31.3). Keratinocyte necrosis, interface change, and ulceration are common (Fig. 31.4). Superficial dermal edema may be seen.
- Cases with subcutaneous involvement may show rimming of adipocytes (resembling subcutaneous panniculitis-like T-cell lymphoma; Fig. 31.5 and Table 31.2).
- *Less common patterns*: Angioinvasion may occur and may be focal or extensive (Fig. 31.6 and Table 31.3). Infarct-like necrosis may be present. Hemophagocytosis may occasionally be seen.
- *Neoplastic cells*: The cell size is variable, but neoplastic cells are usually medium to large with coarsely clumped chromatin. Large blastic cells with vesicular chromatin and large nucleoli are infrequent. Apoptosis and necrosis are common.
- *Reactive cells*: Small reactive lymphocytes and histiocytes.

Immunophenotype

- *Neoplastic cells* (Fig. 31.2): Usually CD3+, CD2+, CD5−, CD7+/−, CD30−, CD56+/−, and betaF1− with strong expression of cytotoxic proteins (e.g., TIA-1). Gamma-delta T cells generally lack CD5 and often express CD56 (Table 31.4). Most cases lack both CD4 and CD8, but some cases are CD8+.

If TCR gamma cannot be obtained (by immunohistochemistry on formalin-fixed tissue or by flow cytometry of fresh tissue), lack of betaF1 may be used for a presumptive diagnosis in the correct clinicopathologic setting. Ki-67 rate is often more than 50%. Epstein-Barr virus (EBV) is negative (Table 31.3).

- *Reactive cells*: Usually CD3+ T cells and CD68+ histiocytes.

Genetics

- Monoclonal rearrangement of T-cell receptor gamma genes in majority of cases. T-cell receptor beta genes may be clonally rearranged or deleted but are not expressed.
- Epstein-Barr virus (EBV) is negative.

Prognosis

- Poor. Median survival is approximately 15 months, but some patients show a prolonged course. Often resistant to multiagent chemotherapy and/or radiation.
- 5-year survival: 0–11%.
- Adverse risk factors: Cases with subcutaneous involvement tend to have a more unfavorable prognosis compared to patients with epidermal or dermal disease only.

Differential Diagnosis

- The category of *subcutaneous panniculitis-like T-cell lymphoma* (SPTCL) is restricted to alpha-beta subcutaneous infiltrates. In addition to expression of betaF1 and CD8, SPTCL is usually CD56-negative. Epidermotropism is not seen. While rimming of fat cells may be observed in both SPTCL and gamma-delta T-cell lymphoma, only the latter would also show dermal and epidermal involvement. Dense diffuse dermal involvement is not seen in SPTCL, though patchy periadnexal adipocyte extension by the pannicular infiltrate may be seen.

- Cutaneous gamma-delta T-cell lymphoma may mimic *lupus panniculitis*, including interface change in the epidermis. The identification of CD56 expression and gamma-delta phenotype is helpful.
- *Mycosis fungoides* (MF) is the most common type of skin lymphoma and classically demonstrates a CD4-positive phenotype. However, a subset of otherwise classical MF cases is cytotoxic, and a gamma-delta phenotype has been documented in rare cases of chronically indolent MF (patch/plaque disease without ulceration or progression). Careful clinical correlation and close follow-up are necessary for accurate classification of cytotoxic infiltrates. The distinction is generally based on the clinical presentation and behavior.
- Other *aggressive cytotoxic cutaneous lymphomas*. Cases with epidermotropism may resemble primary cutaneous aggressive epidermotropic CD8+ T-cell lymphoma (alpha-beta betaF1+ T cells; usually CD2−, CD7+, CD45RA+, CD45RO−, CD56−). Cases with angioinvasion may resemble extranodal NK/T-cell lymphoma nasal type (EBV+).
- Secondary cutaneous involvement by *hepatosplenic T-cell lymphoma* is very rare. Hepatosplenic T-cell lymphoma is generally of gamma-delta T-cell derivation, but some cases have an alpha-beta phenotype. In addition to hepatosplenomegaly, the bone marrow is almost constantly involved (unlike cutaneous gamma-delta lymphoma). Hepatosplenic T-cell lymphoma is usually negative for granzyme B and perforin.

Table 31.2 Differential diagnosis of lymphocytic infiltrates with pannicular involvement

Lymphomas	Benign conditions/indolent lymphoproliferative disorders
Subcutaneous panniculitis-like T-cell lymphoma	Lupus erythematosus panniculitis
Gamma-delta T-cell lymphoma	Rosai-Dorfman disease
Tumor-stage mycosis fungoides	Cold panniculitis
Diffuse large B-cell lymphoma, leg type	Morphea
	Necrobiosis lipoidica

Table 31.3 Differential diagnosis of an atypical angiocentric lymphoid infiltrate in relation to Epstein-Barr virus (EBV) and immunophenotype

EBV	Angiocentric process	Immunophenotype
Positive (+)	Extranodal NK/T-cell lymphoma nasal type	T cell or NK cell
	Hydroa vacciniforme-like lymphoproliferative disorder	T cell or NK cell
	Lymphomatoid granulomatosis (LYG)	B cell
Negative (−)	Cutaneous gamma-delta T-cell lymphoma	Gamma-delta T cell
	Lymphomatoid papulosis (LyP type E)	CD30-positive T cell

Table 31.4 Differential diagnosis of CD56 expression in the skin

Lymphoid/hematopoietic	Nonlymphoid
Rare cases of mycosis fungoides	Merkel cell carcinoma
Rare cases of CD30-positive lymphoproliferative disorders	Schwannoma
Cutaneous gamma-delta T-cell lymphoma	Neuroblastoma
Extranodal NK/T-cell lymphoma, nasal type	Cellular neurothekeoma
Blastic plasmacytoid dendritic cell neoplasm (CD4+/CD56+ hematodermic neoplasm)	Plexiform fibrohistiocytic tumor
Some cases of myeloid leukemia cutis	Metastatic renal cell carcinoma
Most cases of plasma cell myeloma	Damaged muscle fibers

non-MF process, such as gamma-delta T-cell lymphoma.

4. Involvement of all layers of skin (epidermis, dermis, and panniculus) at initial presentation would be unusual for mycosis fungoides and may be a clue for cutaneous gamma-delta T-cell lymphoma.

5. In the past, cases of cutaneous gamma-delta T-cell lymphoma were often classified as Ketron-Goodman (generalized) type of pagetoid reticulosis. Currently, only the localized (Woringer-Kolopp) type of pagetoid reticulosis is used (see Chap. 24).

Pearls and Pitfalls

1. Manuscripts published prior to the 2005 WHO-EORTC classification include gamma-delta T-cell lymphomas in the subcutaneous panniculitis-like T-cell lymphoma category (beware marked differences in prognosis).

2. Subcutaneous lymphomas often demonstrate patchy distribution in the panniculus. Therefore, a large and deep specimen is generally necessary for diagnosis.

3. Ulceration is seen in some cases of advanced, tumor-stage mycosis fungoides (MF). The presence of ulceration at initial presentation would suggest a

Suggested Reading

Guitart J, Weisenburger DD, Subtil A, et al. Cutaneous gamma-delta T cell lymphomas: a spectrum of presentations with overlap with other cytotoxic lymphomas. Am J Surg Pathol. 2012;36(11):1656–65.

Hodak E, David M, Maron L, et al. CD4/CD8 double-negative epidermotropic cutaneous T-cell lymphoma: an immunohistochemical variant of mycosis fungoides. J Am Acad Dermatol. 2006;55:276–84.

Swerdlow SH, et al., editors. WHO classification of tumors of hematopoietic and lymphoid tissues. Lyon: IARC; 2008.

Swerdlow SH, Campo E, Pileri SA, et al. The 2016 revision of the WHO classification of lymphoid neoplasms. Blood. 2016;127(20):2375–90.

Willemze R, Jaffe ES, Burg G, et al. WHO-EORTC classification for cutaneous lymphomas. Blood. 2005;105(10):3768–85.

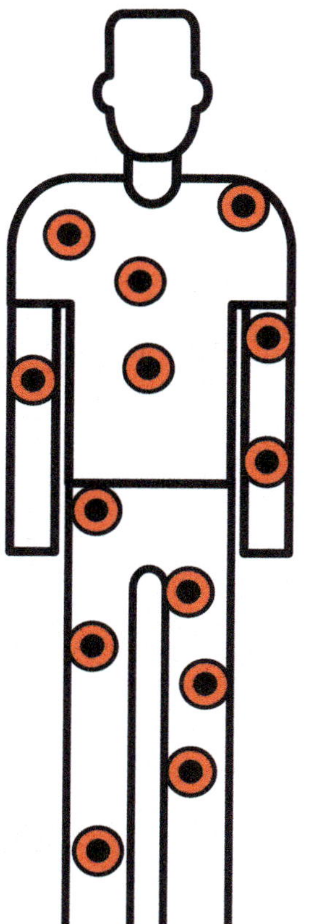

Table 32.1 Key facts

Definition
Primary cutaneous CD8-positive aggressive epidermotropic cytotoxic T-cell lymphoma is a rare cutaneous lymphoma characterized by a proliferation of epidermotropic CD8-positive cytotoxic T cells and aggressive clinical behavior
Prototypic clinical presentation
Extensive annular necrotic plaques or tumor lesions Rapid disease progression
Histopathologic findings
Marked pagetoid epidermotropism. Variable density from band-like lichenoid pattern to dense diffuse dermal infiltrate. Infiltration of adnexal epithelium (particularly folliculotropism) is common. Epidermis may be hyperkeratotic or atrophic but often shows prominent apoptotic keratinocytes, necrosis, and ulceration
Most common immunophenotype (immature cytotoxic alpha-beta T cells): CD3+, CD4−, CD8+, CD2−/+, CD5−/+, CD7+/−, CD30−, CD45RA+/−, CD45RO−, CD56−, TIA1+, granzyme B+, perforin+, and betaF1+. EBV-negative
Prognosis
Poor. Aggressive clinical course

Fig. 32.1 Primary cutaneous CD8-positive aggressive epidermotropic cytotoxic T-cell lymphoma is an aggressive cytotoxic lymphoma. Ulceration and disseminated disease are common

© Springer Nature Switzerland AG 2019
A. Subtil, *Diagnosis of Cutaneous Lymphoid Infiltrates*,
https://doi.org/10.1007/978-3-030-11654-5_32

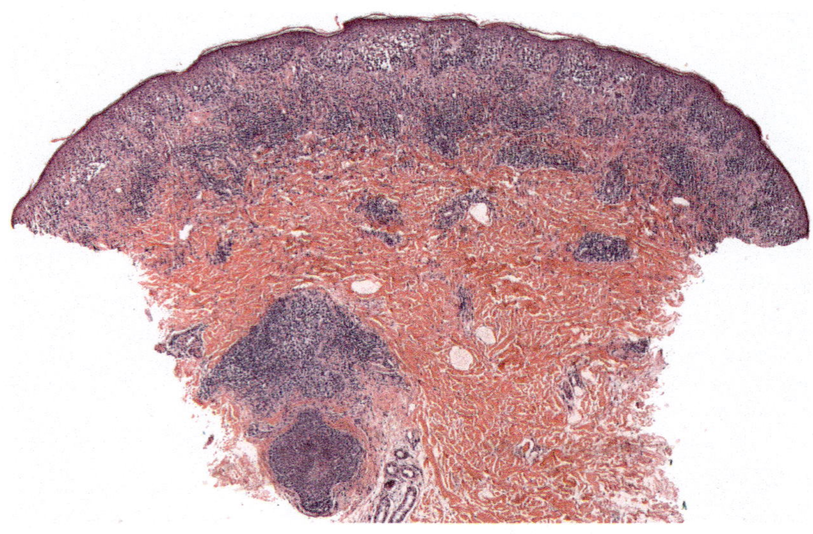

Fig. 32.2 Primary cutaneous CD8-positive aggressive epidermotropic cytotoxic T-cell lymphoma. Biopsy of an early lesion shows a band-like upper dermal lymphocytic infiltrate with infiltration of both epidermis (epidermotropism) and a hair follicle (folliculotropism)

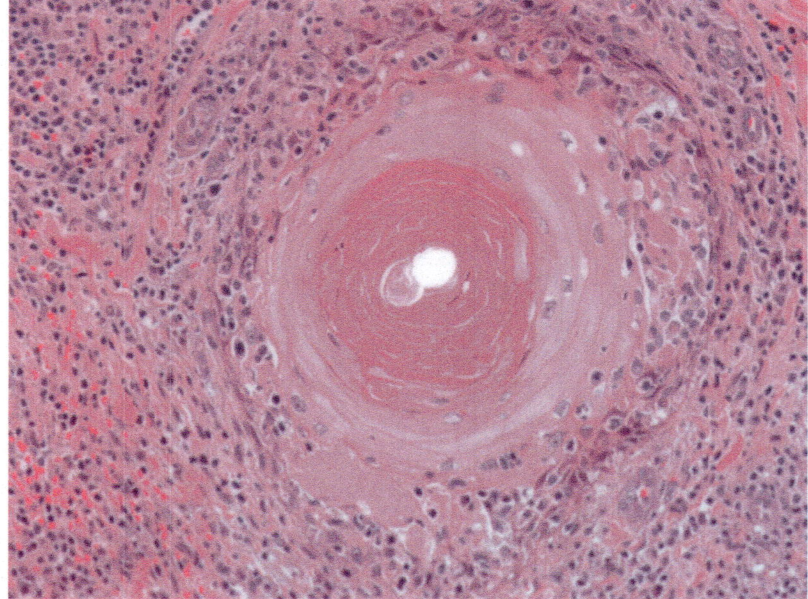

Fig. 32.3 Involvement of hair follicles is a common finding in primary cutaneous CD8-positive aggressive epidermotropic cytotoxic T-cell lymphoma

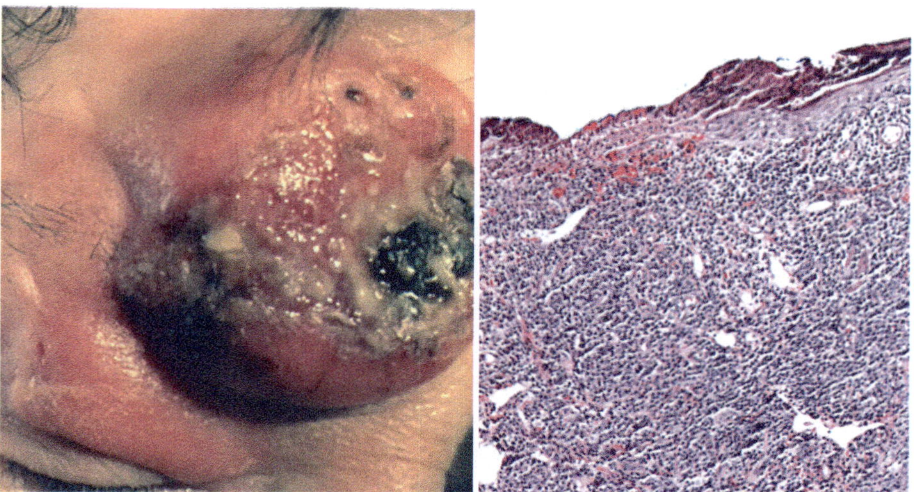

Fig. 32.4 Primary cutaneous CD8-positive aggressive epidermotropic cytotoxic T-cell lymphoma. Ulceration was present in this first skin biopsy of an enlarging nodule of 3-month duration. While the histopathology resembles tumor-stage mycosis fungoides, the patient had no patches or plaques. The presence of tumor-induced ulceration at an early onset is a clue that this cutaneous lymphoma is not mycosis fungoides

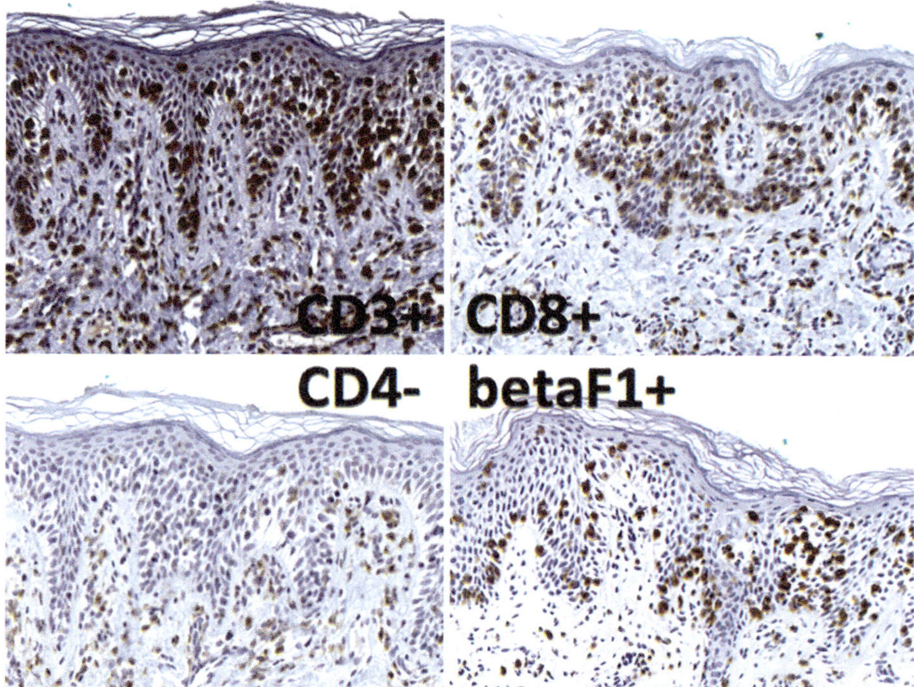

Fig. 32.5 Primary cutaneous CD8-positive aggressive epidermotropic cytotoxic T-cell lymphoma. Epidermotropism by CD8-positive alpha-beta T cells

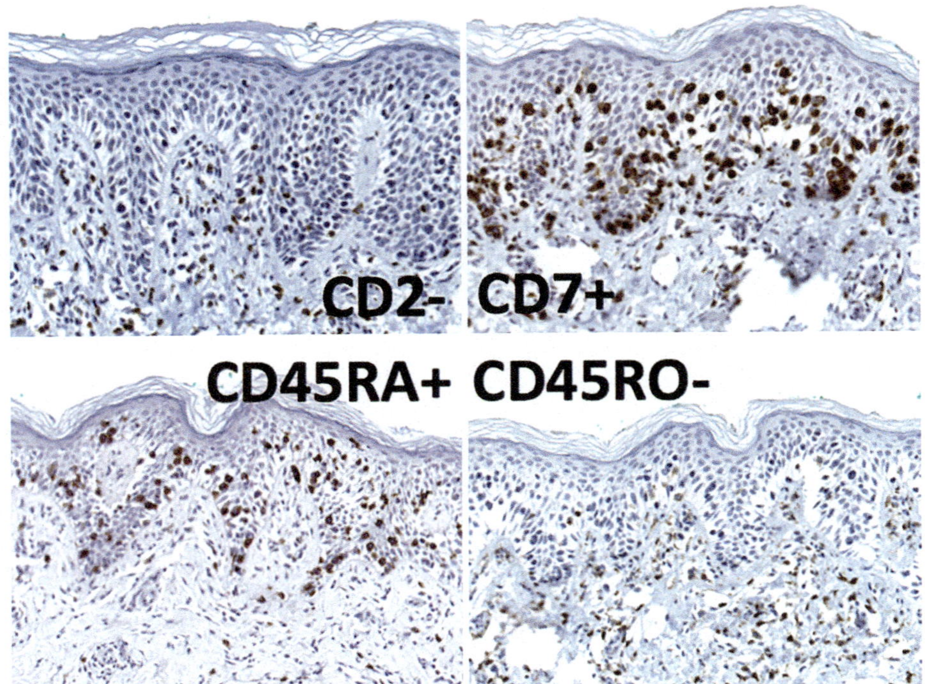

Fig. 32.6 Primary cutaneous CD8-positive aggressive epidermotropic cytotoxic T-cell lymphoma. Comprehensive immunophenotyping can be helpful in the differential diagnosis with mycosis fungoides since the infiltrate is composed of immature CD8-positive T cells (CD2−, CD7+, CD45RA+, CD45RO−). Mycosis fungoides is usually CD2+, CD7−, CD45RA−, and CD45RO+

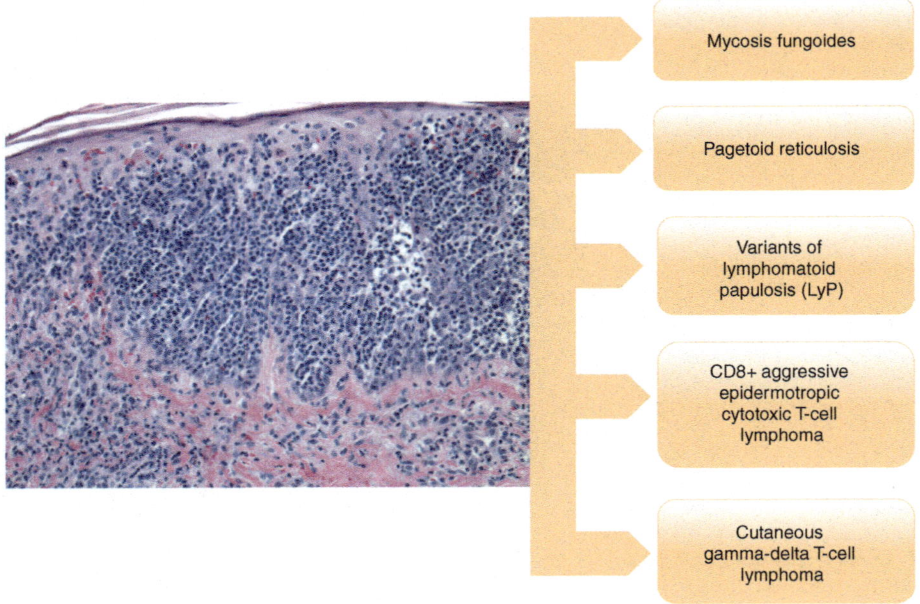

Fig. 32.7 Differential diagnosis of epidermotropism. Several entities may exhibit prominent intraepidermal lymphocytes. Clinical pathologic correlation is essential for proper classification

Disease Definition

- Rare cutaneous lymphoma characterized by a proliferation of epidermotropic CD8-positive cytotoxic T cells and aggressive clinical behavior (Table 32.1)
- Provisional entity in the 2016 WHO classification
- Synonym: Berti lymphoma

Epidemiology

- Rare (less than 1% of all cutaneous lymphomas)
- Usually adults. Median age of 77 (range 19–89)
- Male predominance

Preferential Sites of Involvement

- Generalized skin lesions in most patients (Fig. 32.1). Oral mucosa and genital skin may be involved.
- Visceral dissemination may occur (lung, testis, central nervous system, adrenal glands).
- Lymph nodes and bone marrow are generally spared.
- Hemophagocytic syndrome is generally not seen.

Clinical Features

- Localized or disseminated eruptive papules, nodules, and tumors with central ulceration and necrosis
- Annular necrotic plaques
- Superficial hyperkeratotic or eroded patches and plaques
- Rapid disease progression
- *Less common presentations*: prodrome of chronic patches prior to the development of aggressive ulcerative lesions. May clinically resemble psoriasis, erythema multiforme, and severe pityriasis lichenoides et varioliformis acuta (PLEVA, Mucha-Habermann disease)

Histomorphology

- *Pattern*: Marked pagetoid epidermotropism. Variable density from band-like lichenoid pattern to dense diffuse dermal infiltrate (Fig. 32.2). Infiltration of adnexal epithelium (particularly folliculotropism but also syringotropism) is common (Fig. 32.3). The epidermis may be acanthotic/hyperkeratotic or atrophic but often shows prominent apoptotic keratinocytes, necrosis, and ulceration (Fig. 32.4).
- *Less common patterns*: Subepidermal edema, intraepidermal vesicles, spongiosis, and angioinvasion. Some biopsies may show relatively limited epidermotropism.
- *Neoplastic cells*: Variable cytomorphology (small-medium or medium-large cells; hyperchromatic pleomorphic or blastic nuclei).
- *Reactive cells*: Small reactive lymphocytes, neutrophils (if ulceration is present).

Immunophenotype

- *Neoplastic cells*: Immature cytotoxic alpha-beta T cells. CD3+, CD4−, CD8+, CD2−/+, CD5−/+, CD7+/−, CD30−, CD45RA+/−, CD45RO−, TIA1+, granzyme B+, perforin+, and betaF1+. EBV-negative. CD56 is generally negative (Figs. 32.5 and 32.6).
- *Reactive cells*: Mixed CD3+ T cells; neutrophils stain with TIA1.

Genetics

- Monoclonal rearrangement of T-cell receptor genes in most (but not all) cases.
- EBV (EBER) is negative.

Prognosis

- Poor. Aggressive clinical course. Median survival of 12–32 months. Cell size does not affect survival.
- 5-year survival: 18–32%.

– Adverse risk factors: presence of tumors at the time of diagnosis.

Differential Diagnosis

– Differentiation from other types of CD8-positive lymphomas is primarily based on the clinical presentation and behavior (Table 32.2). Certain histopathologic features (marked epidermotropism, ulceration, immature cytotoxic phenotype) may provide a clue, but clinical correlation is necessary.
– Mycosis fungoides (MF) shows epidermotropism and can occasionally be CD8-positive (Table 32.3). The differential diagnosis may also include folliculotropic MF due to lymphocytic infiltration of hair follicles (Table 32.4). Comprehensive immunophenotyping can be helpful, since the infiltrate is composed of immature CD8-positive T cells (CD2−, CD7+, CD45RA+, CD45RO−). MF is usually CD2+, CD7−, CD45RA− and CD45RO+. The presence of ulceration early in the clinical course would be unusual in MF and would suggest an aggressive cytotoxic lymphoma (Table 32.5).
– Lymphomatoid papulosis (LyP) type D also shows an epidermotropic CD8-positive T-cell infiltrate with frequent ulceration, but the clinical appearance is different (small self-regressing papules).
– Localized pagetoid reticulosis (Woringer-Kolopp disease) may exhibit similar histopathologic features; however, the localized clinical presentation and indolent behavior are distinct.
– Cutaneous gamma-delta T-cell lymphoma may show overlapping clinical and histopathologic features but is composed of gamma-delta T cells (betaF1-negative, often CD56-positive). Angiodestruction and hemophagocytic syndrome are more commonly seen.
– Subcutaneous panniculitis-like T-cell lymphoma is also composed of alpha-beta CD8-positive T cells but involves subcutaneous tissue and lacks epidermotropism.

Table 32.2 Differential diagnosis of CD8-positive cutaneous lymphoid infiltrate

Some cases of otherwise classical or hypopigmented mycosis fungoides
Many cases of localized pagetoid reticulosis
Lymphomatoid papulosis (LyP), type D
Some cases of anaplastic large cell lymphoma (ALCL)
Primary cutaneous CD8+ aggressive epidermotropic cytotoxic T-cell lymphoma
Many cases of cutaneous gamma/delta T-cell lymphoma
Subcutaneous panniculitis-like T-cell lymphoma
Indolent CD8+ lymphoid proliferation of the ear (primary cutaneous acral CD8+ T-cell lymphoma)
Cutaneous pseudolymphoma: CD8-positive infiltrates in the setting of advanced AIDS, many cases of pityriasis lichenoides

Table 32.3 Differential diagnosis of frequent intraepidermal lymphocytes

Lymphomas/lymphoproliferative disorders	Benign dermatoses
Mycosis fungoides	Inflammatory stage of vitiligo
Pagetoid reticulosis	Pityriasis lichenoides
Lymphomatoid papulosis (LyP types B and D and with 6p25.3 rearrangement)	Lymphomatoid lichenoid keratosis
Primary cutaneous aggressive epidermotropic CD8-positive cytotoxic T-cell lymphoma	Early lichen sclerosus
Cutaneous gamma-delta T-cell lymphoma	Pigmented purpuric dermatoses
	Lymphomatoid drug reaction
	Pseudolymphomatous tattoo reaction
	CD8-positive cutaneous infiltrates in the setting of acquired immunodeficiency syndrome

Table 32.4 Differential diagnosis of cutaneous lymphocytic infiltrates with perifollicular accentuation

Lymphomas/lymphoproliferative disorders	Benign dermatoses
Cutaneous marginal zone B-cell lymphoma	Lymphomatoid drug eruption
Folliculotropic mycosis fungoides	Pseudolymphomatous folliculitis
Follicular lymphomatoid papulosis	Primary follicular mucinosis
Primary cutaneous aggressive epidermotropic CD8-positive cytotoxic T-cell lymphoma	Arthropod bite reaction (including persistent nodular scabies)
	Herpes folliculitis
	Lichen striatus
	Lupus erythematosus
	Lichen planopilaris
	Alopecia areata
	Graft-versus-host disease
	Infundibulofolliculitis

Table 32.5 Differential diagnosis of ulceration

Lymphomas/lymphoproliferative disorders	Benign dermatoses/pseudolymphomas
Tumor-stage mycosis fungoides	Pityriasis lichenoides et varioliformis acuta (PLEVA)
CD30-positive lymphoproliferative disorders: lymphomatoid papulosis, cutaneous anaplastic large cell lymphoma	Inflamed molluscum contagiosum
Primary cutaneous aggressive epidermotropic CD8-positive cytotoxic T-cell lymphoma	Herpesvirus infection
Cutaneous gamma-delta T-cell lymphoma	Primary syphilis
Extranodal NK/T-cell lymphoma, nasal type	Leishmania infection

Pearls and Pitfalls

1. Too much epidermotropism would be unusual for classic mycosis fungoides and would raise the possibility of another epidermotropic process, including type D lymphomatoid papulosis (LyP), pagetoid reticulosis, and aggressive epidermotropic CD8-positive cytotoxic T-cell lymphoma (Fig. 32.7).

2. Ulceration is seen in some cases of advanced, tumor-stage mycosis fungoides (MF). The presence of ulceration at initial presentation would suggest a non-MF process.

3. If ulceration is not seen in a skin biopsy, it does not necessarily mean that the patient does not have ulcerated lesions elsewhere, since dermatologists often avoid biopsying lesions with secondary changes. Careful correlation of clinical and histopathologic findings is essential.

4. Ulceration may not be present in the early stage of aggressive cytotoxic skin lymphomas. While immunophenotyping may provide clues to the diagnosis, close follow-up and rebiopsy of changed lesions may prove helpful.

5. In the past, cases of primary cutaneous CD8-positive aggressive epidermotropic cytotoxic T-cell lymphoma were classified as "generalized pagetoid reticulosis, Ketron-Goodman type" (terminology no longer in use).

6. There are rare cases of aggressive skin lymphoma lacking CD8 but with otherwise similar clinicopathologic features of primary cutaneous CD8-positive aggressive epidermotropic cytotoxic T-cell lymphoma. It is conceivable that they might represent the same entity and that this provisional category might be expanded in the next classification to include CD8-negative, EBV-negative, alpha-beta cytotoxic T-cell lymphomas with aggressive behavior.

Suggested Reading

Berti E, Tomasini D, Vermeer MH, et al. Primary cutaneous CD8-positive epidermotropic cytotoxic T cell lymphomas. A distinct clinicopathological entity with an aggressive clinical behavior. Am J Pathol. 1999;155:483–92.

Guitart J, Martinez-Escala ME, Subtil A, et al. Primary cutaneous aggressive epidermotropic cytotoxic T-cell lymphomas: reappraisal of a provisional entity in the 2016 WHO classification of cutaneous lymphomas. Mod Pathol. 2017;30(5):761–72.

Saggini A, Gulia A, Argenyi Z, et al. A variant of lymphomatoid papulosis simulating primary cutaneous aggressive epidermotropic CD8+ cytotoxic T-cell lymphoma. Description of 9 cases. Am J Surg Pathol. 2010;34(8):1168–75.

Swerdlow SH, et al., editors. WHO classification of tumors of hematopoietic and lymphoid tissues. Lyon: IARC; 2008.

Swerdlow SH, Campo E, Pileri SA, et al. The 2016 revision of the WHO classification of lymphoid neoplasms. Blood. 2016;127(20):2375–90.

Willemze R, Jaffe ES, Burg G, et al. WHO-EORTC classification for cutaneous lymphomas. Blood. 2005;105(10):3768–85.

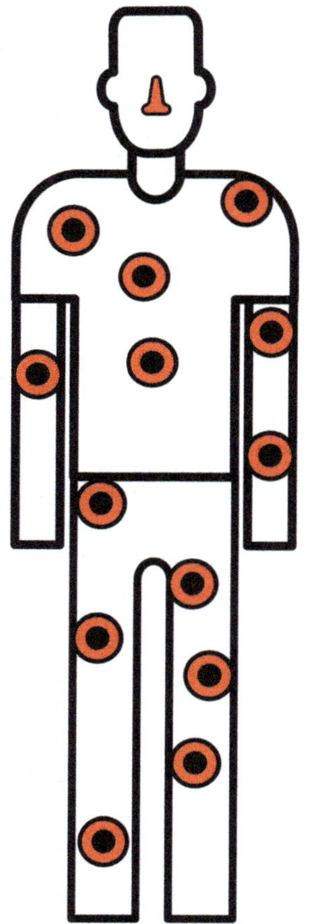

Table 33.1 Key Facts

Definition
Extranodal NK/T-cell lymphoma, nasal type is a primarily extranodal lymphoma characterized by vascular destruction, necrosis, cytotoxic phenotype, and association with Epstein-Barr virus (EBV). Most cases are of NK-cell origin, but a subset shows a cytotoxic T-cell phenotype
Prototypic clinical presentation
Upper aerodigestive tract (particularly nasal cavity): "lethal midline granuloma"   Skin lesions are usually erythematous or violaceous plaques and tumors with frequent ulceration
Histopathologic findings
Dense diffuse lymphoid infiltrate with angiocentric and angiodestructive pattern. Ulceration and necrosis are common. Broad cytologic spectrum and cell size. Most common immunophenotype: CD2+, CD3+, CD56+, EBV+. Positive cytotoxic proteins (TIA-1, granzyme B, perforin). Frequently positive: CD43, CD45RO, CD25. Frequently negative: CD4, CD8, CD5, betaF1, CD16, CD57
Prognosis
Variable but generally poor

Fig. 33.1 Extranodal NK/T-cell lymphoma, nasal type is an aggressive angiodestructive lymphoma that classically involves the upper aerodigestive tract (particularly nasal cavity) but frequently presents in the skin. Ulceration is common

© Springer Nature Switzerland AG 2019

A. Subtil, *Diagnosis of Cutaneous Lymphoid Infiltrates*,

https://doi.org/10.1007/978-3-030-11654-5_33

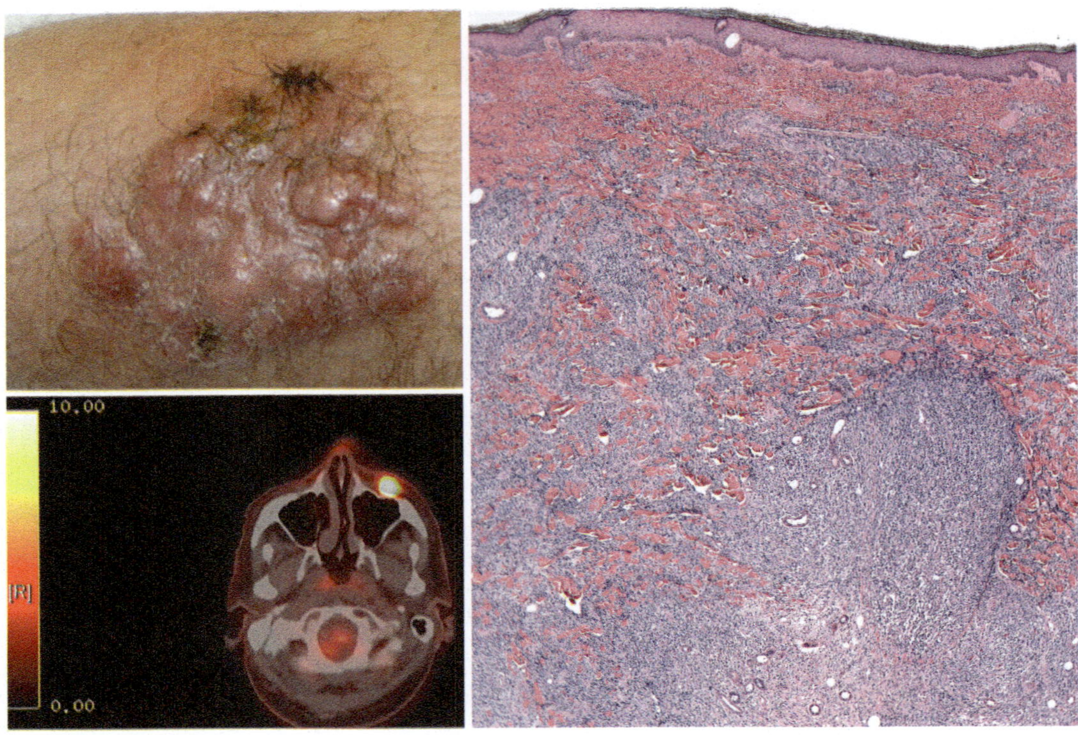

Fig. 33.2 Extranodal NK/T-cell lymphoma, nasal type presenting with both skin and nasal involvement. (Courtesy: Alicia Little, MD). The skin biopsy showed a dense diffuse superficial and deep dermal infiltrate without epidermotropism

Fig. 33.3 Extranodal NK/T-cell lymphoma, nasal type. Atypical dense diffuse dermal lymphoid infiltrate

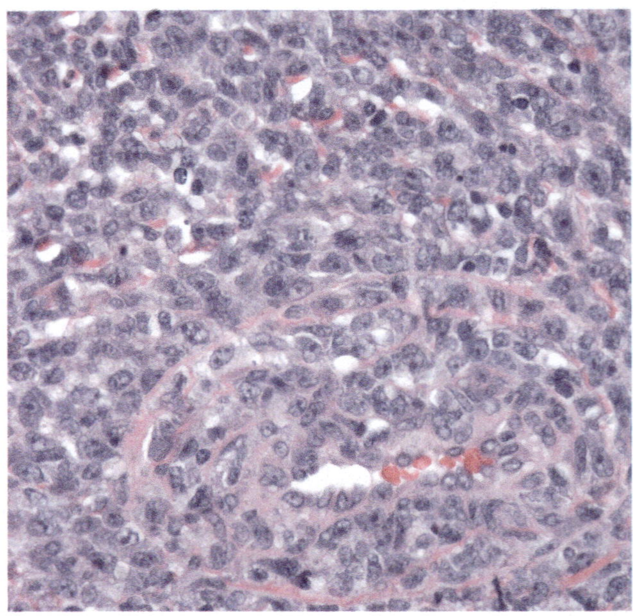

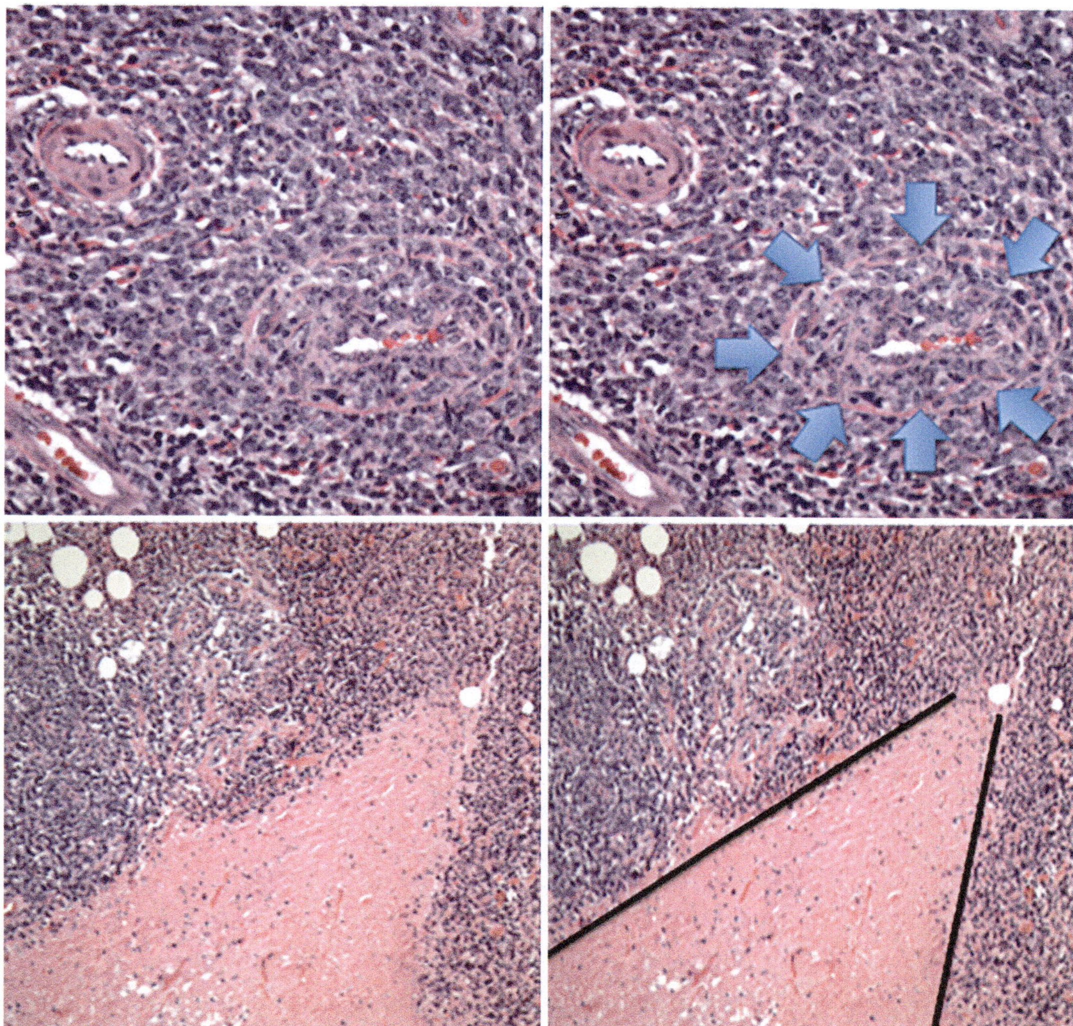

Fig. 33.4 Extranodal NK/T-cell lymphoma, nasal type. Angiocentrism is not always easily recognizable in a biopsy of an angioinvasive lymphoid process. Arrows highlight subtle infiltration of a blood vessel by atypical lymphocytes. An important clue for angiocentrism and angiodestruction is the presence of extensive, infarct-like necrosis (highlighted by lines)

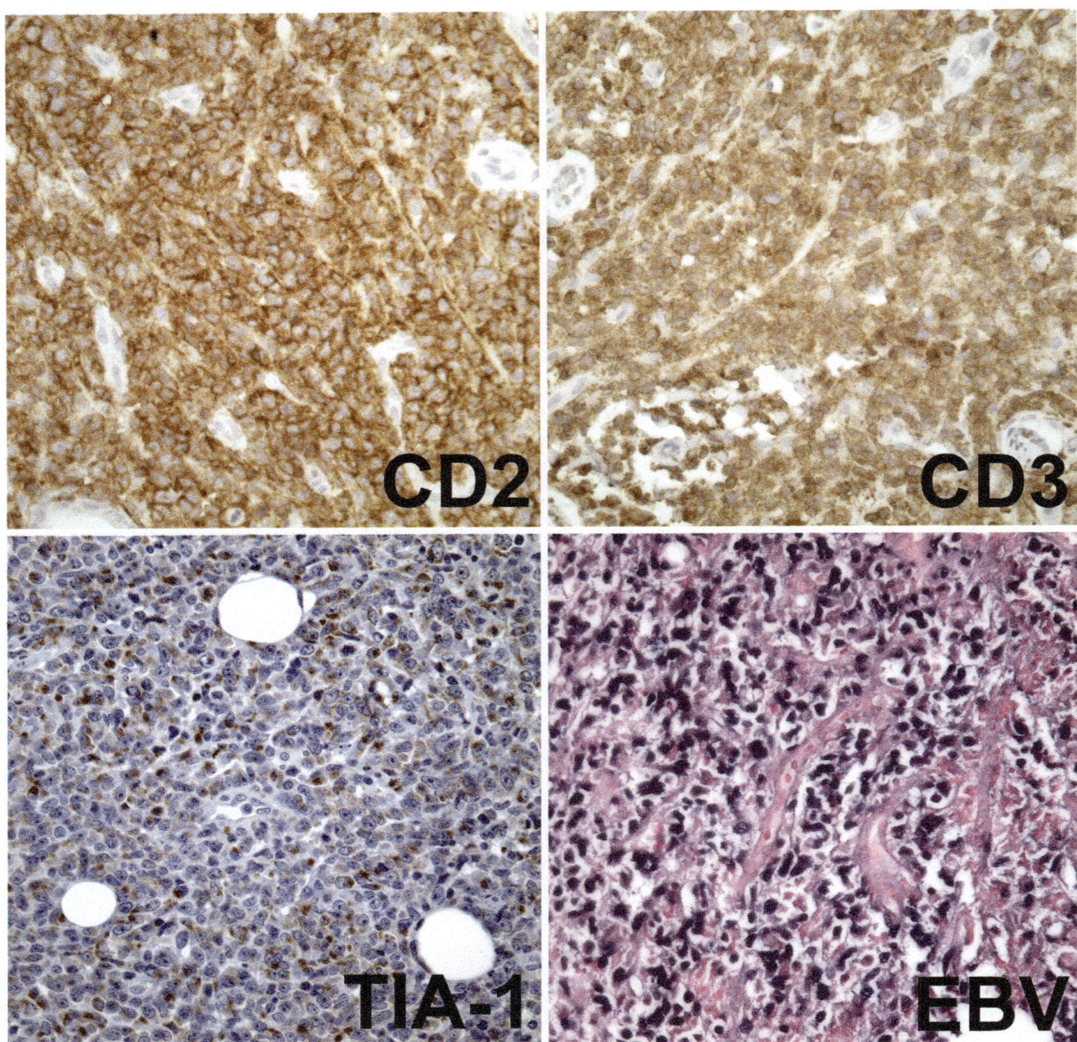

Fig. 33.5 The infiltrate is immunoreactive with T-cell markers CD2 and CD3 and with the cytotoxic marker TIA-1. Positive EBV in situ hybridization (EBER)

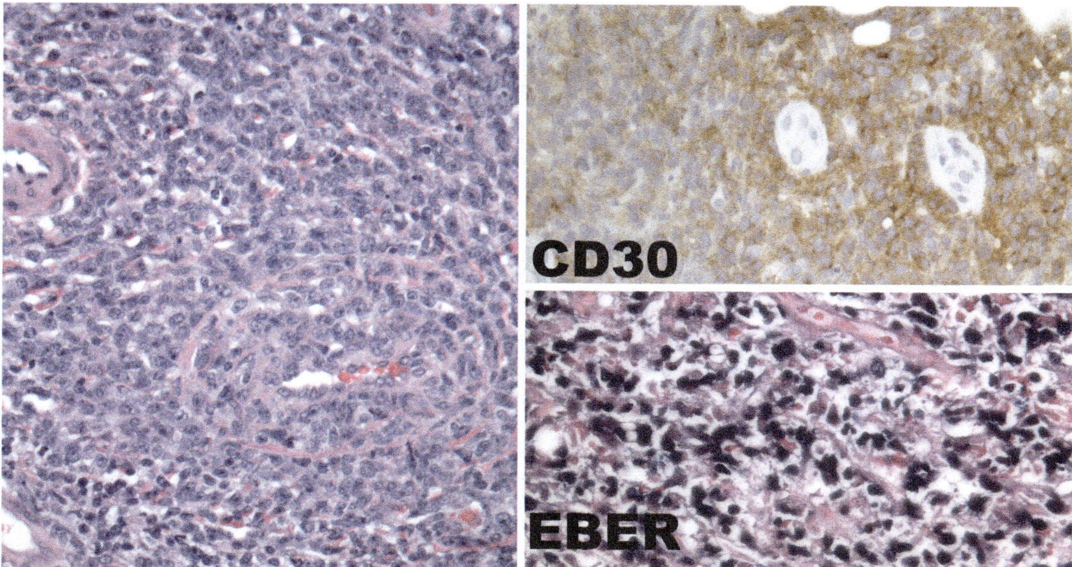

Fig. 33.6 Extranodal NK/T-cell lymphoma, nasal type with partial CD30 expression. Some cases of aggressive cytotoxic lymphomas may exhibit variable CD30 expression. However, the proportion of cells marking with CD30 stain is generally below the positivity threshold of 75% used for anaplastic large cell lymphoma (one of the cutaneous CD30-positive lymphoproliferative disorders). Therefore, this infiltrate is classified as a CD30-negative process, despite the significant level of staining. EBV in situ hybridization (EBER) is positive

Fig. 33.7 Extranodal NK/T-cell lymphoma, nasal type may be of true NK cell origin or of cytotoxic T-cell origin. Depending on the cell of origin, there are minor differences in immunophenotype and molecular results. (IHC, immunohistochemistry; TCR, T-cell receptor)

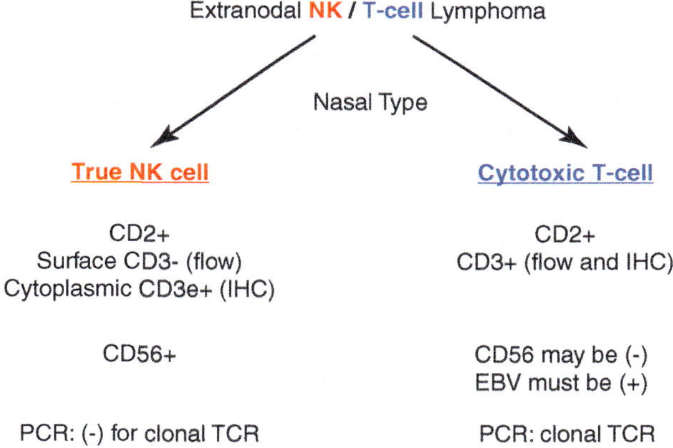

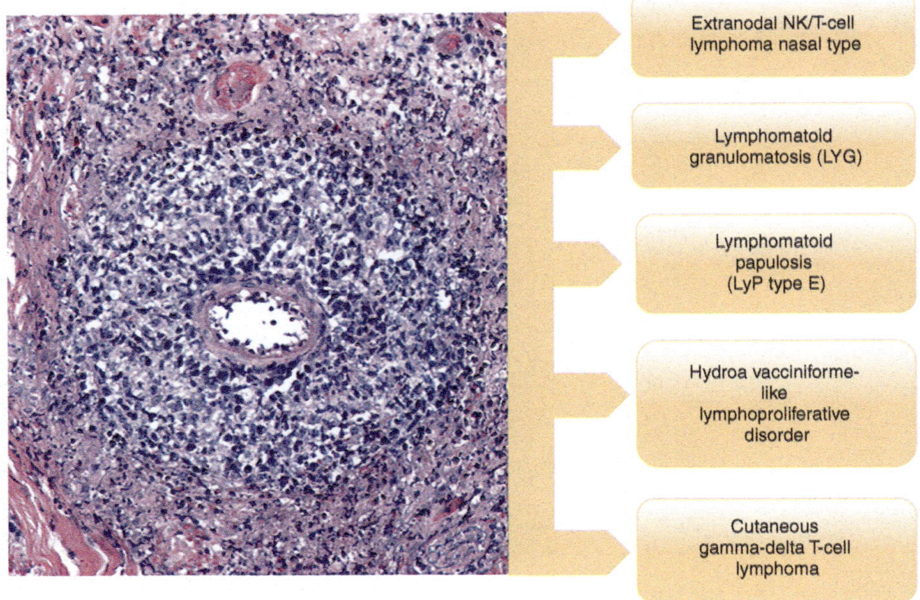

Fig. 33.8 Differential diagnosis of atypical lymphoid infiltrate with angiocentrism

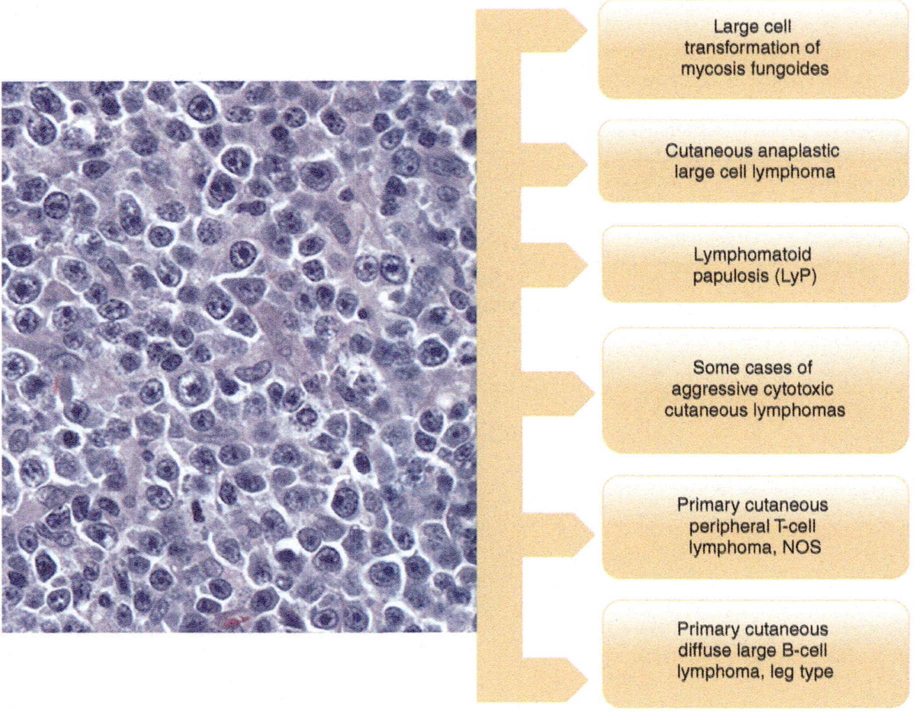

Fig. 33.9 Differential diagnosis of atypical cutaneous large cell lymphoid infiltrate

Disease Definition

- Extranodal NK/T-cell lymphoma, nasal type is an aggressive, primarily extranodal lymphoma characterized by vascular destruction, necrosis, cytotoxic phenotype, and association with Epstein-Barr virus (EBV). Most cases are of NK cell origin, but a subset shows a cytotoxic T-cell phenotype (Table 33.1).

Epidemiology

- More frequent in Asian and native Latin American populations.
- Usually adults. More common in males than females.
- May occur in the setting of immunosuppression (e.g., posttransplant).

Preferential Sites of Involvement

- Upper aerodigestive tract: nasal cavity (prototypic), nasopharynx, paranasal sinuses, and palate ("lethal midline granuloma").
- The skin, soft tissue, gastrointestinal tract, and testis are common sites of involvement.
- Bone marrow involvement is uncommon.
- Secondary lymph node involvement is rare. The WHO 2016 classification recognizes a subtype of nodal peripheral T-cell lymphoma unspecified (PTCL) cases as node-based EBV-positive PTCL. Unlike extranodal NK/T-cell lymphoma, nasal type, these PTCL cases lack angioinvasion and necrosis.

Clinical Features

- Skin lesions are usually nodular, and ulceration is common (Fig. 33.1). Erythematous or violaceous plaques and tumors.
- If nasal involvement: symptoms of nasal obstruction or epistaxis. Eventually, extensive midfacial destructive lesions with large ulcers (Fig. 33.2).
- High-stage disease (involvement of multiple sites) at presentation is common.
- B symptoms may be present.
- Hemophagocytic syndrome may occur.
- *Less common presentations*: Cutaneous presentation with subtle macular lesions or with patches resembling mycosis fungoides has been reported. Persistent prominent facial swelling. Intestinal lesions may present with perforation. Other involved sites may present with mass lesions.

Histomorphology

- *Pattern*: Dense diffuse lymphoid infiltrate in the dermis with frequent pannicular extension (Fig. 33.3). Angiocentric and angiodestructive pattern is characteristic (Fig. 33.4), though not always present in every biopsy. Ulceration and necrosis are common (Table 33.2). Apoptosis is frequent.
- *Less common patterns*: Epidermotropism and Pautrier microabscesses may be seen. Interface change at the dermal-epidermal junction. Vascular fibrinoid changes without angioinvasive infiltration. Pseudoepitheliomatous hyperplasia.
- *Neoplastic cells*: Broad cytologic spectrum (small-, intermediate-sized, large or anaplastic). Admixture of small and large cells is common. Nuclei may be irregularly folded or elongated. Usually granular chromatin (but vesicular in large cells). Inconspicuous to small nucleoli. Moderate cytoplasm (often pale or clear). Frequent mitotic figures.
- *Reactive cells*: Neutrophils are common if ulceration is present. Some cases may have mixed inflammatory infiltrate (small lymphocytes, plasma cells, eosinophils, and histiocytes) or granulomatous inflammation.

Immunophenotype

- Most typical pattern: CD2+, CD3+, CD56+, and EBV+. Positive cytotoxic proteins (TIA-1, granzyme B, perforin) (Fig. 33.5). Frequently positive: CD43, CD45RO, HLA-DR, and CD25. CD7 and CD30 may be expressed (Fig. 33.6). Frequently negative: CD4, CD8, CD5, betaF1, CD16, and CD57.
- As the name indicates, extranodal NK/T-cell lymphoma, nasal type may be of NK-cell origin (more common) or T-cell origin. Depending on the cell of origin, there may be some differences in immunophenotype (Fig. 33.7).
- Unlike T cells, NK cells lack surface CD3. Therefore, NK cells are CD3-negative by flow cytometry (since flow generally analyzes surface membrane proteins). However, NK cells express the epsilon chain of CD3 within the cytoplasm. Since the epitope of CD3 antibody targets the epsilon chain, NK cells stain positive with CD3 immunohistochemistry.
- While CD56 expression is generally present, some cases of cytotoxic T-cell origin may be CD56-negative. Therefore, in the setting of angiocentrism and cytotoxic phenotype, EBV in situ hybridization (EBER) should be obtained.
- If an atypical infiltrate is both CD56- and EBV-negative, the process is likely not extranodal NK/T-cell lymphoma, nasal type.

Genetics

- As the name indicates, extranodal NK/T-cell lymphoma, nasal type may be of NK-cell origin or T-cell origin. Depending on the cell of origin, PCR results will be different. NK-cell origin (most common type) will be associated with negative T-cell clonality (germline configuration). Monoclonal rearrangement of T-cell receptor genes occurs in a minority of cases (cytotoxic T-cell origin).
- EBV in situ hybridization (EBER) is positive.

Prognosis

- Variable but generally poor. Prolonged survival reported in rare cases.
- 5-year survival: <30–40%.
- Adverse risk factors: high titer of circulating EBV DNA, advanced stage disease, unfavorable International Prognostic Index (IPI), invasion of bone and skin, presence of EBV-positive cells in the bone marrow.

Differential Diagnosis

- Angioinvasion may be a feature of aggressive lymphomas, such as extranodal NK/T-cell lymphoma nasal type, lymphomatoid granulomatosis, and gamma-delta T-cell lymphoma (Table 33.3). However, some cases of lymphomatoid papulosis show angioinvasion (LyP type E) (Fig. 33.8).
- Hydroa vacciniforme-like T-cell lymphoproliferative disorder is also EBV-positive but occurs in children and shows photo-distributed lesions at presentation.
- CD56 expression is not specific for extranodal NK/T-cell lymphoma, nasal type and may occur in other processes, including gamma-delta T-cell lymphoma and some cases of lymphomatoid papulosis.
- Cases with involvement of subcutaneous tissue may resemble subcutaneous panniculitis-like T-cell lymphoma (SPTCL). While both are composed of cytotoxic TIA1-positive cells, SPTCL is CD56-negative and EBV-negative and lacks dermal involvement.
- Extranodal NK/T-cell lymphoma nasal type may show a broad cytologic spectrum (small-, intermediate-sized and/or large). Cases composed of large cells may cause diagnostic confusion with other lymphomas, including indolent ones such as anaplastic large cell lymphoma (Fig. 33.9). Comprehensive immunophenotyping and EBV testing are essential for proper classification of cytotoxic infiltrates.

Table 33.2 Differential diagnosis of ulceration

Lymphomas/lymphoproliferative disorders	Benign dermatoses/pseudolymphomas
Tumor-stage mycosis fungoides	Pityriasis lichenoides et varioliformis acuta (PLEVA)
CD30-positive lymphoproliferative disorders: lymphomatoid papulosis, cutaneous anaplastic large cell lymphoma	Inflamed molluscum contagiosum
Primary cutaneous aggressive epidermotropic CD8-positive cytotoxic T-cell lymphoma	Herpesvirus infection
Cutaneous gamma-delta T-cell lymphoma	Primary syphilis
Extranodal NK/T-cell lymphoma, nasal type	Leishmania infection

Table 33.3 Differential diagnosis of an atypical angiocentric lymphoid infiltrate in relation to Epstein-Barr virus (EBV) and immunophenotype

EBV	Angiocentric process	Immunophenotype
Positive (+)	Extranodal NK/T-cell lymphoma nasal type	T cell or NK cell
	Hydroa vacciniforme-like lymphoproliferative disorder	T cell or NK cell
	Lymphomatoid granulomatosis (LYG)	B cell
Negative (−)	Cutaneous gamma-delta T-cell lymphoma	Gamma-delta T cell
	Lymphomatoid papulosis (LyP type E)	CD30-positive T cell

Table 33.4 Differential diagnosis of CD56 expression in the skin

Lymphoid/hematopoietic	Nonlymphoid
Rare cases of mycosis fungoides	Merkel cell carcinoma
Rare cases of CD30-positive lymphoproliferative disorders	Schwannoma
Cutaneous gamma-delta T-cell lymphoma	Neuroblastoma
Extranodal NK/T-cell lymphoma, nasal type	Cellular neurothekeoma
Blastic plasmacytoid dendritic cell neoplasm (CD4+/CD56+ hematodermic neoplasm)	Plexiform fibrohistiocytic tumor
Some cases of myeloid leukemia cutis	Metastatic renal cell carcinoma
Most cases of plasma cell myeloma	Damaged muscle fibers

Table 33.5 Lymphoproliferative diseases with frequent EBV expression

Extranodal NK/T-cell lymphoma, nasal type
EBV+ diffuse large B-cell lymphoma
Systemic EBV+ T-cell lymphoma of childhood
Hydroa vacciniforme-like lymphoproliferative disorder
Lymphomatoid granulomatosis (LYG)
EBV+ mucocutaneous ulcer
Aggressive NK-cell leukemia
Posttransplant lymphoproliferative disorders
Plasmablastic lymphoma
Primary effusion lymphoma
Diffuse large B-cell lymphoma associated with chronic inflammation
Angioimmunoblastic T-cell lymphoma
Classical Hodgkin lymphoma
Burkitt lymphoma

Table 33.6 When to check EBV in situ hybridization (EBER)

Presence of angioinvasion/angiodestruction
Presence of extensive, infarct-like necrosis
Infiltrate with prominent CD56 expression
Infiltrate with cytotoxic immunophenotype
Patient with both skin and lung lesions
Young patients with facial edema and lesions on sun-exposed skin
Elderly patients
History of congenital or acquired immunodeficiency
History of transplant

Pearls and Pitfalls

1. Ulceration is seen in some cases of advanced, tumor-stage mycosis fungoides (MF). The presence of ulceration at initial presentation would suggest a non-MF process.
2. Some pseudolymphomas may also demonstrate ulceration. These include pityriasis lichenoides and infectious processes, such as leishmaniasis and inflamed molluscum contagiosum.
3. If ulceration is not seen in a skin biopsy, it does not necessarily mean that the patient does not have ulcerated lesions elsewhere, since dermatologists often avoid biopsying lesions with secondary changes. Careful correlation of clinical and histopathologic findings is essential.
4. Angiocentrism is not always present in every biopsy of an angioinvasive lymphoid process. Clues for the diagnosis would include infarct-like necrosis and cytotoxic immunophenotype. EBV in situ hybridization (EBER) and careful clinical pathologic correlation would be essential for proper classification.
5. Infiltration and destruction of blood vessel walls is generally not a feature of intravascular lymphomas (atypical lymphocytes within vessel lumens).
6. The threshold of positivity is variable for different markers. For example, for anaplastic large cell lymphoma (ALCL; one of the cutaneous CD30-positive lymphoproliferative disorders), CD30 must be positive in at least 75% of atypical cells (i.e., even if 60% of an infiltrate marks with CD30, that level of staining is not sufficient for ALCL, and other entities should be considered in the differential diagnosis). A high cutoff is also used for CD56 (i.e., if only a small subset of cells stain with CD56 in a lymphoid infiltrate, that process is considered CD56-negative) (Table 33.4).
7. While several lymphomas may express EBV, the identification of EBV may or may not be part of the minimum diagnostic criteria for a particular lymphoma (Tables 33.5 and 33.6). For example, Burkitt lymphoma is frequently EBV-positive, but if a case of Burkitt lymphoma were EBV-negative, this would not change the diagnosis. In contrast, a nasal T-cell lymphoma that is CD3-positive and CD56-negative but negative for EBV would not be classified as extranodal NK/T-cell lymphoma nasal type.
8. In situ hybridization for Epstein-Barr encoded RNA (EBER) is the most reliable method to demonstrate the presence of EBV. Immunohistochemical stains for LMP1 are inconsistent.

Suggested Reading

Li S, Feng X, Li T, et al. Extranodal NK/T-cell lymphoma, nasal type: a report of 73 cases at MD Anderson Cancer Center. Am J Surg Pathol. 2013;37(1):14–23.

Swerdlow SH, Campo E, Pileri SA, et al. The 2016 revision of the WHO classification of lymphoid neoplasms. Blood. 2016;127(20):2375–90.

Swerdlow SH, et al., editors. WHO classification of tumors of hematopoietic and lymphoid tissues. Lyon: IARC; 2008.

Willemze R, Jaffe ES, Burg G, et al. WHO-EORTC classification for cutaneous lymphomas. Blood. 2005;105(10):3768–85.

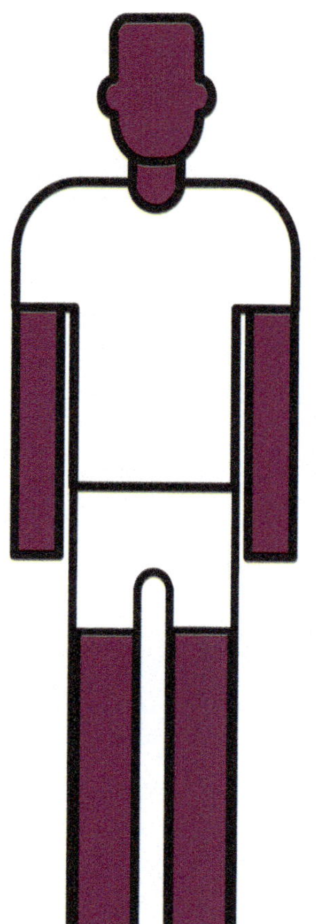

Fig. 34.1 Hydroa vacciniforme-like lymphoproliferative disorder is a rare EBV-positive condition that usually presents with necrotic lesions on sun-exposed skin of young patients

Table 34.1 Key Facts

Definition
Hydroa vacciniforme-like lymphoproliferative disorder is a primarily cutaneous disorder of polyclonal or (most often) monoclonal T cells or NK cells with a broad spectrum of clinical aggressiveness and disease progression. Classic HV, severe HV, and HV-like T-cell lymphoma constitute a continuous spectrum
Prototypic clinical presentation
Children and adolescents. Asians and Native Americans from Central and South America. Papulovesicular eruption with ulceration and scarring on sun-exposed skin. Edema and involvement of non-exposed skin in more severe cases
Histopathologic findings
Mild to moderate superficial and mid-dermal lymphoid infiltrate with variable deep dermal/pannicular extension. Perivascular and periadnexal accentuation. Angiodestruction, epidermal necrosis, and ulceration are common
Most common immunophenotype: EBV-positive cytotoxic T- or NK-cell dermal infiltrate. CD30 may be positive
Prognosis
Variable clinical course

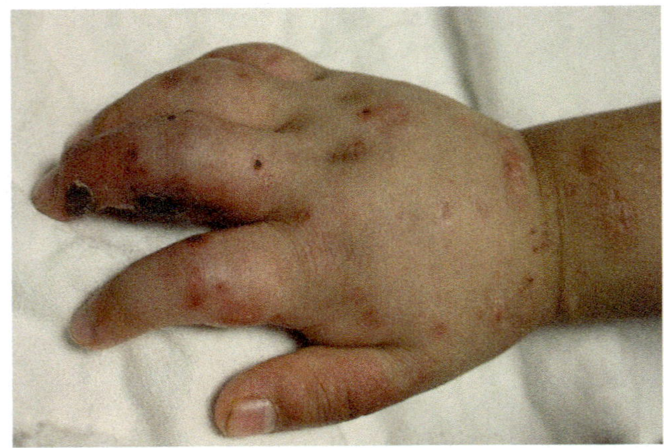

Fig. 34.2 Edema and multiple skin lesions with ulceration on sun-exposed skin of a young patient with hydroa vacciniforme-like lymphoproliferative disorder

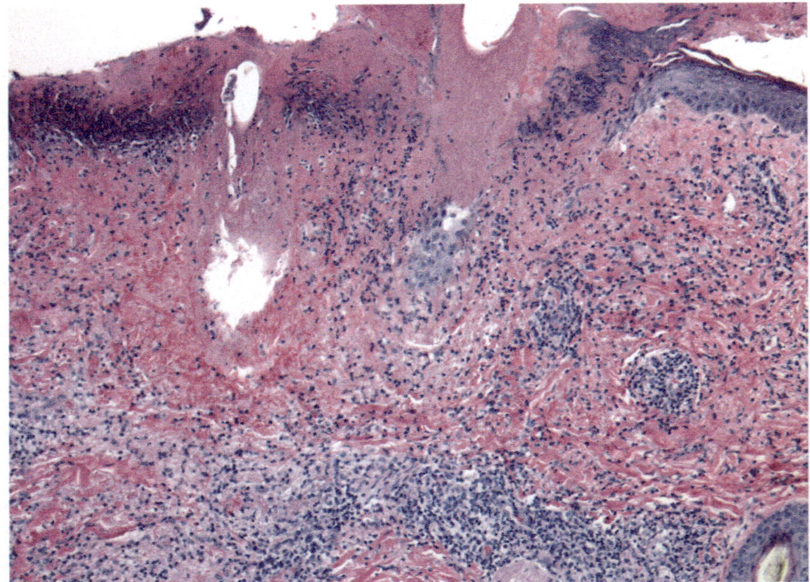

Fig. 34.3 Skin biopsy of hydroa vacciniforme-like lymphoproliferative disorder showing abrupt, full-thickness epidermal necrosis and dermal lymphoid infiltrate

Fig. 34.4 Hydroa vacciniforme-like lymphoproliferative disorder. The atypical lymphoid infiltrate shows angiocentrism with infiltration of a blood vessel wall

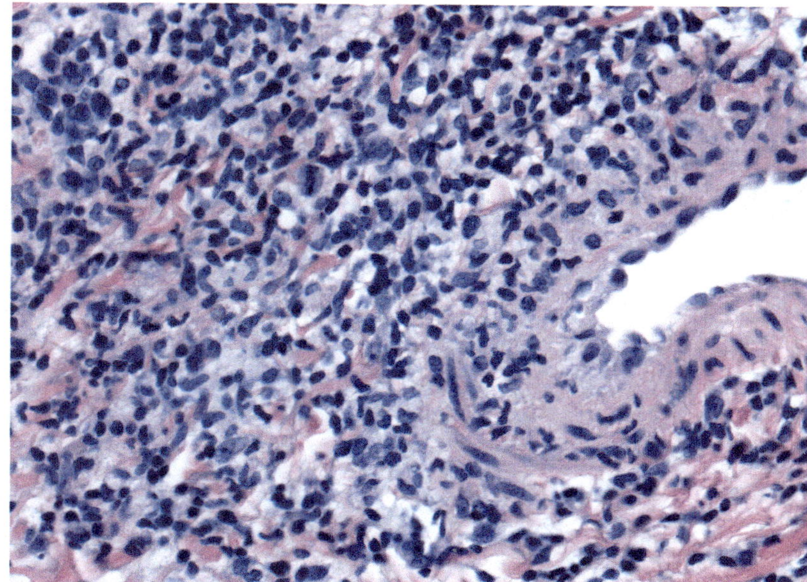

Fig. 34.5 Hydroa vacciniforme-like lymphoproliferative disorder. The atypical lymphoid infiltrate is angiocentric and angiodestructive. Hemorrhage, fibrin deposition, and necrosis are present

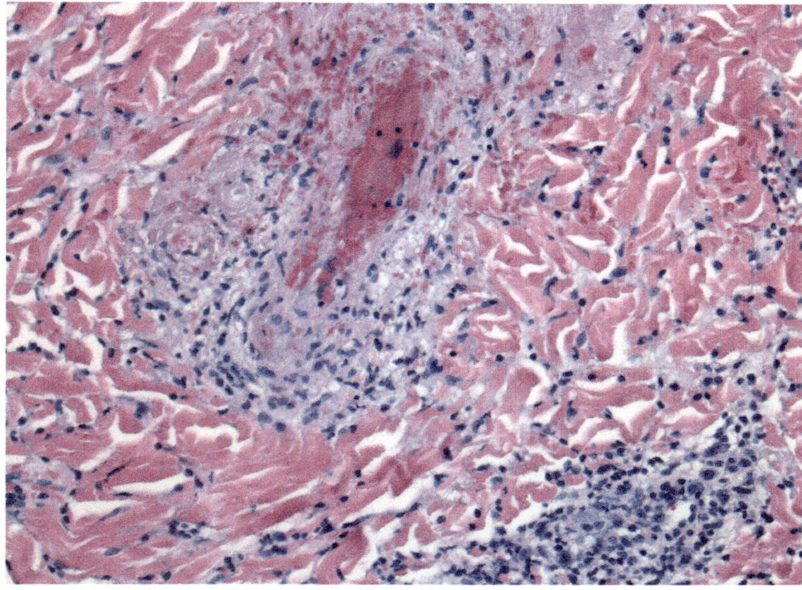

Fig. 34.6 Hydroa vacciniforme-like lymphoproliferative disorder. The atypical dermal lymphoid infiltrate is EBV-positive (Epstein-Barr virus in situ hybridization)

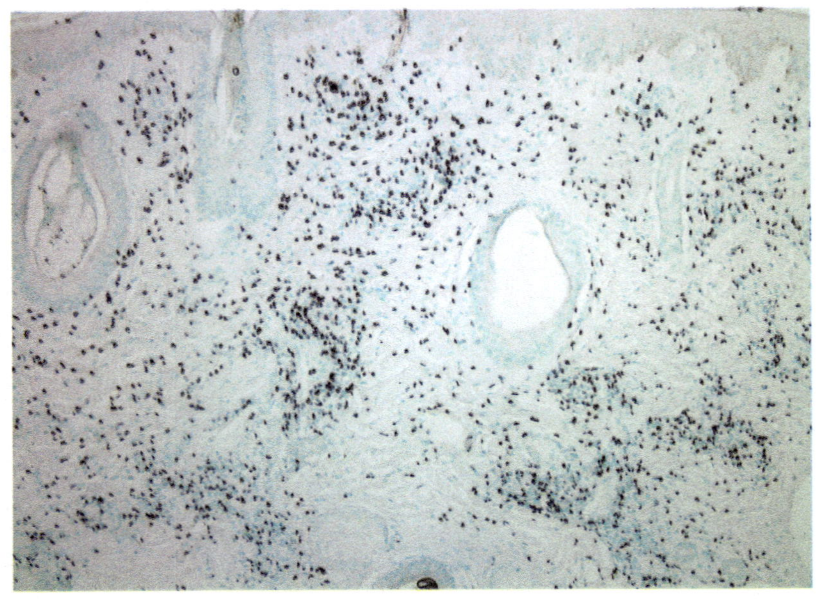

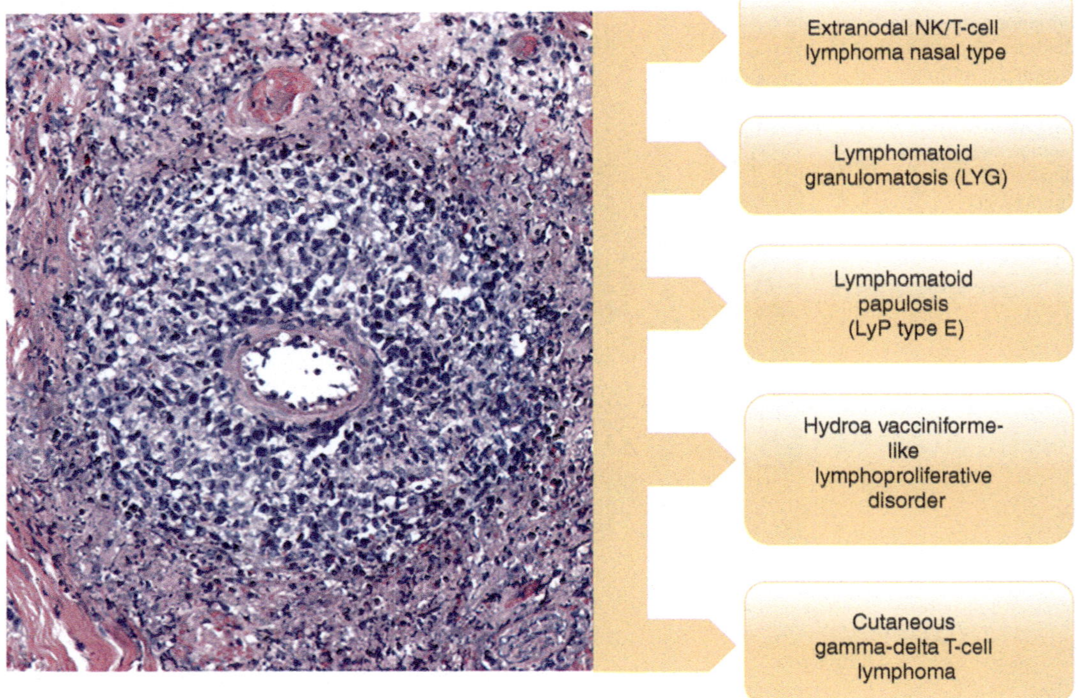

Fig. 34.7 Differential diagnosis of atypical lymphoid infiltrate with angiocentrism

Disease Definition

- Hydroa vacciniforme-like lymphoproliferative disorder is part of the group of EBV (Epstein-Barr virus)-positive T-cell and NK-cell lymphoproliferative diseases of childhood. It is a form of cutaneous chronic active EBV infection and is associated with a risk of developing systemic lymphoma.
- Hydroa vacciniforme-like lymphoproliferative disorder is a primarily cutaneous disorder of polyclonal or (most often) monoclonal T cells or NK cells with a broad spectrum of clinical aggressiveness. The clinical course is usually long. Fever, hepatosplenomegaly, and lymphadenopathy may develop. Classic hydroa vacciniforme (HV), severe HV, and HV-like T-cell lymphoma constitute a continuous spectrum (Table 34.1).

Epidemiology

- Asians and Native Americans from Central and South America. Children and adolescents (rare in adults). Slight male predominance.
- Age range at diagnosis: 1–15 years.

Preferential Sites of Involvement

- Sun-exposed and non-exposed skin. Early disease: face, earlobes, and dorsal hands (Fig. 34.1). It can become generalized with advanced disease.

Clinical Features

- Papulovesicular eruption usually proceeding to ulceration and scarring (varioliform scars). Umbilication and crust formation. Broad spectrum of clinical severity.
- Classic HV pattern: indolent clinical course with localized lesions on sun-exposed skin and no systemic symptoms. While spontaneous remission and clearing after photoprotec-tion may occur, many cases show prolonged course with remissions and recurrences over time and variable progression to more severe disease. Seasonal variation (spring and summer recurrences).
- More severe disease: extensive skin lesions, including in non-exposed areas, and edema (Fig. 34.2). Systemic symptoms may occur and include fever, lymphadenopathy, and hepatosplenomegaly.
- *Less common presentations*: tumors, periorbital swelling, severe mosquito bite allergy, adults.

Histomorphology

- *Pattern*: Epidermis: reticular degeneration, spongiotic vesiculation, and abrupt full-thickness necrosis (Fig. 34.3). Mild to moderate superficial and mid-dermal lymphoid infiltrate with variable deep dermal/pannicular extension. Perivascular and periadnexal accentuation. Angiodestruction, necrosis, and ulceration are common (Figs. 34.4 and 34.5).
- *Neoplastic cells*: Usually small- to intermediate-sized lymphoid cells. Cytologic atypia is variable and may not be significant.
- *Reactive cells*: Scattered histiocytes. Neutrophils in the presence of ulceration.

Immunophenotype

- *Neoplastic cells*: T- or NK-cell dermal infiltrate positive with EBER (Epstein-Barr virus encoded small RNA) in situ hybridization (variable number of positive cells; Fig. 34.6). LMP1 is generally negative. Variable phenotype: usually CD8-positive cytotoxic T cell, often NK cell (CD56-positive) or gamma-delta T cell, and occasionally CD4-positive. May be CD4−/CD8−. CD2+, CD3+, TIA1+. CD30 expression is common.
- *Reactive cells*: Scattered CD68-positive histiocytes. TIA-1 marks cytotoxic lymphocytes as well as neutrophils.

Genetics

- Monoclonal rearrangement of T-cell receptor genes in a subset of cases (germline configuration in NK-cell cases).

Prognosis

- Variable. Clinical course often prolonged with variable disease progression.
- Adverse risk factors: systemic involvement.

Differential Diagnosis

- The group of EBV-positive T-cell and NK-cell lymphoproliferative diseases of childhood shows significant overlap in histomorphologic features. Therefore, clinical correlation is necessary to differentiate hydroa vacciniforme-like lymphoproliferative disorder from other conditions in this group, such as severe mosquito bite allergy. Systemic EBV-positive T-cell lymphoma of childhood has a very fulminant clinical course and is usually associated with hemophagocytic syndrome. Other angiocentric and/or EBV-positive conditions should also be considered (Table 34.2).
- Because CD30 is often positive and ulceration is common in hydroa vacciniforme-like lymphoproliferative disorder, some cases may resemble lymphomatoid papulosis (LyP), though the degree of cytologic atypia is less prominent. Careful clinical correlation and EBV in situ hybridization are advised.

Table 34.2 Differential diagnosis of an atypical angiocentric lymphoid infiltrate in relation to Epstein-Barr virus (EBV) and immunophenotype

EBV	Angiocentric process	Immunophenotype
Positive (+)	Extranodal NK/T-cell lymphoma nasal type	T cell or NK cell
	Hydroa vacciniforme-like lymphoproliferative disorder	T cell or NK cell
	Lymphomatoid granulomatosis (LYG)	B cell
Negative (−)	Cutaneous gamma-delta T-cell lymphoma	Gamma-delta T cell
	Lymphomatoid papulosis (LyP type E)	CD30-positive T cell

Table 34.3 When to check EBV in situ hybridization (EBER)

Presence of angioinvasion/angiodestruction
Presence of extensive, infarct-like necrosis
Infiltrate with prominent CD56 expression
Infiltrate with cytotoxic immunophenotype
Patient with both skin and lung lesions
Young patients with facial edema and lesions on sun-exposed skin
Elderly patients
History of congenital or acquired immunodeficiency
History of transplant

Table 34.4 Lymphoproliferative diseases with frequent EBV expression

Extranodal NK/T-cell lymphoma, nasal type
EBV+ diffuse large B-cell lymphoma
Systemic EBV+ T-cell lymphoma of childhood
Hydroa vacciniforme-like lymphoproliferative disorder
Lymphomatoid granulomatosis (LYG)
EBV+ mucocutaneous ulcer
Aggressive NK-cell leukemia
Posttransplant lymphoproliferative disorders
Plasmablastic lymphoma
Primary effusion lymphoma
Diffuse large B-cell lymphoma associated with chronic inflammation
Angioimmunoblastic T-cell lymphoma
Classical Hodgkin lymphoma
Burkitt lymphoma

Pearls and Pitfalls

1. Angiocentrism is not always identifiable in a biopsy of an angioinvasive lymphoid process (Fig. 34.7). Clues for angiodestruction would include infarct-like necrosis. EBV in situ hybridization and careful clinical pathologic correlation would be essential for proper classification.
2. Since EBV expression is an uncommon finding in most geographic regions, most laboratories do not routinely check EBV in situ hybridization (EBER). Therefore, it is important to determine scenarios to consider EBV testing (Table 34.3).
3. Infiltration and destruction of blood vessel walls (angiodestruction) is generally not a feature of intravascular lymphomas (atypical lymphocytes within vessel lumens).
4. While several lymphoproliferative conditions may express EBV, the identification of EBV may or may not be part of the minimum diagnostic criteria for a particular disease. For example, Burkitt lymphoma is frequently EBV-positive, but if a case of Burkitt lymphoma were EBV-negative, this would not change the diagnosis. In contrast, a nasal T-cell lymphoma that is CD3-positive and CD56-negative but negative for EBV would not be classified as extranodal NK/T-cell lymphoma nasal type (Table 34.4).
5. In situ hybridization for Epstein-Barr encoded RNA (EBER) is the most reliable method to demonstrate the presence of EBV. Immunohistochemical stains for EBV yield variable and inconsistent results.

Suggested Reading

Magaña M, Massone C, Magaña P, Cerroni L. Clinicopathologic features of hydroa vacciniforme-like lymphoma: a series of 9 patients. Am J Dermatopathol. 2016;38(1):20–5.

Quintanilla-Martinez L, Ridaura C, Nagl F, Sáez-de-Ocariz M, Durán-McKinster C, Ruiz-Maldonado R, Alderete G, Grube P, Lome-Maldonado C, Bonzheim I, Fend F. Hydroa vacciniforme-like lymphoma: a chronic EBV+ lymphoproliferative disorder with risk to develop a systemic lymphoma. Blood. 2013;122(18):3101–10.

Swerdlow SH, Campo E, Pileri SA, et al. The 2016 revision of the WHO classification of lymphoid neoplasms. Blood. 2016;127(20):2375–90.

Swerdlow SH, et al., editors. WHO classification of tumors of hematopoietic and lymphoid tissues. Lyon: IARC; 2008.

Swerdlow SH, et al., editors. WHO Classification of tumors of hematopoietic and lymphoid tissues (Revised 4th edition). Lyon: IARC; 2017.

Willemze R, Jaffe ES, Burg G, et al. WHO-EORTC classification for cutaneous lymphomas. Blood. 2005;105(10):3768–85.

Table 35.1 Key Facts

Definition
Adult T-cell leukemia/lymphoma (ATLL) is a mature T-cell neoplasm caused by the human retrovirus HTLV-1
Prototypic clinical presentation
Variable (erythematous patches, plaques, multipapular, tumors/nodules, erythroderma, or purpuric). Skin involvement may be seen in different clinical subtypes of ATLL
Histopathologic findings
Variable with different degrees of infiltration by pleomorphic neoplastic cells (epidermal, dermal and/or pannicular). Frequent epidermotropism
Most common immunophenotype: CD3+, CD4+, CD8-, CD2+, CD5+, CD7-, CD25+, CD45RO+, CD20-, ALK-, variable CD30 expression
Prognosis
Variable (short survival in acute and lymphomatous clinical subtypes but protracted clinical course in chronic and smoldering forms)

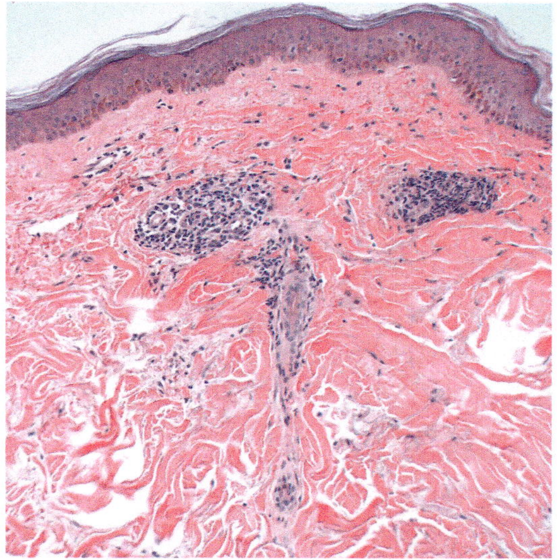

Fig. 35.1 Low-power magnification of smoldering variant of adult T-cell leukemia/lymphoma with perivascular dermal lymphoid infiltrate

© Springer Nature Switzerland AG 2019
A. Subtil, *Diagnosis of Cutaneous Lymphoid Infiltrates*,
https://doi.org/10.1007/978-3-030-11654-5_35

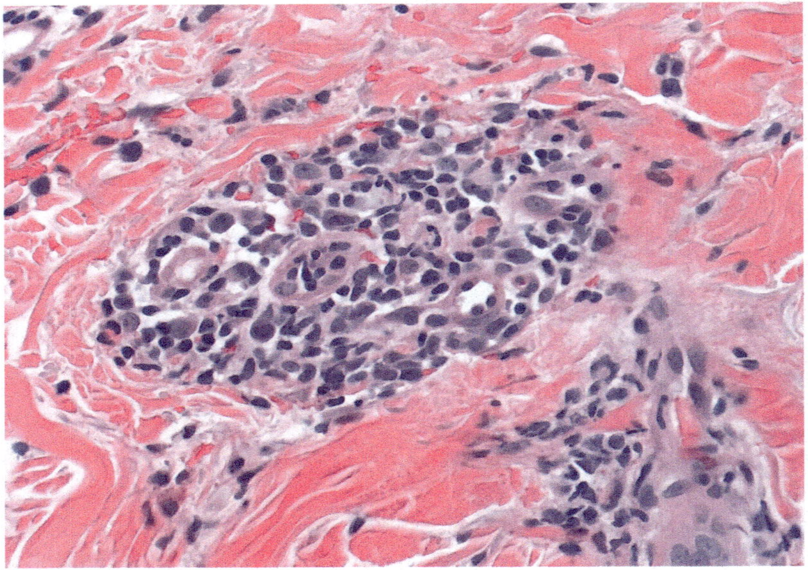

Fig. 35.2 Cutaneous adult T-cell leukemia/lymphoma with pleomorphic neoplastic lymphoid cells

Disease Definition

- Adult T-cell leukemia/lymphoma (ATLL) is a mature T-cell neoplasm caused by the retrovirus human T-cell leukemia virus type 1 (HTLV-1) (Table 35.1).

Epidemiology

- Endemic in certain geographic regions (Japan, Caribbean, and parts of Central Africa and South America) but rare elsewhere.
- Disease distribution related to prevalence of HTLV-1 virus in the population.
- Occurs only in adults.
- Slight male predominance.

Preferential Sites of Involvement

- ATLL is usually widely disseminated (lymph nodes, peripheral blood, and extranodal sites).
- The skin is the most common extralymphatic involved organ (>50% of cases).
- Skin lesions are usually a manifestation of widely disseminated disease.
- Smoldering ATLL is a slowly progressive variant that may have only skin involvement.

Clinical Features

- Four clinical subtypes of ATLL depending on severity and organ involvement: smoldering (no lymphocytosis but >5% circulating neoplastic cells; frequent skin lesions), chronic (frequently associated with exfoliative skin rash and lymphocytosis), acute (leukemic phase with marked leukocytosis and frequent hepatosplenomegaly, lymphadenopathy, hypercalcemia, and skin rash), and lymphomatous (prominent lymphadenopathy but without blood involvement). Progression to acute phase may occur over time in a subset of patients.
- Skin involvement may be seen in all clinical forms of ATLL, and staging workup is necessary for subtype classification.
- Variable clinical morphology. Most common: plaques, multipapular, and/or tumors/nodules.
- *Less common presentations*: erythematous patches, erythroderma, or purpuric.

Histomorphology

- *Pattern*: variable with different degrees of infiltration by pleomorphic neoplastic cells (epidermal, dermal, and/or pannicular).

Frequent epidermotropism (including Pautrier microabscesses). Skin lesions in the smoldering variant may show sparse perivascular dermal infiltrates (Fig. 35.1).
- *Neoplastic cells*: highly pleomorphic lymphoid cells with intermediate-sized to large nuclei. Marked nuclear irregularity (multilobed flower cells) and prominent nucleoli are frequent (Fig. 35.2).
- *Less common patterns*: small lymphocytes with slight nuclear abnormalities. Follicular mucinosis.
- *Reactive cells*: usually sparse inflammatory background but may see eosinophils, small lymphocytes and/or a few scattered histiocytes.

Immunophenotype

- *Neoplastic cells*: CD3+, CD4+, CD8−, CD2+, CD5+, CD7−, CD25+, CD45RO+, CD20−, ALK−, and variable CD30 expression. Rare cases may be CD4−/CD8+ or CD4+/CD8+.

Genetics

- Monoclonal rearrangement of T-cell receptor genes in the majority of cases.
- Monoclonal integration of HTLV-1 in neoplastic cells.

Prognosis

- Variable (short survival in acute and lymphomatous clinical subtypes, but protracted clinical course in chronic and smoldering forms).
- Adverse risk factors: clinical subtype, age, performance status, and hypercalcemia.

Differential Diagnosis

- ATLL shows frequent epidermotropism (including Pautrier microabscesses) and may histologically resemble mycosis fungoides and Sézary syndrome. In addition, some cases of ATLL may show dense infiltrates of large lymphoid cells with CD30 expression and may mimic cutaneous CD30-positive lymphoproliferative disorders (anaplastic large cell lymphoma and lymphomatoid papulosis). Careful clinical correlation and HTLV-1 testing in patients from endemic regions are necessary.

Pearls and Pitfalls
1. After more than 20 years of persistent viral infection, 5% of carriers develop HTLV-1-related diseases: neoplastic (adult T-cell leukemia/lymphoma in 2.5% of carriers) and nonneoplastic (tropical spastic paraparesis/HTLV-1-associated myelopathy; infective dermatitis; uveitis; pneumonitis).
2. Immunosuppression is common in ATLL, and opportunistic infections may occur.

Suggested Reading

Elder DE, Massi D, Scolyer RA. In: Willemze R, editor. WHO classification of skin tumors. 4th ed. Lyon: IARC; 2018.

Gonçalves DU, Proietti FA, Ribas JG, Araújo MG, Pinheiro SR, Guedes AC, Carneiro-Proietti AB. Epidemiology, treatment, and prevention of human T-cell leukemia virus type 1-associated diseases. Clin Microbiol Rev. 2010;23(3):577–89.

Swerdlow SH, Campo E, Harris NL, Jaffe ES, Pileri SA, Stein H, Thiele J, editors. WHO classification of tumours of haematopoietic and lymphoid tissues (revised 4th edition). Lyon: IARC; 2017.

Willemze R, Jaffe ES, Burg G, et al. WHO-EORTC classification for cutaneous lymphomas. Blood. 2005;105(10):3768–85.

Primary Cutaneous Acral CD8-Positive T-Cell Lymphoma (Indolent CD8-Positive Lymphoid Proliferation of the Ear)

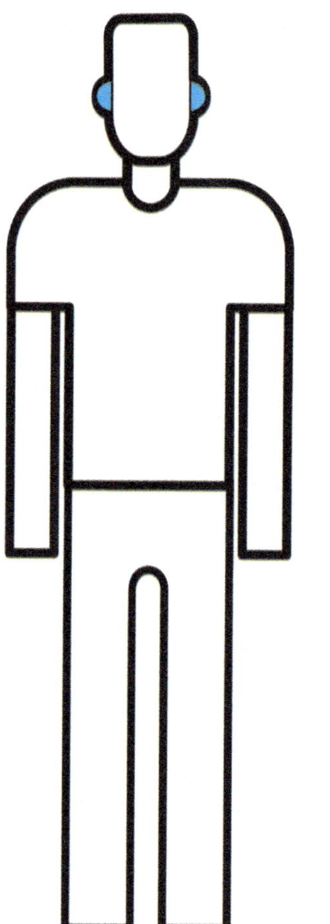

Table 36.1 Key facts

Definition	
Primary cutaneous acral CD8-positive T-cell lymphoma (indolent CD8-positive lymphoid proliferation of the ear) is a rare, nonaggressive lymphoproliferative disorder classically presenting with a solitary lesion on the ear or another acral site	
Prototypic clinical presentation	
Slowly growing or stable asymptomatic papule, plaque, or nodule on the ear (occasionally bilateral or another acral site). Ulceration is absent	
Histopathologic findings	
Dense diffuse dermal lymphoid infiltrate with variable pannicular extension. Grenz zone between infiltrate and epithelium. Absence of epidermotropism, folliculotropism, ulceration, necrosis, interface change, prominent mitotic activity, or angiodestruction. Most common immunophenotype: CD3+, CD4-, CD8+, CD2+, CD5+/−, CD7+/−, CD20-, CD30-, CD56-, CD45RA-, betaF1+, TIA1+, granzyme B-, EBV (EBER)-, and PD1-. Low proliferative index (Ki-67 <30%)	
Prognosis	
Excellent (5-year survival of 100%)	

Fig. 36.1 Primary cutaneous acral CD8-positive T-cell lymphoma (indolent CD8-positive lymphoid proliferation of the ear) is a rare lymphoproliferative disorder classically presenting with a solitary nodular lesion on the ear (occasionally bilateral)

© Springer Nature Switzerland AG 2019

A. Subtil, *Diagnosis of Cutaneous Lymphoid Infiltrates*,

https://doi.org/10.1007/978-3-030-11654-5_36

Fig. 36.2 Primary cutaneous acral CD8-positive T-cell lymphoma (indolent CD8-positive lymphoid proliferation of the ear). Low-power magnification of a biopsy of a solitary nodular lesion on the ear showing a dense diffuse dermal-based lymphoid infiltrate

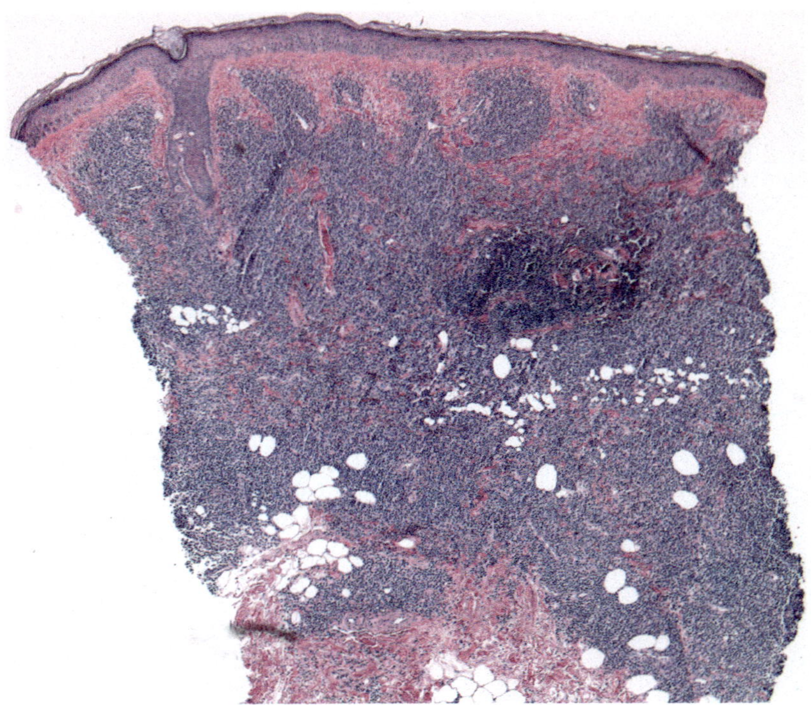

Fig. 36.3 Grenz zone of uninvolved epidermis and adnexa

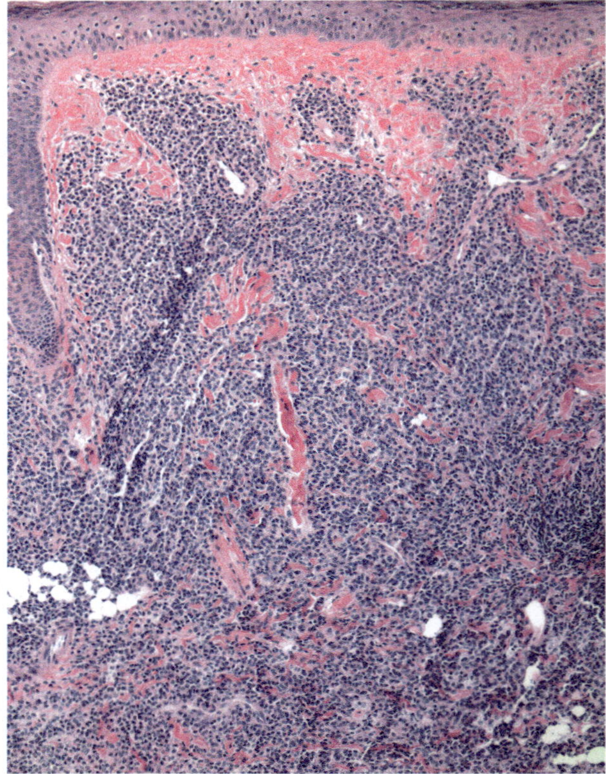

Fig. 36.4 The infiltrate does not involve the epidermis (epidermotropism or ulceration is not present)

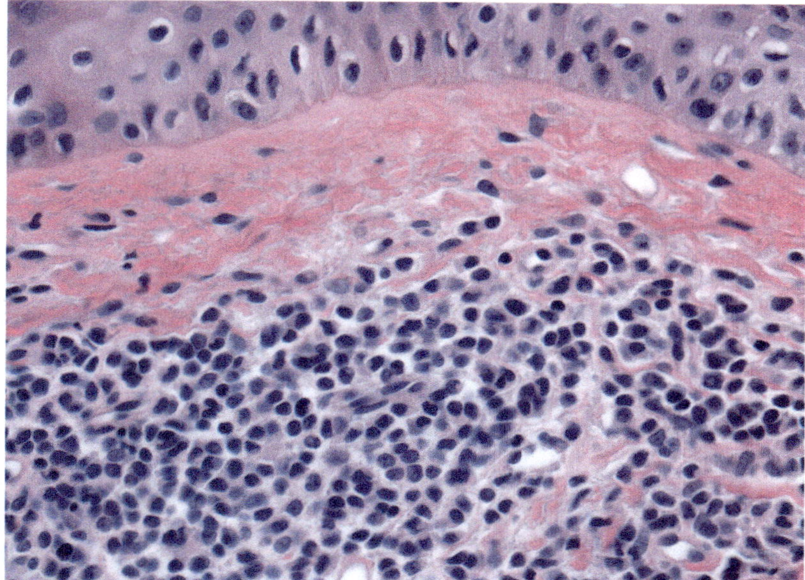

Fig. 36.5 The infiltrate does not involve hair follicles (folliculotropism is not present)

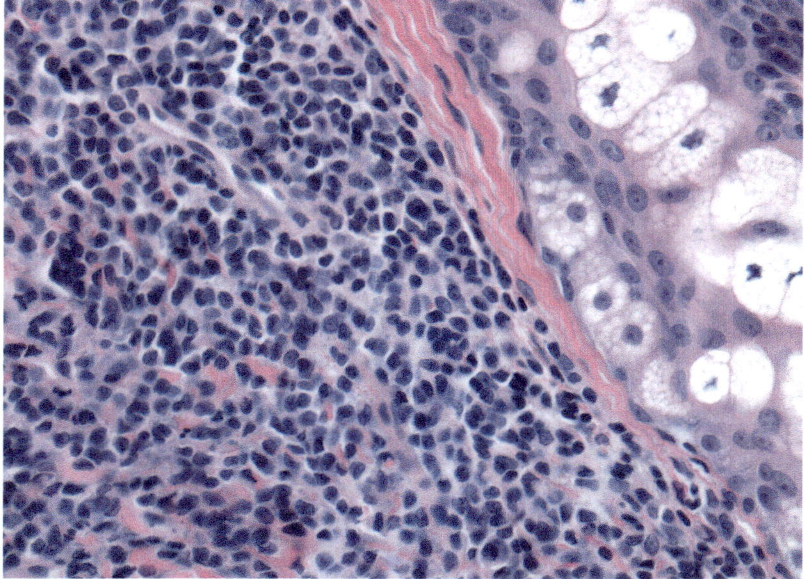

Fig. 36.6
Cytomorphology of primary cutaneous acral CD8-positive T-cell lymphoma (indolent CD8-positive lymphoid proliferation of the ear). Medium-sized, monomorphic lymphoid cells with blastoid features. Angiodestruction, necrosis, or prominent mitotic activity is not identified

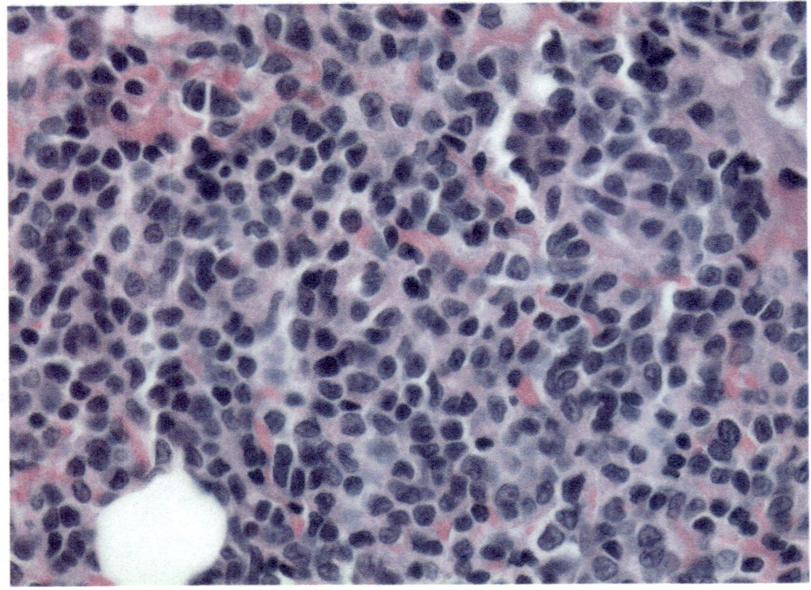

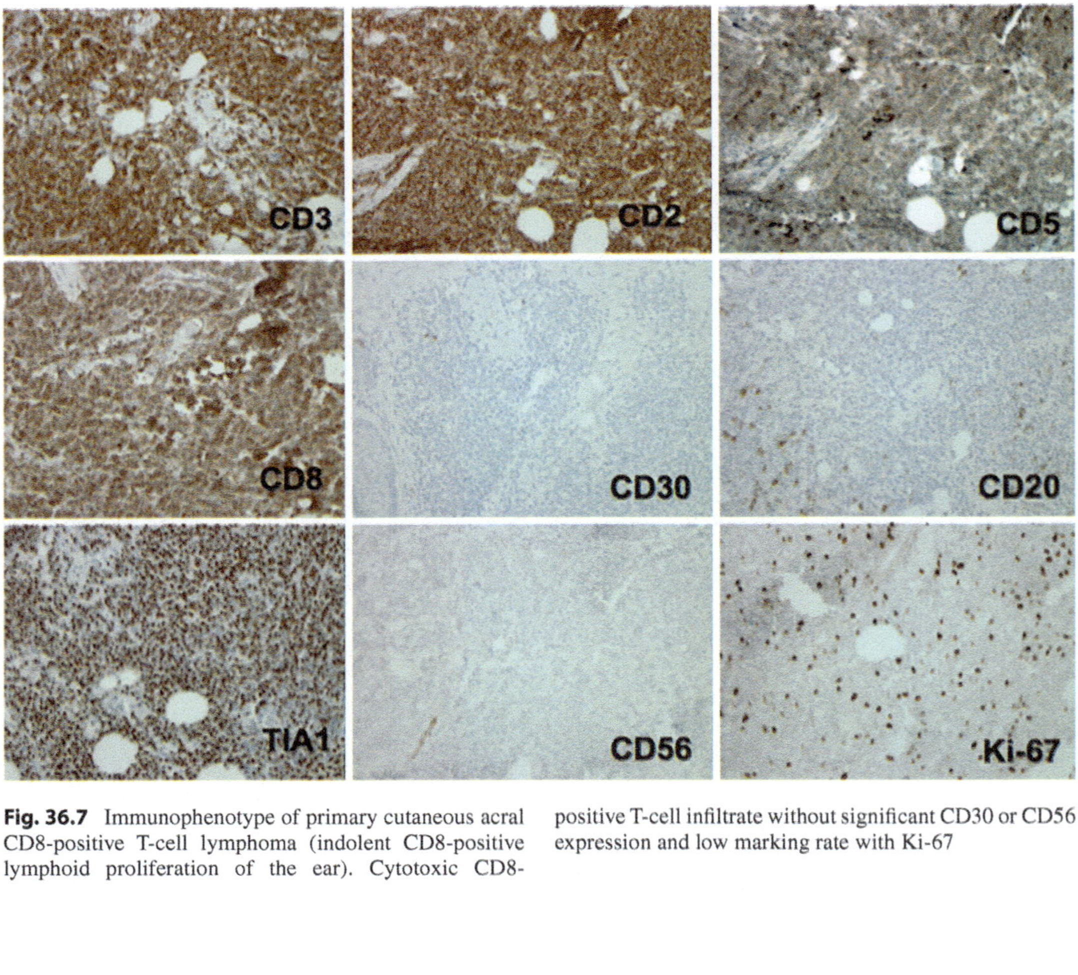

Fig. 36.7 Immunophenotype of primary cutaneous acral CD8-positive T-cell lymphoma (indolent CD8-positive lymphoid proliferation of the ear). Cytotoxic CD8-positive T-cell infiltrate without significant CD30 or CD56 expression and low marking rate with Ki-67

Disease Definition

- Indolent CD8-positive lymphoid proliferation of the ear is a rare, nonaggressive lymphoproliferative disorder classically presenting with a solitary nodular lesion on the ear (occasionally bilateral) (Fig. 36.1). This entity is now included in the 2016 WHO classification under provisional status and has been renamed primary cutaneous acral CD8-positive T-cell lymphoma, since it may occasionally involve other acral sites (Table 36.1).

Epidemiology

- Very rare

Preferential Sites of Involvement

- Ear is the prototypic site.
- Face (e.g., nose, eyelid).
- Extrafacial skin lesions (e.g., foot, hand) may occur rarely.
- Negative systemic staging (skin-only disease).

Clinical Features

- Usually solitary, but bilateral ear involvement may occur.
- Slowly growing or stable asymptomatic papule, plaque, or nodule. Lesion may be erythematous or violaceous. Ulceration is absent.
- *Less common presentations*: disease relapse at another cutaneous site has rarely been reported.

Histomorphology

- *Pattern*: dense diffuse dermal lymphoid infiltrate with variable pannicular extension (Figs. 36.2 and 36.3). Grenz zone between infiltrate and uninvolved epithelium (Fig. 36.4). Absence of epidermotropism, folliculotropism, ulceration, necrosis, interface change, prominent mitotic activity, or angiodestruction (Fig. 36.5).
- *Less common patterns*: rare reports of mild exocytosis of lymphocytes in the overlying epidermis.
- *Neoplastic cells*: monomorphic medium-sized blastoid cells. Delicate chromatin with small inconspicuous nucleoli. Scant to moderate cytoplasm (Fig. 36.6).
- *Reactive cells*: small noncleaved lymphocytes with dense chromatin. Scattered plasma cells. Eosinophils or histiocytes are not usually seen.

Immunophenotype

- *Neoplastic cells* (Fig. 36.7): CD3+, CD4−, CD8+, CD2+, CD5+/−, CD7+/−, CD20−, CD30−, CD56−, CD45RA−, betaF1+, TIA1+, granzyme B−, EBV (EBER)−, and PD1−. Low proliferative index (Ki-67 usually <30%). Absence of gamma-delta markers
- *Reactive cells*: CD20-positive B cells and scattered CD79a-positive plasma cells

Genetics

- Monoclonal rearrangement of T-cell receptor genes in majority of cases

Prognosis

- Indolent
- 5-year survival: 100%

Differential Diagnosis

- Differentiation from other types of CD8-positive lymphomas is primarily based on the clinical presentation and staging results (Table 36.2). Certain histopathologic features (lack of epidermotropism or ulceration) may provide a clue, but clinical correlation is necessary.
- Subcutaneous panniculitis-like T-cell lymphoma is also composed of alpha-beta CD8-positive T cells but specifically involves subcutaneous tissue and lacks significant dermal involvement.

- Cutaneous gamma-delta T-cell lymphoma is often CD8-positive but is composed of gamma-delta T cells (betaF1-negative, often CD56-positive). Angiodestruction, ulceration, hemophagocytic syndrome, and aggressive behavior are commonly seen.
- CD8 expression may be seen in primary cutaneous aggressive epidermotropic cytotoxic T-cell lymphoma, lymphomatoid papulosis type D, some cases of mycosis fungoides, and many cases of pagetoid reticulosis, but these entities demonstrate prominent epidermotropism. Primary cutaneous acral CD8-positive T-cell lymphoma (indolent CD8-positive lymphoid proliferation of the ear) is a non-epitheliotropic process.
- Some cases of cutaneous anaplastic large cell lymphoma (ALCL) may be CD8-positive and show dense non-epitheliotropic dermal infiltrates; however, the cytomorphology is different (large anaplastic cells in ALCL as opposed to medium-sized blastoid cells), and CD30 is strongly expressed (>75% of atypical cells).
- Secondary cutaneous involvement by a systemic CD8-positive T-cell lymphoma may closely mimic primary cutaneous acral CD8-positive T-cell lymphoma (indolent CD8-positive lymphoid proliferation of the ear). Staging is necessary to rule out this possibility.

Table 36.2 Differential diagnosis of CD8-positive cutaneous lymphoid infiltrate

Some cases of otherwise classical or hypopigmented mycosis fungoides
Many cases of localized pagetoid reticulosis
Lymphomatoid papulosis (LyP), type D
Some cases of anaplastic large cell lymphoma (ALCL)
Primary cutaneous CD8+ aggressive epidermotropic cytotoxic T-cell lymphoma
Many cases of cutaneous gamma-delta T-cell lymphoma
Subcutaneous panniculitis-like T-cell lymphoma
Indolent CD8+ lymphoid proliferation of the ear (primary cutaneous acral CD8+ T-cell lymphoma)
Cutaneous pseudolymphoma: CD8-positive infiltrates in the setting of advanced AIDS, many cases of pityriasis lichenoides

Pearls and Pitfalls

1. Clinical correlation and staging are essential for proper classification of atypical cutaneous lymphoid infiltrates. Despite the worrisome histopathology (dense tumoral infiltrate of cytotoxic T cells), primary cutaneous acral CD8-positive T-cell lymphoma (indolent CD8-positive lymphoid proliferation of the ear) is an indolent lymphoproliferative disorder.
2. Some have considered this entity as a phenotypic variant of primary cutaneous CD4-positive small-/medium-sized pleomorphic T-cell lymphoproliferative disorder, since both are indolent and generally present with solitary lesions (often on the head and neck region). However, the cytomorphology is distinct (monomorphic versus pleomorphic), and some epitheliotropism and PD1 expression are generally present in the CD4-positive cases.

Suggested Reading

Li JY, Guitart J, Pulitzer MP, et al. Multicenter case series of indolent small/medium-sized CD8+ lymphoid proliferations with predilection for the ear and face. Am J Dermatopathol. 2014;36:402–8.

Petrella T, Maubec E, Cornillet-Lefebvre P, et al. Indolent CD8-positive lymphoid proliferation of the ear. A distinct primary cutaneous T-cell lymphoma. Am J Surg Pathol. 2007;31:1887–92.

Swerdlow SH, et al., editors. WHO classification of tumors of hematopoietic and lymphoid tissues. Lyon: IARC; 2008.

Swerdlow SH, Campo E, Pileri SA, et al. The 2016 revision of the WHO classification of lymphoid neoplasms. Blood. 2016;127(20):2375–90.

Willemze R, Jaffe ES, Burg G, et al. WHO-EORTC classification for cutaneous lymphomas. Blood. 2005;105(10):3768–85.

Table 37.1 Key facts

Definition	
Primary cutaneous peripheral T-cell lymphoma, NOS, is a diagnosis of exclusion used for rare primary cutaneous T-cell lymphomas that do not fit into any of the well-defined types of T-cell lymphomas	
Prototypic clinical presentation	
Generalized or regionally localized tumors and nodules with variable ulceration	
Histopathologic findings	
Dense diffuse or nodular dermal-based infiltrates with variable pannicular extension. Epidermotropism is generally absent or minimal	
Most common immunophenotype: CD3+, CD4+, CD8−, CD30−, ALK−, and betaF1+ large cell infiltrate with variable loss of pan-T-cell markers. EBV is negative	
Prognosis	
Generally poor, but some cases may show indolent behavior	

Table 37.2 Criteria for diagnosis of primary cutaneous peripheral T-cell lymphoma, NOS (diagnosis of exclusion)

	Primary cutaneous peripheral T-cell lymphoma, NOS	Alternative diagnoses to be excluded:
Patches and plaques (either prior history or concurrent at the time of diagnosis)	Absent	If patches and plaques are present, consider mycosis fungoides
CD30	Negative CD30 or rare positive cells	If CD30+ infiltrate, consider cutaneous CD30+ T-cell lymphoproliferative disorders
Alpha-beta vs. gamma-delta status	Alpha-beta	If gamma-delta infiltrate, consider cutaneous gamma-delta T-cell lymphoma or secondary skin involvement by systemic lymphoma
Epidermotropism if CD8+	Absent	If a significant component of epidermotropic CD8+ cells is present, consider primary cutaneous CD8+ aggressive epidermotropic cytotoxic T-cell lymphoma, CD8+ mycosis fungoides, CD8+ cutaneous gamma-delta T-cell lymphoma, CD8+ pagetoid reticulosis, and lymphomatoid papulosis type D
EBV (EBER in situ hybridization)	Negative	If positive, consider extranodal NK/T-cell lymphoma nasal type, lymphomatoid granulomatosis, hydroa vacciniforme-like lymphoproliferative disorder, and other cutaneous manifestations of active EBV infection

(continued)

© Springer Nature Switzerland AG 2019
A. Subtil, *Diagnosis of Cutaneous Lymphoid Infiltrates*,
https://doi.org/10.1007/978-3-030-11654-5_37

Table 37.2 (continued)

	Primary cutaneous peripheral T-cell lymphoma, NOS	Alternative diagnoses to be excluded:
Cell size if CD4+	Large (>30% large cells in infiltrate)	If the infiltrate is composed of small-/intermediate-sized CD4+ cells, consider primary cutaneous CD4+ small/medium T-cell lymphoproliferative disorder (particularly if solitary/localized disease and low proliferation rate)
Staging workup	Skin-only process (no evidence of systemic disease)	If prior history of systemic T-cell lymphoma or if systemic disease is identified at the time of diagnosis, consider secondary cutaneous involvement by systemic peripheral T-cell lymphoma

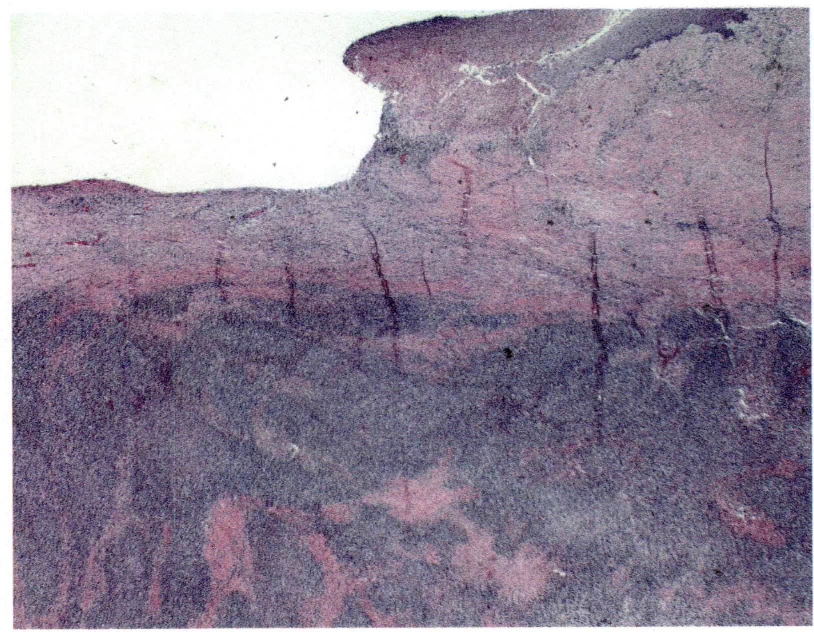

Fig. 37.1 Primary cutaneous peripheral T-cell lymphoma, NOS. Low-power magnification showing a dense diffuse dermal lymphoid infiltrate with overlying ulceration

Fig. 37.2
Epidermotropism is not identified in this case of primary cutaneous peripheral T-cell lymphoma, NOS

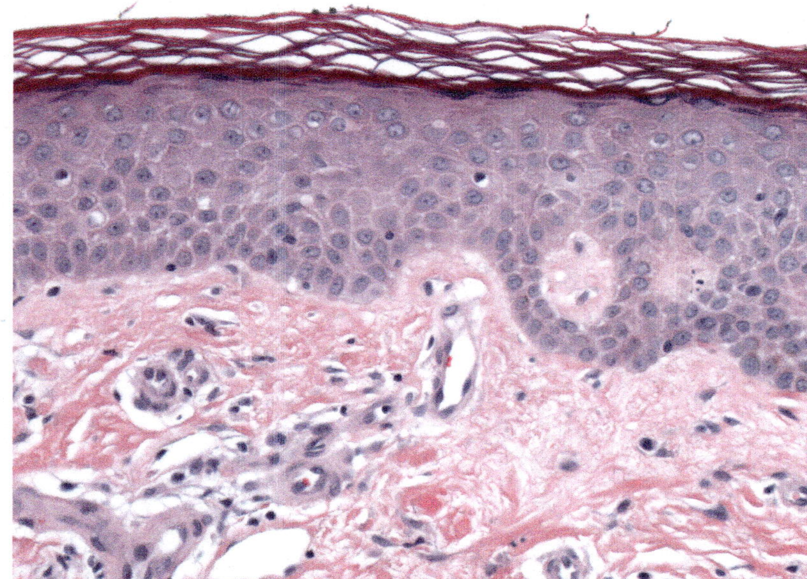

Fig. 37.3 Primary cutaneous peripheral T-cell lymphoma, NOS. Dense diffuse dermal infiltrate composed predominantly of large lymphoid cells admixed with histiocytes and small reactive lymphocytes

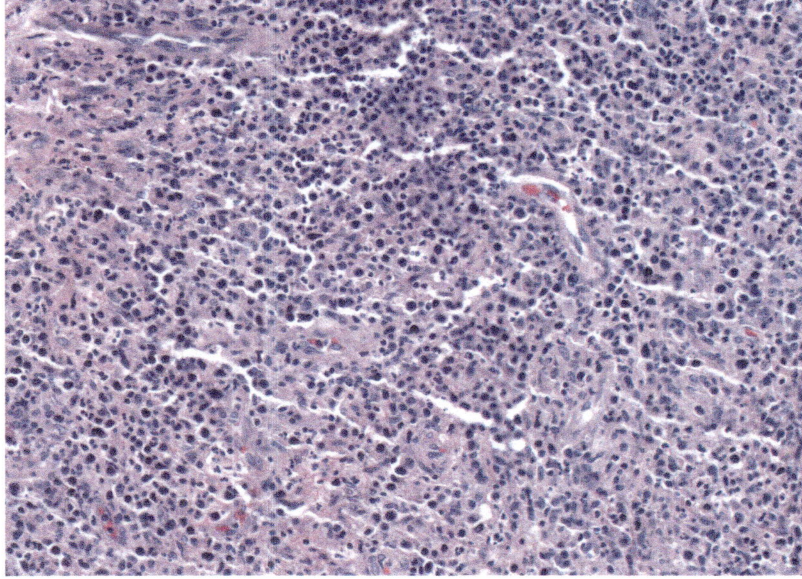

Fig. 37.4 Primary cutaneous peripheral T-cell lymphoma, NOS. High-power magnification demonstrates that the majority of atypical cells are large lymphocytes with prominent nucleoli. Scattered histiocytes and small reactive lymphocytes are also present

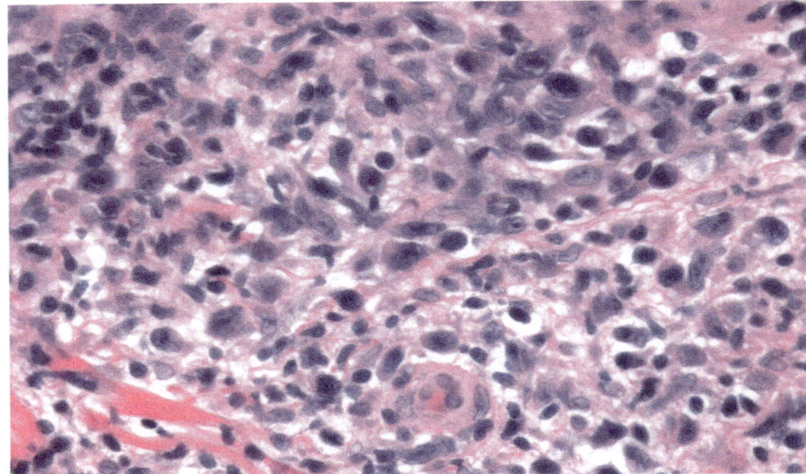

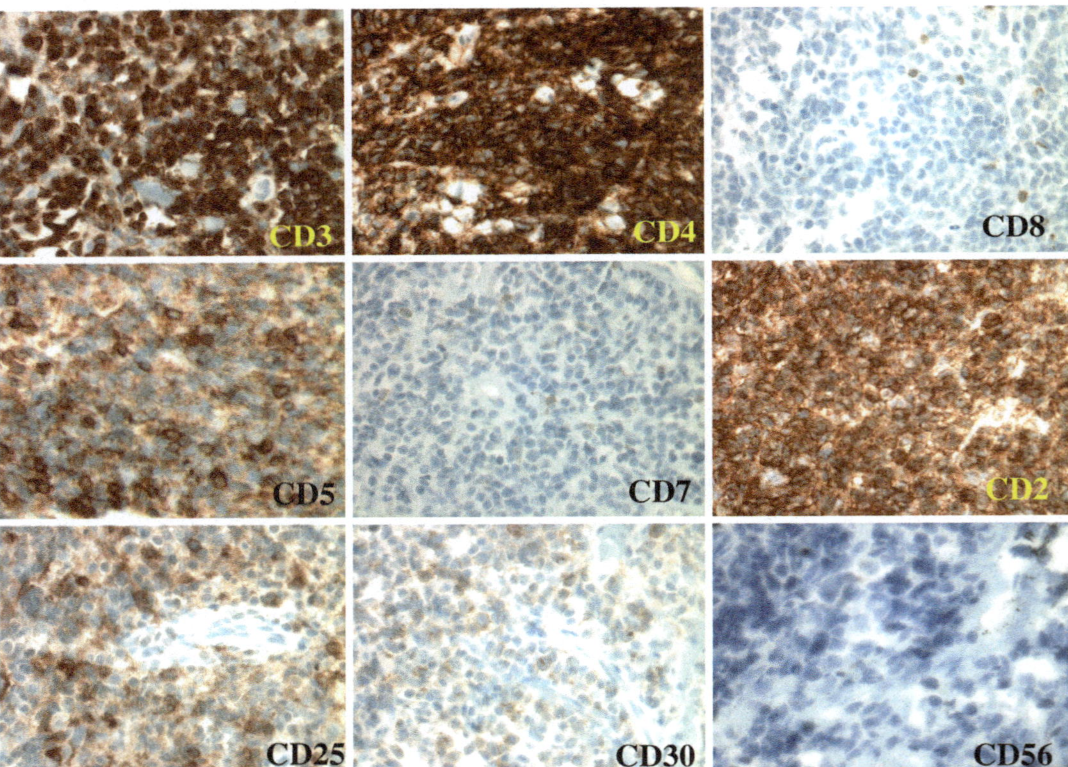

Fig. 37.5 Primary cutaneous peripheral T-cell lymphoma, NOS. This large cell infiltrate is CD2+, CD3+, CD4+, and CD8−. There is loss of CD7 and CD5 (partial). Significant CD30 or CD56 expression is not seen

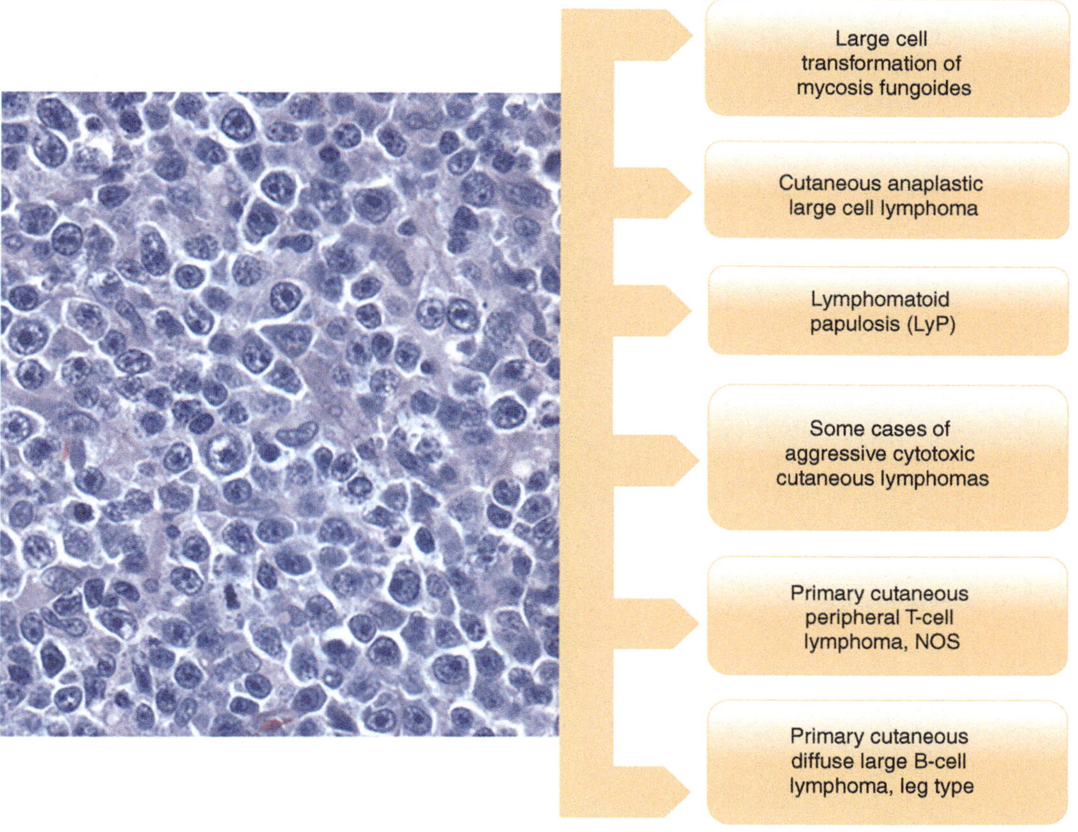

Fig. 37.6 Differential diagnosis of atypical cutaneous large cell lymphoid infiltrate

Disease Definition

- Primary cutaneous peripheral T-cell lymphoma, not otherwise specified is a diagnosis of exclusion used for rare primary cutaneous T-cell lymphomas that do not fit into any of the well-defined types of T-cell lymphomas (Table 37.1). Therefore, mycosis fungoides and other T-cell lymphomas must be ruled out (Table 37.2).

Epidemiology

- Usually adults

Preferential Sites of Involvement

- No preferential sites of involvement; however, localized disease in the head and neck region would be unusual.

Clinical Features

- Generalized or regionally localized tumors and nodules.
- Ulceration may occur.
- Absence of patches and plaques.
- Absence of systemic disease at the time of diagnosis.

Histomorphology

- *Pattern*: dense diffuse or nodular dermal-based infiltrates with variable pannicular extension. Ulceration may be present (Fig. 37.1). Epidermotropism is generally absent but may be focally present (Fig. 37.2). High mitotic rate is common. Infarct-like necrosis, angiocentrism, or pannicular-based infiltrates would be unusual.

- *Neoplastic cells*: most cases are CD4+ and show >30% large cells in the infiltrate (Figs. 37.3 and 37.4). Neoplastic cells are often pleomorphic or immunoblast-like with prominent nucleoli and variable cytoplasm.
- *Less common patterns*: rare cases are composed of a dermal-based CD8+ infiltrate without epidermotropism (and with variable cell size). Another subset of cases may rarely exhibit a small-/medium-sized CD4+ infiltrate (<30% large cells) histologically resembling primary cutaneous CD4+ small/medium T-cell lymphoproliferative disorder but with a disseminated/generalized/fast-progressing clinical picture.
- *Reactive cells*: small lymphocytes, histiocytes (may be prominent), and/or eosinophils.

Immunophenotype

- *Neoplastic cells*: Most cases are composed of a CD3+, CD4+, CD8−, CD30−, ALK−, and betaF1+ large cell infiltrate with variable loss of pan-T-cell markers (Fig. 37.5). CD56 or cytotoxic protein (TIA1, granzyme B, perforin) expression may be occasionally observed. EBV is negative.
- *Less common patterns*: Rare cases may show a dermal-based CD8+ alpha-beta T-cell infiltrate without epidermotropism.
- *Reactive cells*: Small CD3+ T cells, CD68+ histiocytes.

Genetics

- Monoclonal rearrangement of T-cell receptor genes in the majority of cases.

Prognosis

- Generally poor, but some cases may show indolent behavior.
- 5-year survival: less than 20%.

Differential Diagnosis

- Mycosis fungoides (tumor stage with large cell transformation) must be ruled out by complete clinical examination and careful clinical history. Patients with prior history of patches and plaques (or their concurrent presence at the time of the initial biopsy) should be classified as mycosis fungoides.
- Primary cutaneous CD4+ small/medium T-cell lymphoproliferative disorder has less than 30% large cells and is solitary/localized (Fig. 37.6).
- Cutaneous gamma-delta T-cell lymphoma is composed of gamma-delta T cells, while primary cutaneous peripheral T-cell lymphoma NOS is composed of alpha-beta T cells.
- Primary cutaneous CD8+ aggressive epidermotropic cytotoxic T-cell lymphoma shows prominent epitheliotropism, which is largely absent in primary cutaneous peripheral T-cell lymphoma.
- Primary cutaneous CD30+ T-cell lymphoproliferative disorders express CD30 and are generally indolent, while primary cutaneous peripheral T-cell lymphoma NOS lacks significant CD30 expression and is usually aggressive.
- Extranodal NK/T-cell lymphoma nasal type is EBV-positive, while primary cutaneous peripheral T-cell lymphoma NOS is EBV-negative.
- Secondary cutaneous involvement by systemic peripheral T-cell lymphoma should be ruled out. The distinction is made by prior history of systemic T-cell lymphoma or identification of systemic disease at the time of initial staging workup.

Pearls and Pitfalls

1. Some cases of primary cutaneous peripheral T-cell lymphoma NOS are composed of small/medium cells and may histologically resemble primary cutaneous CD4+ small/medium T-cell lymphoproliferative disorder. The latter diagnosis should be restricted to cases with solitary/localized disease. If disseminated/generalized/fast-progressing clinical presentation and/or unusual histopathology (high proliferation rate, >30% large cells), cutaneous peripheral T-cell lymphoma NOS should be considered.

Suggested Reading

Bekkenk MW, Vermeer MH, Jansen PM, et al. Peripheral T-cell lymphomas unspecified presenting in the skin: analysis of prognostic factors in a group of 82 patients. Blood. 2003;102:2213–9.

Elder DE, Massi D, Scolyer RA, Willemze R, editors. WHO classification of skin tumors. 4th ed. Lyon: IARC; 2018.

Swerdlow SH, et al., editors. WHO classification of tumors of hematopoietic and lymphoid tissues. Lyon: IARC; 2008.

Swerdlow SH, Campo E, Harris NL, Jaffe ES, Pileri SA, Stein H, Thiele J, editors. WHO classification of tumours of haematopoietic and lymphoid tissues (revised 4th edition). Lyon: IARC; 2017.

Willemze R, Jaffe ES, Burg G, et al. WHO-EORTC classification for cutaneous lymphomas. Blood. 2005;105(10):3768–85.

Primary Cutaneous Diffuse Large B-Cell Lymphoma, Leg Type

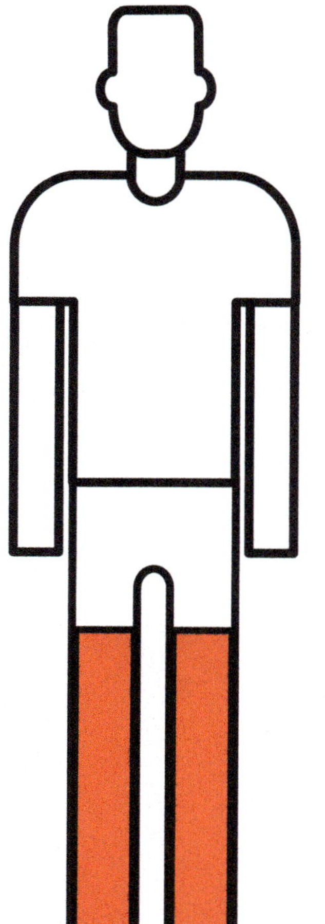

Fig. 38.1 The lower extremities are the preferential sites of involvement by primary cutaneous diffuse large B-cell lymphoma, leg type

Table 38.1 Key Facts

Definition
Primary cutaneous diffuse large B-cell lymphoma, leg type (DLBCL-LT), is a primary cutaneous diffuse large B-cell lymphoma composed exclusively of large B cells (immunoblasts and centroblasts), most commonly arising in the leg(s)
Prototypic clinical presentation
Tumors on one or both lower extremities of elderly women
Histopathologic findings
Dense, diffuse, non-epitheliotropic infiltrate of large round cells: immunoblasts (large noncleaved nuclei with prominent central nucleolus) and centroblasts (large noncleaved nuclei and multiple peripheral nucleoli)
Most common immunophenotype: CD3−, CD20+, CD79a+, BCL2+, MUM1+, BCL6+/−, CD10−, CyclinD1−, TdT−, high Ki-67
Prognosis
Intermediate (5-year survival: 50%)

A. Subtil, *Diagnosis of Cutaneous Lymphoid Infiltrates*,
https://doi.org/10.1007/978-3-030-11654-5_38

Fig. 38.2 Main types of lymphoid morphology. Primary cutaneous diffuse large B-cell lymphoma, leg type is composed of an admixture of immunoblasts and centroblasts. Unlike primary cutaneous follicle center lymphoma, follicular dendritic cells and centrocytes are absent

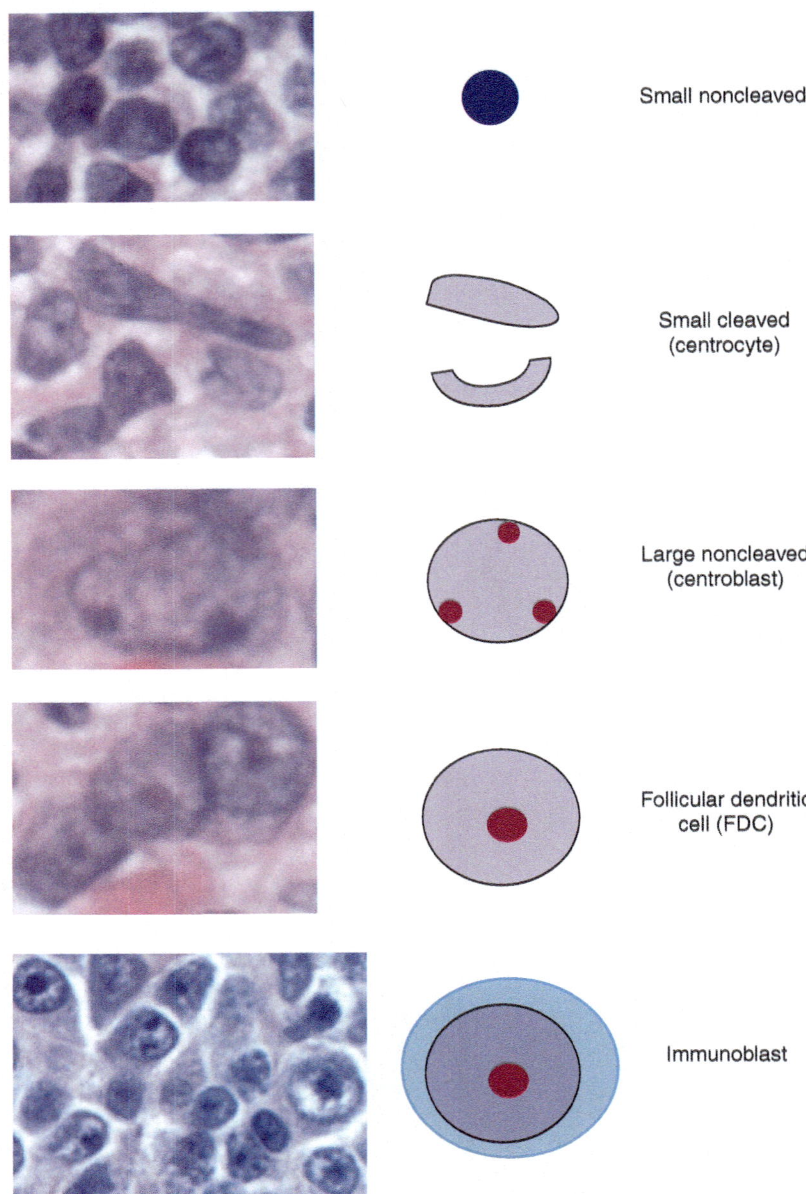

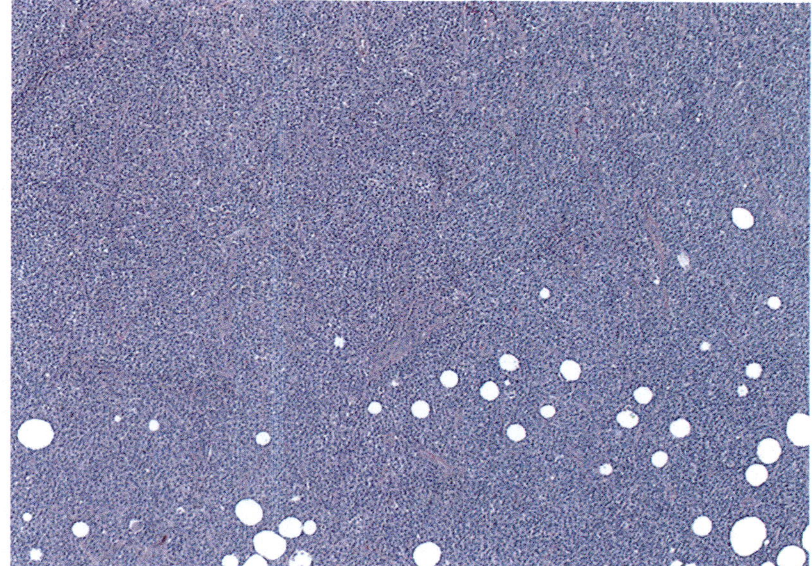

Fig. 38.3 Primary cutaneous diffuse large B-cell lymphoma, leg type. Dense diffuse infiltrate of lymphocytes in the dermis and panniculus. A nodular pattern is not seen because lymphoid follicles are not present

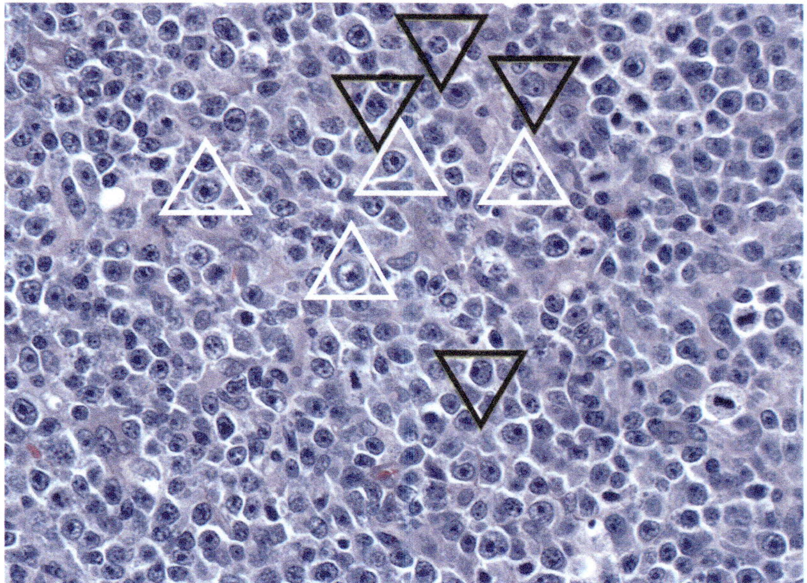

Fig. 38.4 Primary cutaneous diffuse large B-cell lymphoma, leg type. The dense diffuse infiltrate of large lymphocytes is composed of an admixture of immunoblasts (highlighted within white triangles: cells with large noncleaved nucleus, prominent central nucleolus, and moderate cytoplasm) and centroblasts (within black triangles: cells with large noncleaved nucleus, multiple peripheral nucleoli, and scant cytoplasm). Centrocytes are not present. Mitotic figures are frequent

Fig. 38.5 Primary cutaneous diffuse large B-cell lymphoma, leg type. Dense diffuse dermal infiltrate of large CD20-positive B cells with cytoplasmic BCL2 expression

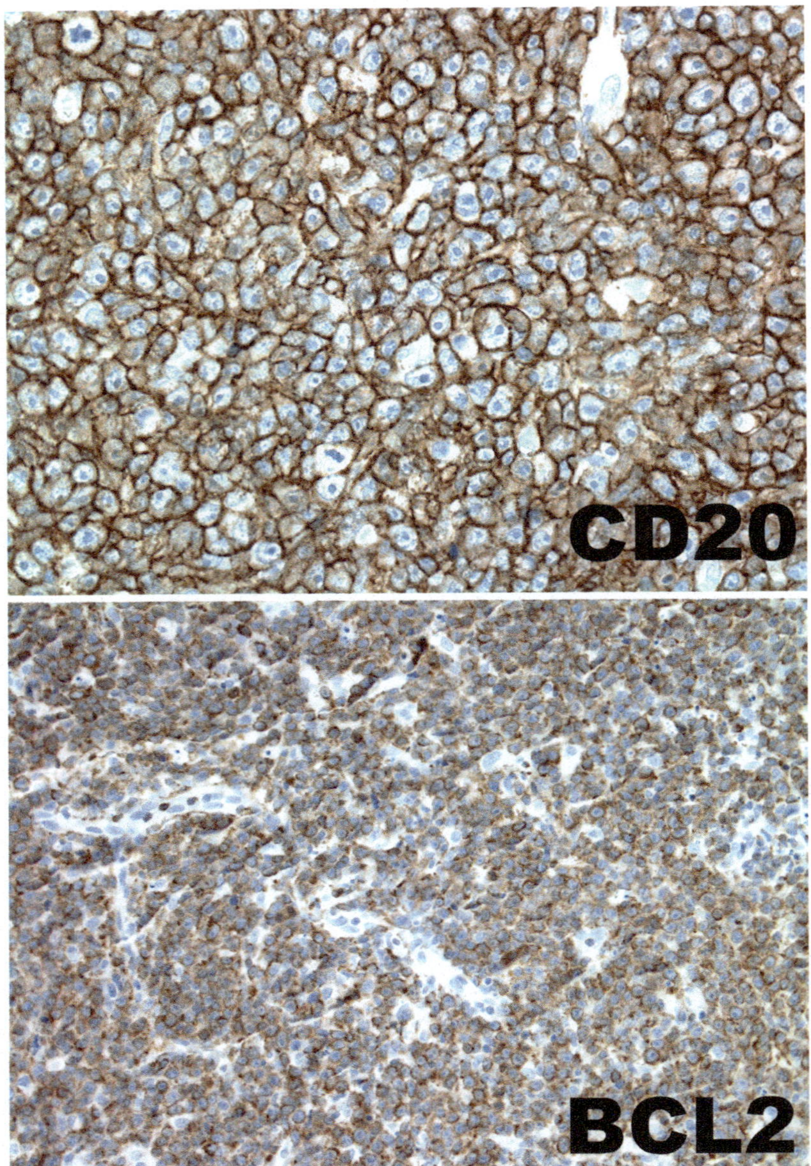

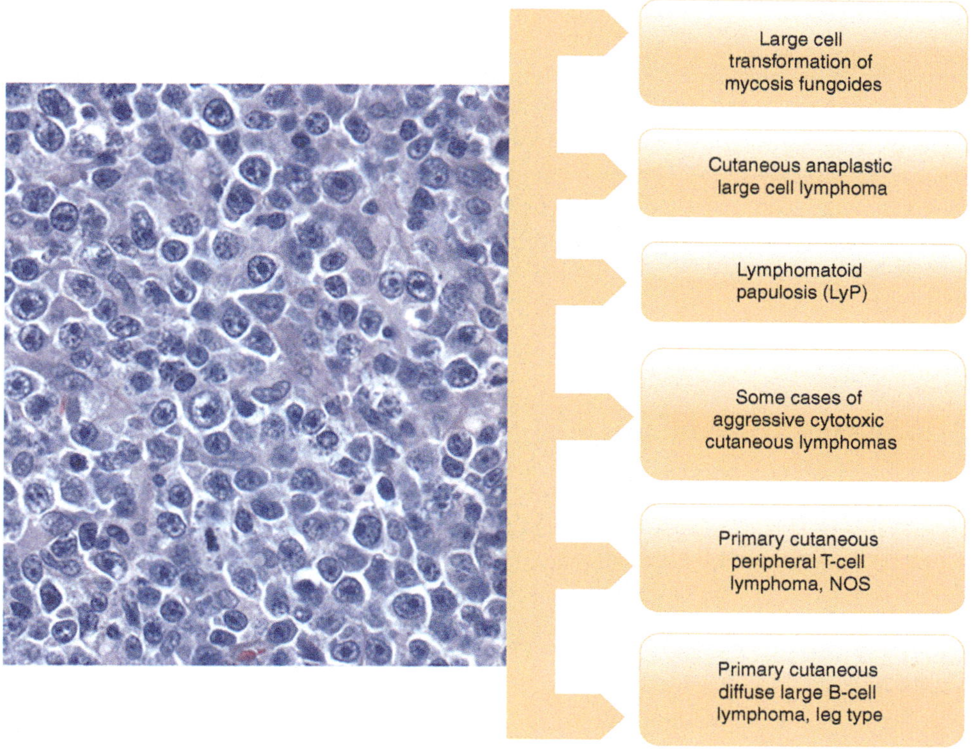

Fig. 38.6 Differential diagnosis of an atypical cutaneous large cell lymphoid infiltrate

Fig. 38.7 Comparison of cytomorphologic features of diffuse large B-cell lymphoma (immunoblasts and centroblasts) and cutaneous follicle center lymphoma (centroblasts and centrocytes)

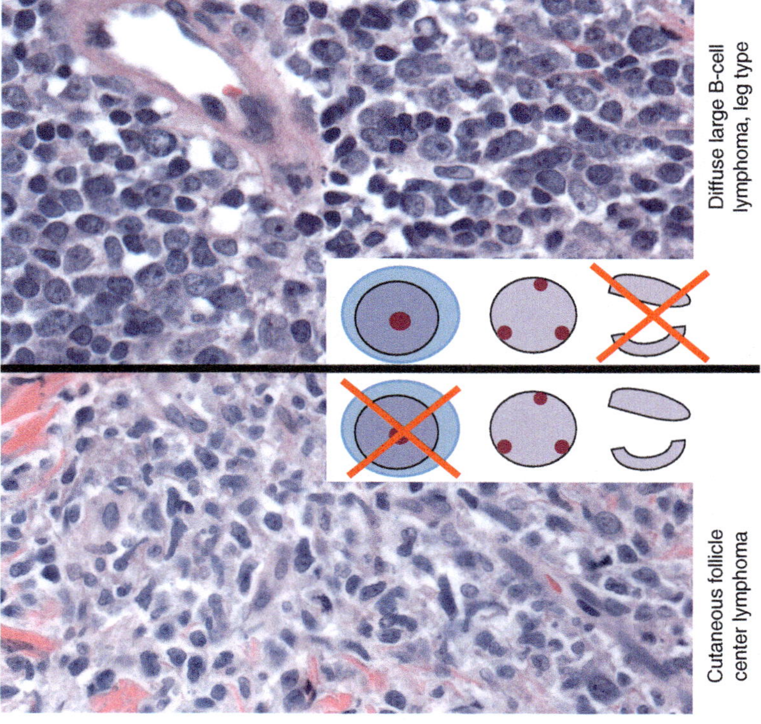

Disease Definition

- Primary cutaneous diffuse large B-cell lymphoma, leg type (DLBCL-LT), is a primary cutaneous diffuse large B-cell lymphoma composed exclusively of large B cells (immunoblasts and centroblasts), most commonly arising in the leg(s) (Figs. 38.1 and 38.2; Table 38.1).

Epidemiology

- 4% of all primary skin lymphomas
- 20% of all primary CBCLs (cutaneous B-cell lymphomas)
- Typically lower legs of elderly women (M:F ratio of 1:3; median age in the 7th decade)

Preferential Sites of Involvement

- Lower leg(s) (unilateral or bilateral)
- 10–15% arise elsewhere

Clinical Features

- Red or bluish-red tumors on one or both lower extremities. Lesions may be solitary or multiple at presentation.
- Ulceration may occur.
- Less common presentations: papules, plaques, and annular lesions.
- Frequent dissemination to extracutaneous sites.

Histomorphology

- Pattern: dense, diffuse, monotonous, and non-epitheliotropic infiltrate in reticular dermis and panniculus (Fig. 38.3). A nodular pattern is not seen because lymphoid follicles are not present.
- Less common patterns: incidental epidermal extension is rare. Occasionally, a dense band-like infiltrate is present in the upper and mid dermis. Angioinvasion is uncommon. Early lesions may show relatively sparse infiltrates with perivascular collections of large atypical lymphoid cells.
- Neoplastic cells: admixture of large round cells—immunoblasts (cells with large non-cleaved nucleus and prominent central nucleolus) and centroblasts (cells with large noncleaved nucleus and multiple peripheral nucleoli) (Fig. 38.4 and Table 38.2). Frequent mitotic figures.
- Reactive cells: relatively few reactive T cells (predominantly perivascular). Absent: centrocytes (small cleaved germinal center B cells) and follicular dendritic cells (large noncleaved cells with round nucleus with single central nucleolus, scant cytoplasm, often in small overlapping clusters).

Immunophenotype

- Neoplastic cells: CD3−, CD20+, CD79a+, BCL2+ (cytoplasmic), MUM1+ (nuclear), FOX-P1+, BCL6+/− (nuclear), CD10−, CyclinD1−, TdT−, HHV8−, CD138−, and high Ki-67 (>50%) (Fig. 38.5). BCL2 or MUM1 is negative in 10% of cases.
- Reactive cells: relatively few CD3+ T cells. Negative CD21 stain (absent follicular dendritic cell meshworks).

Genetics

- Monoclonal rearrangement of immunoglobulin genes in majority of cases
- Gene expression profile of activated B-cell-like diffuse large B-cell lymphoma

Prognosis

- Intermediate.
- 5-year survival: 50%.
- Adverse risk factors: multiple skin lesions at diagnosis, inactivation of CDKN2A (by deletion or promoter hypermethylation).
- BCL2- cases have the same prognosis of BCL2+ cases.

Differential Diagnosis

- Other lymphomas may show infiltrates composed of large cells (Fig. 38.6). However, the immunophenotype is different (i.e., T or NK cell), and the cytomorphology does not show the admixture of immunoblasts and centroblasts.
- Primary cutaneous follicle center lymphoma: centrocytes (small cleaved germinal center B cells) are present (Fig. 38.7). CD21+ follicular dendritic cell meshworks of lymphoid follicles are generally present. BCL2 is often negative. MUM1 is generally negative. Usually on the scalp or upper back of middle-aged men.
- Secondary cutaneous involvement by systemic high-grade B-cell lymphoma: clinical history and staging results. Cyclin D1 expression in mantle cell lymphoma. TdT expression in B lymphoblastic lymphoma. Burkitt lymphoma is usually CD10+ and BCL2− and shows nearly 100% Ki-67 expression.

Table 38.2 Comparison of types of lymphocyte morphology and cellular composition of primary cutaneous diffuse large B-cell lymphoma, leg type (DLBCL-LT)

Lymphoid cell morphology	Dense chromatin	Nuclear shape	Prominent nucleolus	Cytoplasm	Presence in DLBCL-LT
Small noncleaved	Yes (dark blue)	Round	No	Scant	Present (reactive T cells)
Centrocyte (Small cleaved)	No	Elongated, spindle-like (cleaved)	No	Scant	Absent
Centroblast (Large noncleaved)	No	Round	Yes (multiple and peripheral)	Scant	Present (neoplastic)
Immunoblast	No	Round	Yes (single and central)	Moderate	Present (neoplastic)
Follicular dendritic cell	No	Round	Yes (single and central)	Scant	Absent

Pearls and Pitfalls

1. Immunoblasts (large noncleaved lymphocytes with central nucleolus) are often seen in inflammatory infiltrates due to viral infection, such as herpes folliculitis and inflamed molluscum contagiosum. However, the proportion of large cells in this setting is generally small. Identification of viral cytopathic effect would facilitate the diagnosis.
2. High-grade B-cell lymphomas are uncommon in young patients. In this setting, consider the possibility of a mimic as well as viral-associated lymphoproliferative processes (e.g., Epstein-Barr virus, human immunodeficiency virus).
3. The "leg type" terminology is similar to the "nasal type" terminology used for extranodal NK/T-cell lymphoma. Both terms describe the most common site of involvement and emphasize the prototypic clinical presentation. However, if either process initially presents in another site, the diagnosis is the same.

Suggested Reading

Grange F, Beylot-Barry M, Courville P, et al. Primary cutaneous diffuse large B-cell lymphoma, leg type: clinicopathologic features and prognostic analysis in 60 cases. Arch Dermatol. 2007;143(9):1144–50.

Swerdlow SH, et al., editors. WHO classification of tumors of hematopoietic and lymphoid tissues. Lyon: IARC; 2008.

Swerdlow SH, Campo E, Pileri SA, et al. The 2016 revision of the WHO classification of lymphoid neoplasms. Blood. 2016;127(20):2375–90.

Willemze R, Jaffe ES, Burg G, et al. WHO-EORTC classification for cutaneous lymphomas. Blood. 2005;105(10):3768–85.

Table 39.1 Key facts. Intravascular large B-cell lymphoma

Definition
Intravascular large B-cell lymphoma is an extranodal lymphoma with a proliferation of neoplastic B cells within the lumina of blood vessels and without an obvious extravascular tumor mass
Prototypic clinical presentation
Erythematous patches and plaques with telangiectasia. May involve normal-looking skin and hemangiomas
Histopathologic findings
Large atypical lymphocytes with prominent nucleoli (often with immunoblastic features) confined to the lumina of small- and intermediate-sized blood vessels Most common immunophenotype: CD3−, CD20+, CD79a+, MUM1+, BCL2+, CD5−/+, and CD10−/+
Prognosis
Variable (usually poor, but isolated cutaneous variant has better survival)

Table 39.2 Key facts. Cutaneous plasmablastic lymphoma

Definition
Plasmablastic lymphoma is a predominantly extranodal lymphoma composed of a diffuse proliferation of large cells resembling immunoblasts and/or plasmablasts with a CD20-negative plasma cell phenotype
Prototypic clinical presentation
Tumors, nodules
Histopathologic findings
Dense dermal diffuse infiltrate of large atypical lymphoid cells with features of immunoblasts (large noncleaved nucleus with prominent central nucleolus and moderately abundant cytoplasm) and/or plasmablasts (abundant cytoplasm and eccentric nuclei with atypical features) Most common immunophenotype: CD3−, CD20−, PAX5−, CD79a+/−, CD138+, MUM1+, CD30+/−, EMA+/−, CD10−/+, CD56−/+, BCL2−, BCL6−, Cyclin D1−, HHV8− and ALK−. High proliferation index (Ki-67 >90%). EBV (EBER) in situ hybridization often positive
Prognosis
Usually poor

© Springer Nature Switzerland AG 2019
A. Subtil, *Diagnosis of Cutaneous Lymphoid Infiltrates*,
https://doi.org/10.1007/978-3-030-11654-5_39

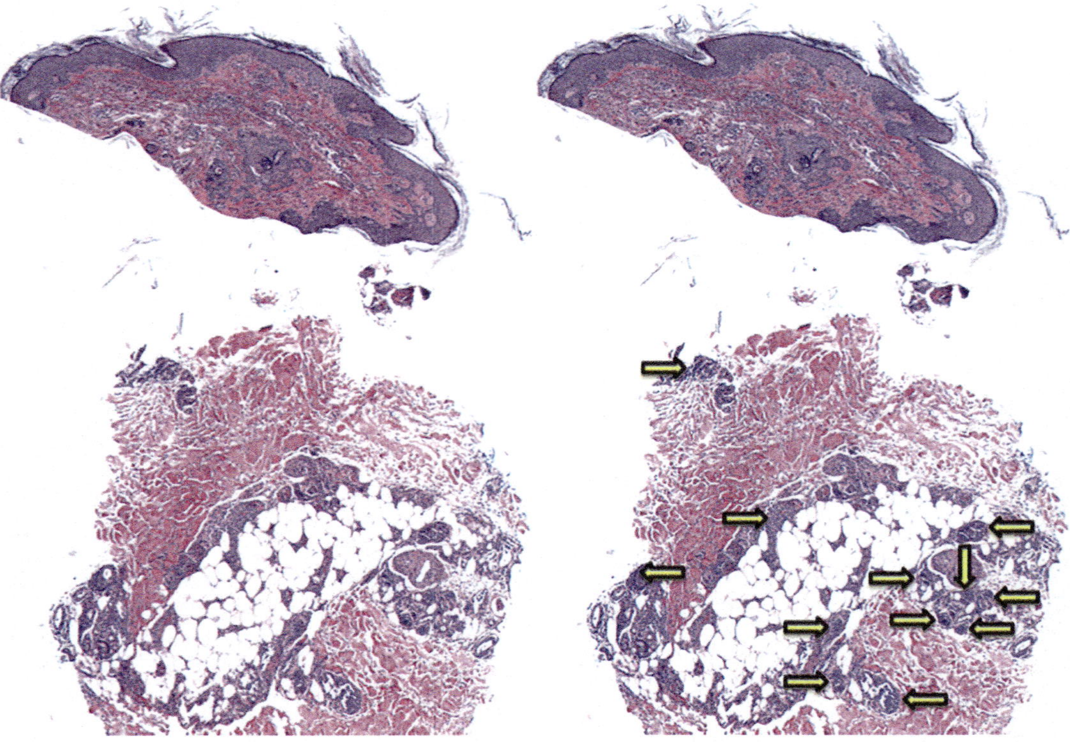

Fig. 39.1 Intravascular large B-cell lymphoma may be very subtle microscopically, particularly at low-power magnification. Affected vessels are highlighted by arrows

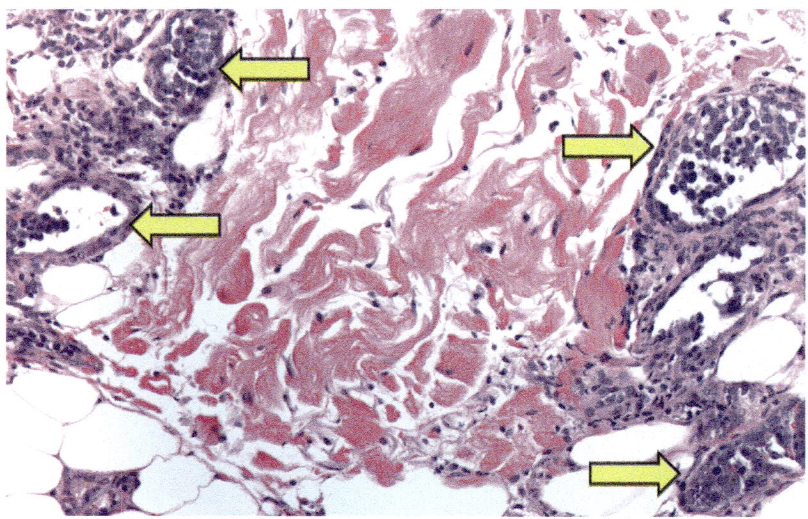

Fig. 39.2 Intravascular large B-cell lymphoma exhibits atypical lymphocytes within the lumen of dilated blood vessels (arrows)

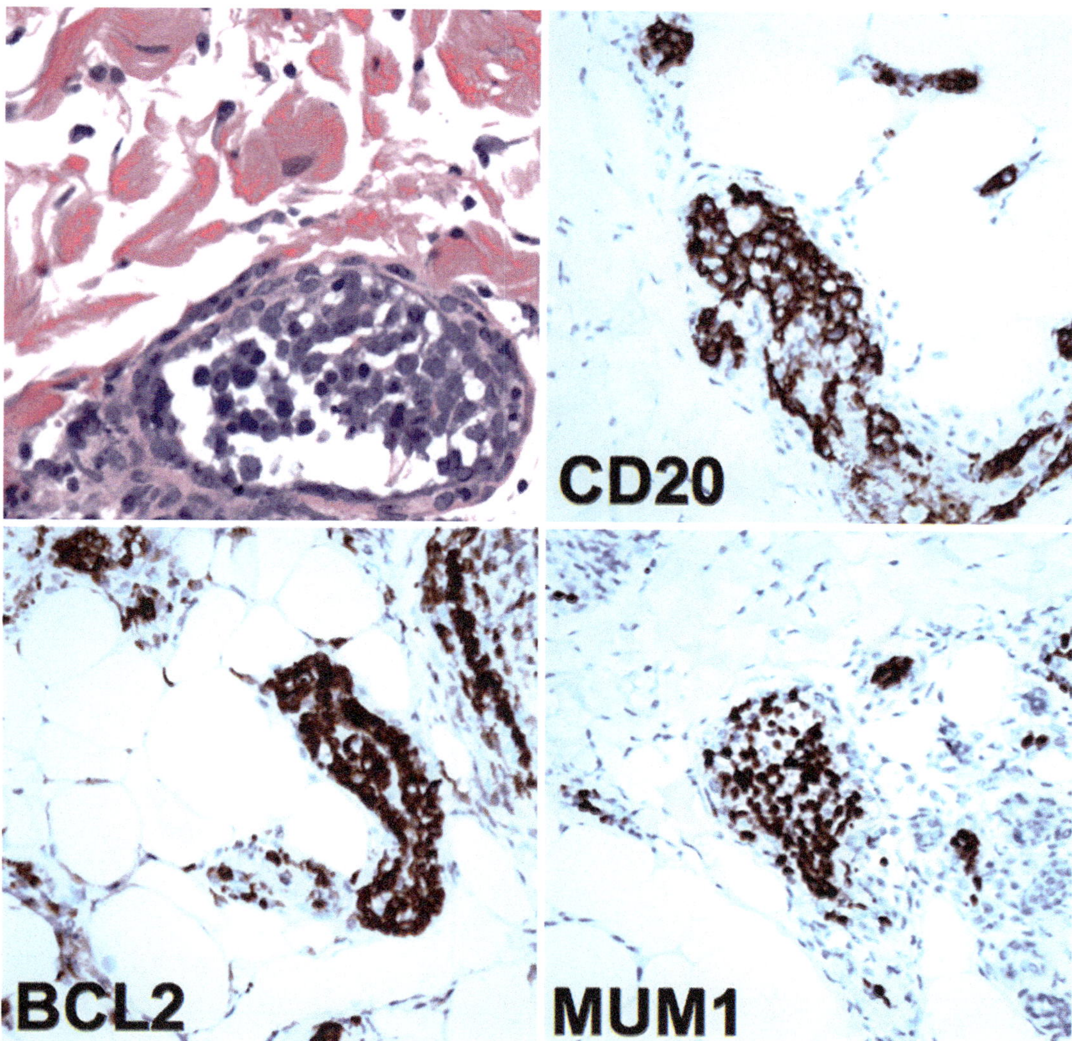

Fig. 39.3 Immunophenotype of intravascular large B-cell lymphoma

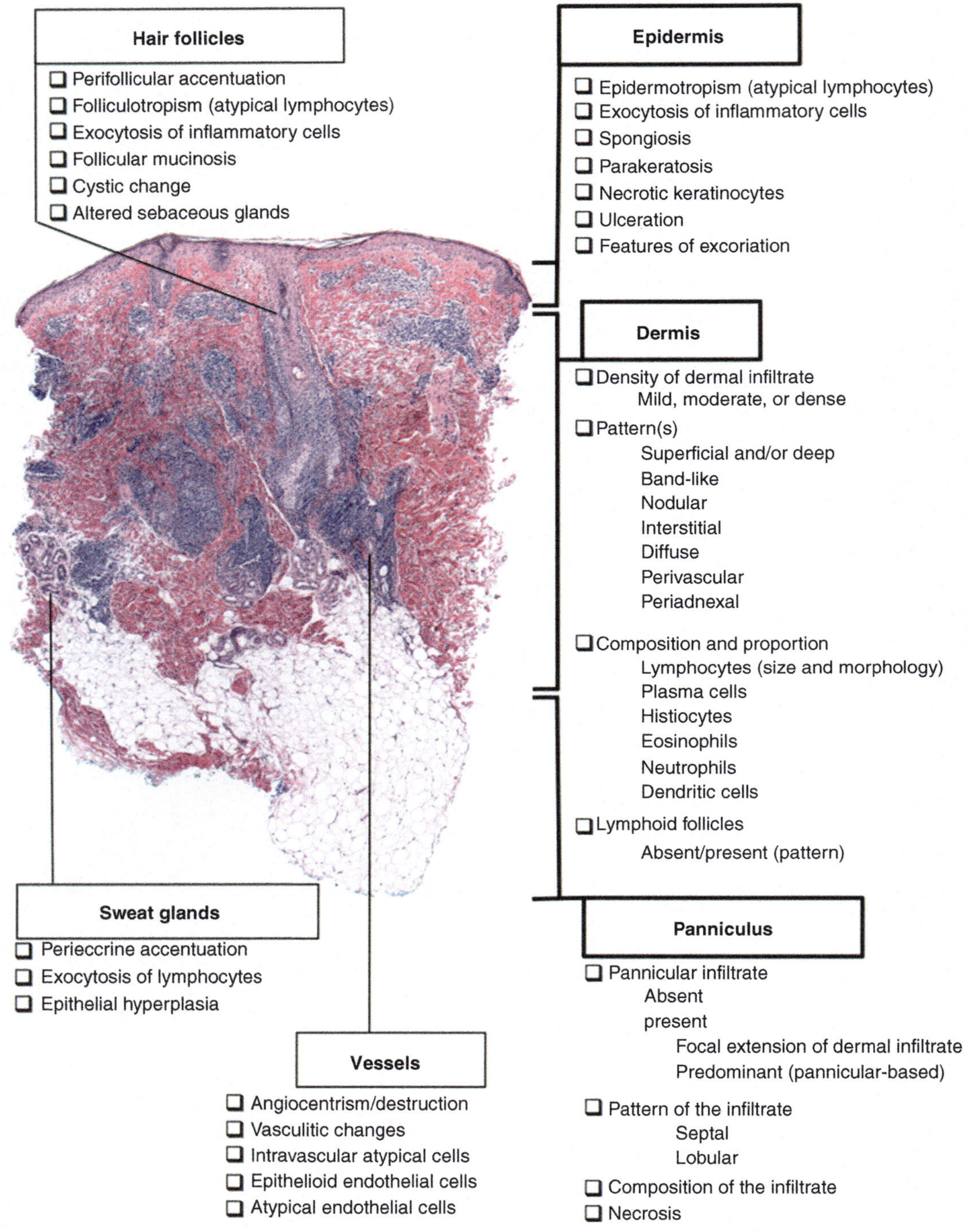

Fig. 39.4 Checklist of possible histomorphologic findings in the initial evaluation of cutaneous lymphoid infiltrates

Fig. 39.5 Cutaneous plasmablastic lymphoma. Dense diffuse atypical lymphoid infiltrate in the dermis

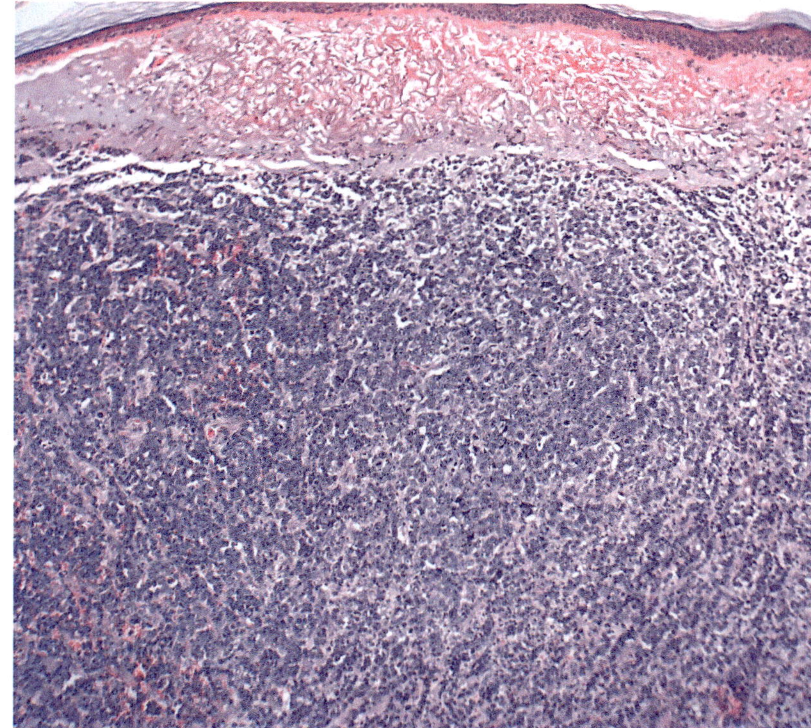

Fig. 39.6 Dense dermal infiltrate of cutaneous plasmablastic lymphoma with predominantly immunoblastic cytomorphology: large noncleaved nucleus with prominent central nucleolus and moderately abundant cytoplasm

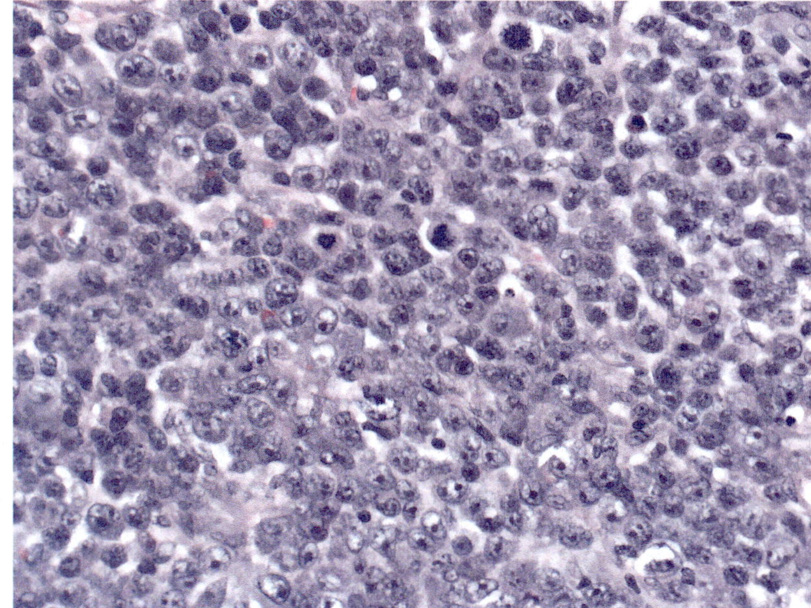

Fig. 39.7 Cutaneous plasmablastic lymphoma with plasmablastic cytomorphology: abundant cytoplasm and eccentric nuclei. The dermis shows solar elastosis

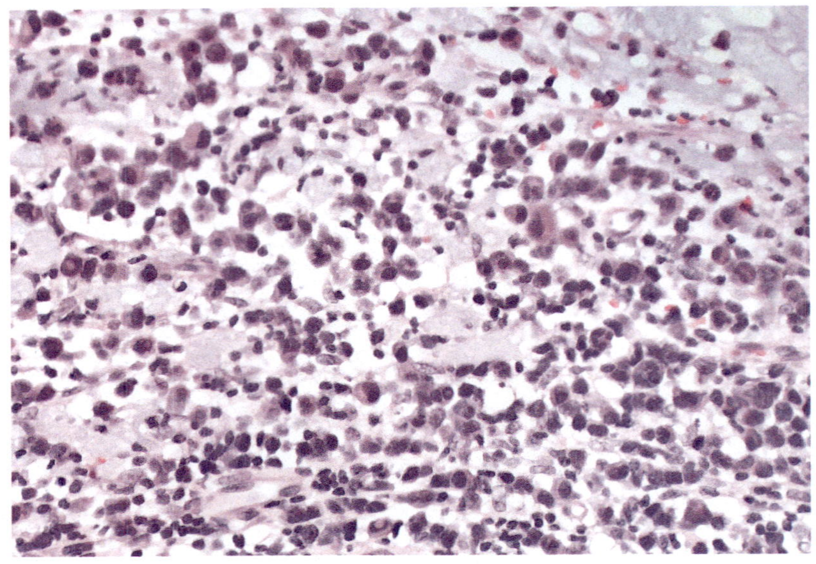

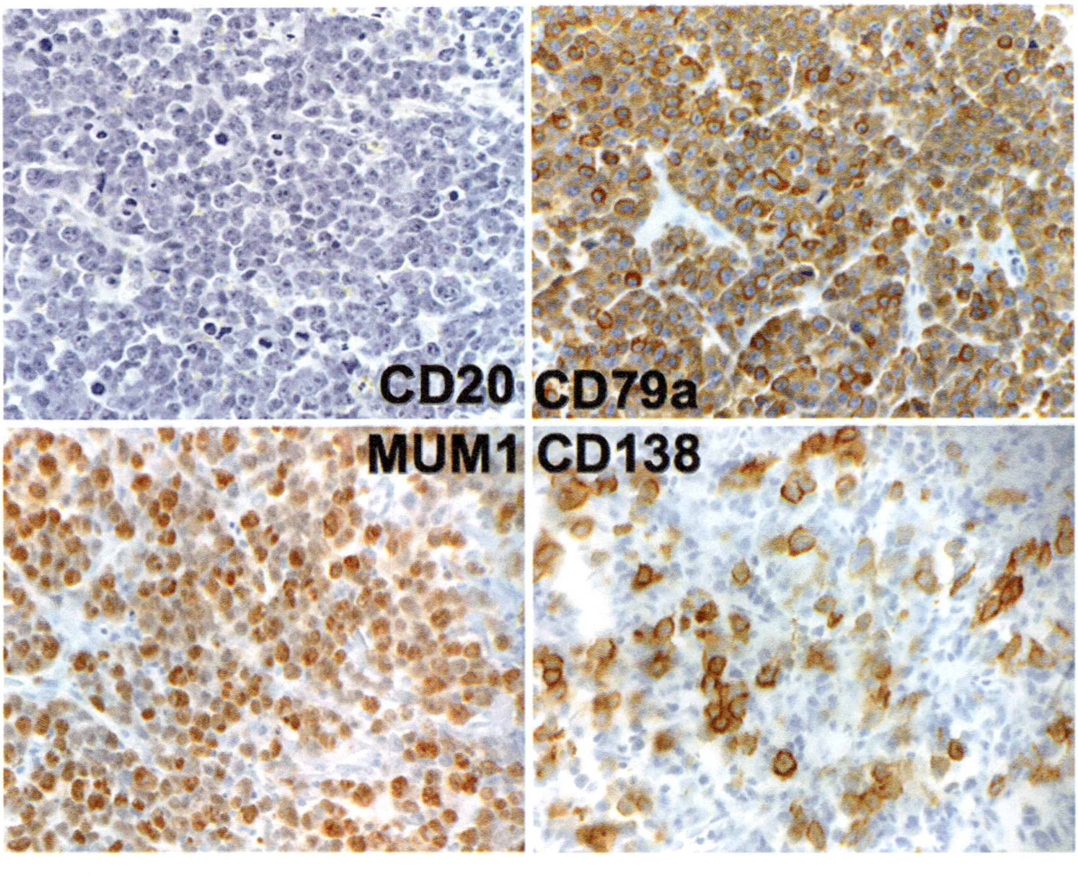

Fig. 39.8 Immunophenotype of cutaneous plasmablastic lymphoma with classic absence of CD20 and expression of plasma cell markers

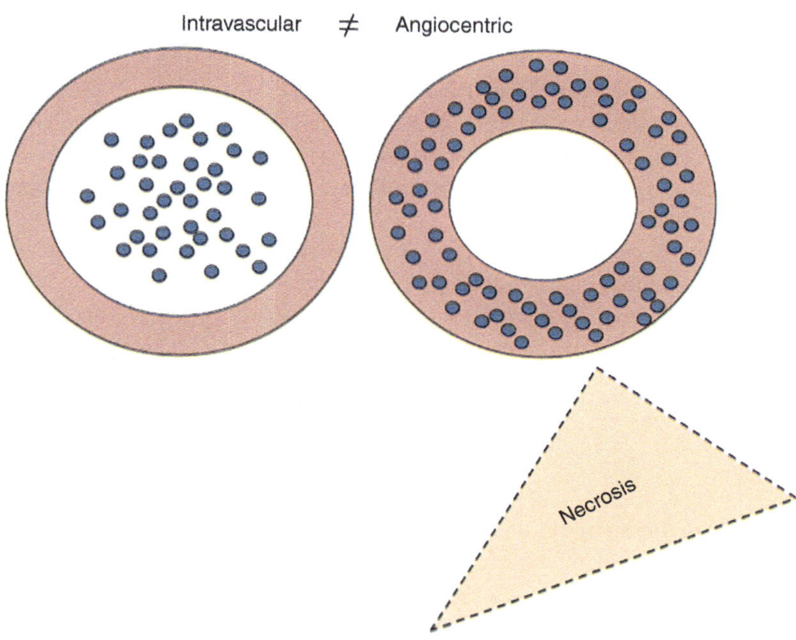

Fig. 39.9 Comparison of intravascular and angiocentric/angiodestructive lymphomas. Angiocentric lymphomas show infiltration and destruction of blood vessel walls (which results in infarct-like necrosis), while intravascular lymphomas exhibit atypical lymphocytes within the lumen of preserved blood vessels

Intravascular Large B-Cell Lymphoma

Disease Definition

- Intravascular large B-cell lymphoma is characterized by extranodal involvement, proliferation of lymphoma cells within the lumina of blood vessels, and lack of an extravascular tumor mass (Table 39.1 and Fig. 39.1).

Epidemiology

- Median age: seventh decade
- No gender predilection but female predominance in isolated cutaneous variant

Preferential Sites of Involvement

- Widely disseminated in extranodal sites.
- Can present in any organ.
- May be identified in normal-appearing skin.
- Lymph nodes are usually spared, but bone marrow may be involved.
- Colonization of pre-existing hemangioma may occur.

Clinical Features

- Variable clinical patterns

(a) Classic type:
  - Usually seen in Western countries
  - Predominantly skin and nervous system involvement
(b) Hemophagocytic syndrome-associated form:
  - Usually seen in Asian patients
  - Multi-organ failure, hepatosplenomegaly, and peripheral blood cytopenias
(c) Isolated cutaneous variant:
  - Tumor cells confined to the skin.
  - Female predominance.
  - More common in Western countries (24% of all cases) than in Asia (3% of all cases).
  - Skin lesions: erythematous or violaceous macules, patches, and plaques; livedoid plaques. Telangiectasia, edema, and pain may be observed. May be present in normal-looking skin. Upper arms, legs, trunk, and inframammary region.

Histomorphology

- *Pattern*: Dilated vessels are filled with densely packed atypical lymphoid cells. Panniculus is more commonly involved than dermis.
- *Less common patterns*: Minimal extravascular involvement may occur.
- *Neoplastic cells*: Large atypical lymphocytes with prominent nucleoli (often with immunoblastic features) confined to the lumina of small- and intermediate-sized blood vessels (Fig. 39.2). Mitotic figures are frequent.
- *Reactive cells*: Normal peripheral blood cells.

Immunophenotype

- *Neoplastic cells* (Fig. 39.3): B-cell antigens (CD20+, CD79a+), usually MUM1+ and BCL2+, occasionally CD5+ (38% of cases), infrequently CD10+ (13% of cases).

Genetics

- Monoclonal immunoglobulin rearrangement may be identified.

Prognosis

- Variable (usually poor, but isolated cutaneous variant has better prognosis).
- 3-year survival: 60–81%.
- Adverse risk factors: central nervous system relapse and neurolymphomatosis.

Differential Diagnosis

- Other intravascular lymphomas (including NK/T cell and CD30+). Immunophenotyping is required for proper classification of intravascular infiltrates.
- Intralymphatic histiocytosis. The intraluminal cells are histiocytes with abundant cytoplasm and demonstrate CD68/CD163 expression. Dilated lymphatic vessels are not completely filled with cells.

Pearls and Pitfalls

1. Blood vessels are frequently overlooked in the evaluation of cutaneous lymphoid infiltrates but may show critical diagnostic features. Features such as angiocentrism, angiodestruction, or intravascular atypical cells are uncommon but have critical diagnostic value (Fig. 39.4).
2. The dermis may be spared, while the subcutaneous tissue is more commonly involved in intravascular large B-cell lymphoma. Therefore, a deep biopsy including panniculus is recommended.
3. The intravascular growth pattern appears to be secondary to defects in homing receptors and adhesion molecules (CD29/integrin beta-1, CD54/ICAM1).

Cutaneous Plasmablastic Lymphoma

Disease Definition

- Plasmablastic lymphoma is a predominantly extranodal lymphoma composed of a diffuse proliferation of large cells resembling immunoblasts and/or plasmablasts with a CD20-negative plasmacytic phenotype (Table 39.2). This category excludes cases with ALK or HHV8 expression.

Epidemiology

- Usually adults and elderly patients
- May occur in association with HIV infection or other causes of immunodeficiency (post-transplant, autoimmune disease, age-related immunosenescence)

Preferential Sites of Involvement

- Oral mucosa, head, and neck.
- Cutaneous cases are rare.

Clinical Features

- Nodules, tumors.
- *Less common presentations*: nodal involvement is rare.

Histomorphology

- *Pattern*: Dense diffuse dermal infiltrate of large atypical lymphoid cells (Fig. 39.5). Frequent mitotic figures and apoptosis.
- *Neoplastic cells*: large cells resembling immunoblasts (large noncleaved nucleus with prominent central nucleolus and moderately abundant cytoplasm; Fig. 39.6) and/or plasmablasts (abundant cytoplasm and eccentric nuclei with atypical features; Fig. 39.7).
- *Reactive cells*: sparse small reactive lymphocytes.

Immunophenotype

- *Neoplastic cells* (Fig. 39.8): plasma cell phenotype (CD20−, PAX5−, CD79a+/−, CD138+, MUM1+). Common expression of cytoplasmic immunoglobulin (either kappa or lambda), CD30, and EMA. CD10 and CD56 occasionally expressed. BCL2 and BCL6 usually negative. Negative cyclin D1. High proliferation index (Ki-67 > 90%). EBV (EBER) in situ hybridization is often positive (60–75% of cases). HHV8 and ALK are negative by definition.
- *Reactive cells*: sparse small CD3+ T cells.

Genetics

- Monoclonal IGH rearrangement may be demonstrated.

Prognosis

- Usually poor
- Adverse risk factors: MYC translocation

Differential Diagnosis

- Plasmablastic transformation of myeloma in patients with prior plasma cell neoplasms.
- Diffuse large B-cell lymphoma with predominant immunoblastic morphology is strongly positive with CD20 and PAX5, while plasmablastic lymphoma is negative with these markers and shows a plasma cell phenotype.
- Cutaneous marginal zone lymphoma, plasmacytic variant is a low-grade process and is composed of mature plasma cells. Plasmablastic lymphoma is a high-grade lymphoma composed of immunoblasts and/or plasmablasts.

Pearls and Pitfalls

1. Angiocentric lymphomas show infiltration and destruction of blood vessel walls, while intravascular lymphomas exhibit atypical lymphocytes within the lumen of preserved blood vessels (Fig. 39.9). Angiocentrism and angiodestruction are a feature of extranodal NK/T-cell lymphoma nasal type, lymphomatoid granulomatosis, lymphomatoid papulosis type E, and some cases of gamma-delta T-cell lymphoma.

Suggested Reading

Elder DE, Massi D, Scolyer RA, Willemze R, editors. WHO classification of skin tumors. 4th ed. Lyon: IARC; 2018.

Swerdlow SH et al. (Eds.). WHO classification of tumors of hematopoietic and lymphoid tissues. IARC: Lyon 2008.

Swerdlow SH, Campo E, Pileri SA, et al. The 2016 revision of the WHO classification of lymphoid neoplasms. Blood. 2016;127(20):2375–90.

Swerdlow SH, Campo E, Harris NL, Jaffe ES, Pileri SA, Stein H, Thiele J (Eds). WHO classification of tumours of haematopoietic and lymphoid tissues (revised 4th edition). IARC: Lyon 2017.

Willemze R, Jaffe ES, Burg G, et al. WHO-EORTC classification for cutaneous lymphomas. Blood. 2005;105(10):3768–85.

Table 40.1 Key facts

Definition
Primary cutaneous follicle center lymphoma is a tumor of neoplastic follicle center cells (centrocytes and a variable number of centroblasts) with a follicular, follicular and diffuse, or diffuse growth pattern
Prototypic clinical presentation
Middle-aged adults with grouped papules, plaques, and/or tumors on the scalp or back
Histopathologic findings
Nodular (follicular) and/or diffuse interstitial growth pattern. Abnormal follicular architecture: crowding of germinal centers (back to back follicles), diminished to absent mantle zones, usually diminished proliferation rate with few mitotic figures, and usually scant tingible-body macrophages
Most common immunophenotype: CD20+, CD79a+, CD3−, BCL6+, MUM1−, CD5−, and CD43−. Variable CD10 and BCL2
Prognosis
Good

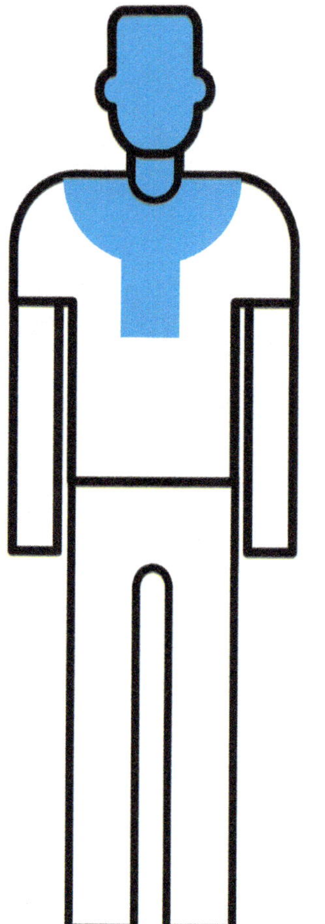

Fig. 40.1 Primary cutaneous follicle center lymphoma is an indolent skin lymphoma with preferential involvement of the scalp or upper trunk

© Springer Nature Switzerland AG 2019

A. Subtil, *Diagnosis of Cutaneous Lymphoid Infiltrates*,

https://doi.org/10.1007/978-3-030-11654-5_40

Fig. 40.2 Main types of lymphoid morphology

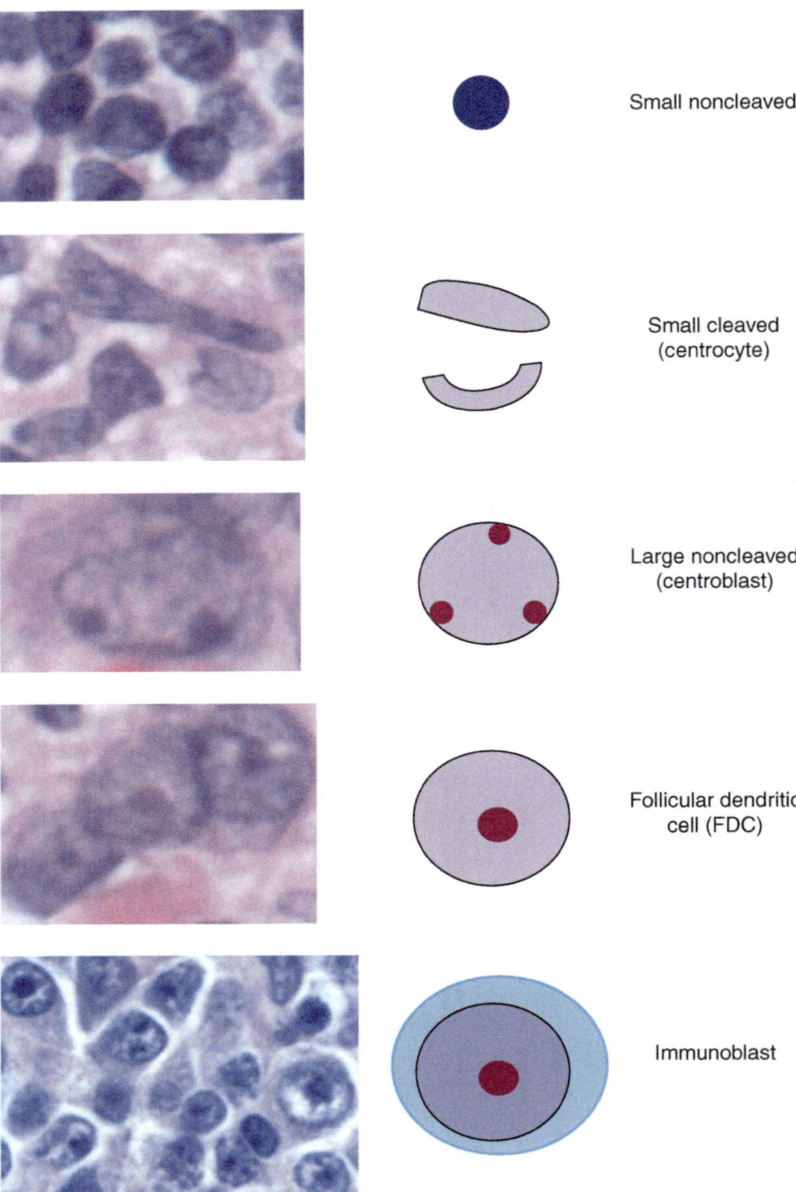

Fig. 40.3 Main compartments of the lymphoid follicle: mantle zone and germinal center

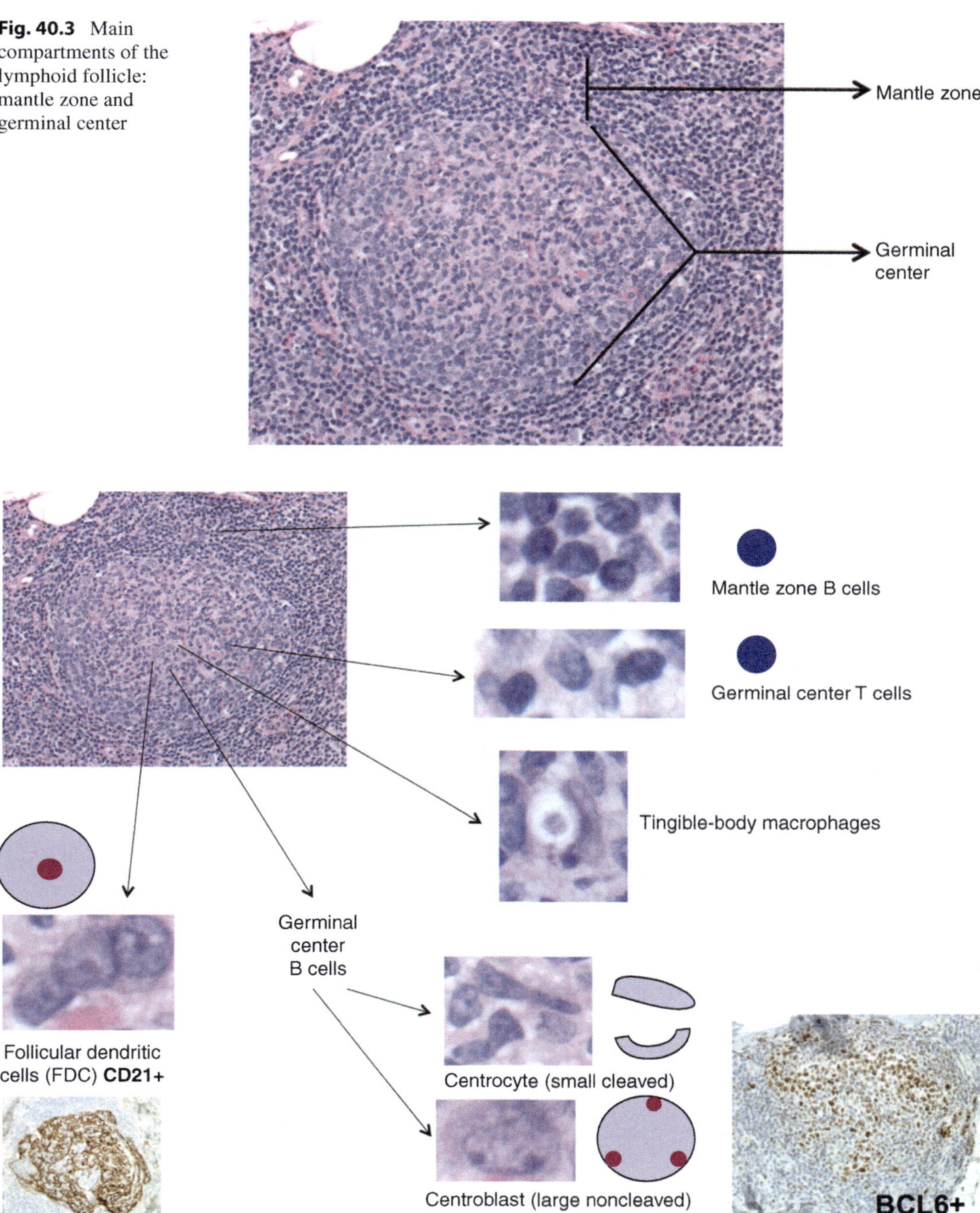

Fig. 40.4 Cellular components of the lymphoid follicle

Fig. 40.5 Comparison of the histomorphologic features of reactive and neoplastic lymphoid follicles in pseudolymphoma (reactive lymphoid hyperplasia) and cutaneous follicle center lymphoma, respectively

- Well spaced lymphoid follicles
- Mantle zones generally well preserved
- Frequent mitoses
- Tingible-body macrophages
- Germinal centers often polarized

- Back to back follicles (crowding)
- Mantle zones diminished to absent
- Less frequent mitoses (exception: high grade)
- Less frequent tingible-body macrophages

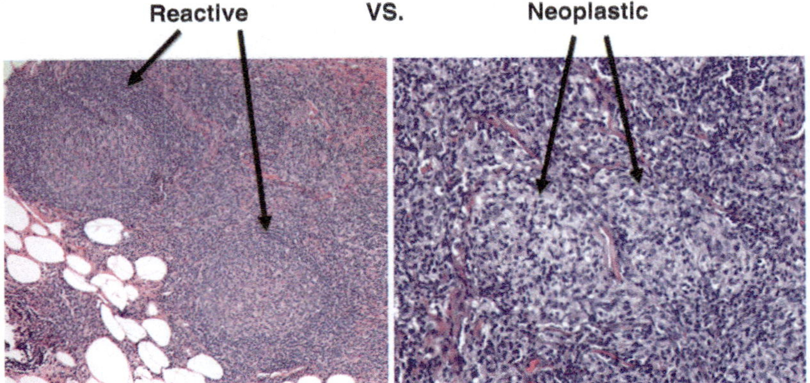

Fig. 40.6 Primary cutaneous follicle center lymphoma. Low-power magnification shows a predominantly nodular dermal infiltrate due to the presence of lymphoid follicle formation (round light areas)

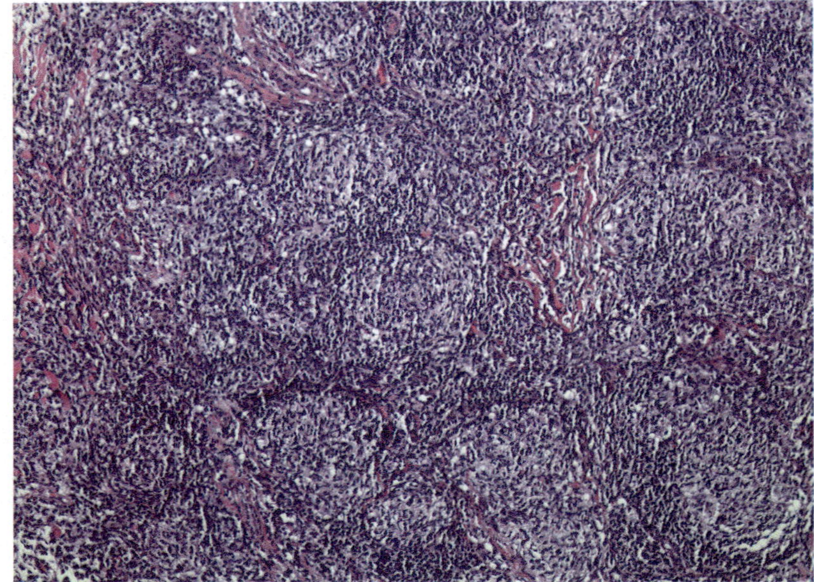

Fig. 40.7 Primary cutaneous follicle center lymphoma. High-power magnification demonstrates atypical lymphoid follicles (crowded, irregular outlines, and absent mantle zones)

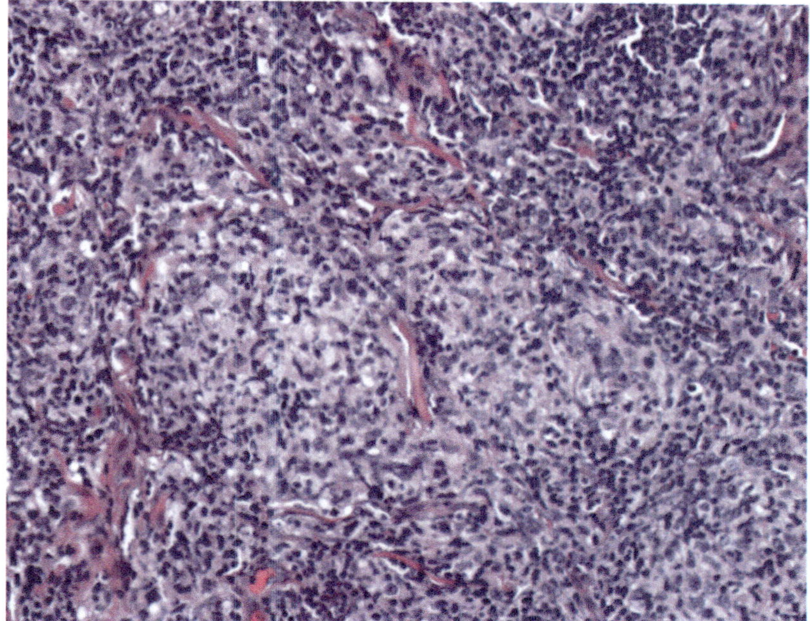

Fig. 40.8 Primary cutaneous follicle center lymphoma. Extensive staining with CD20 in the infiltrate

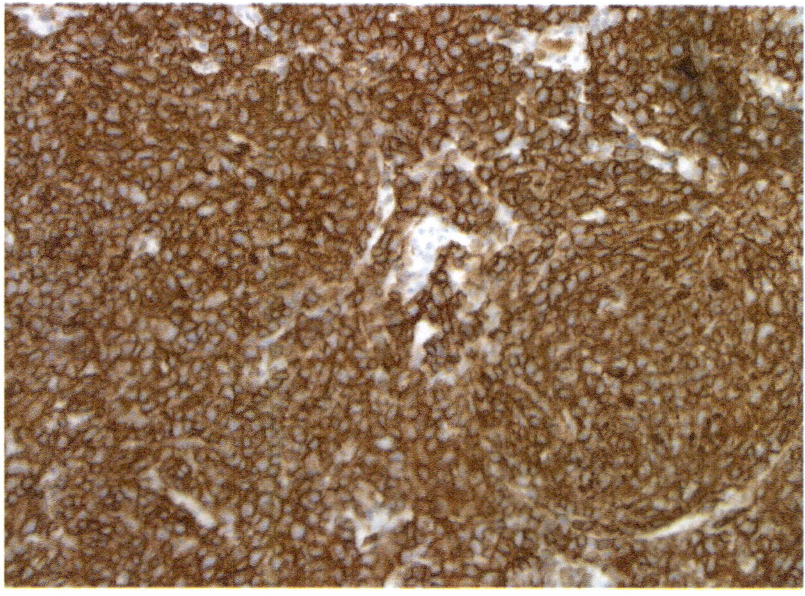

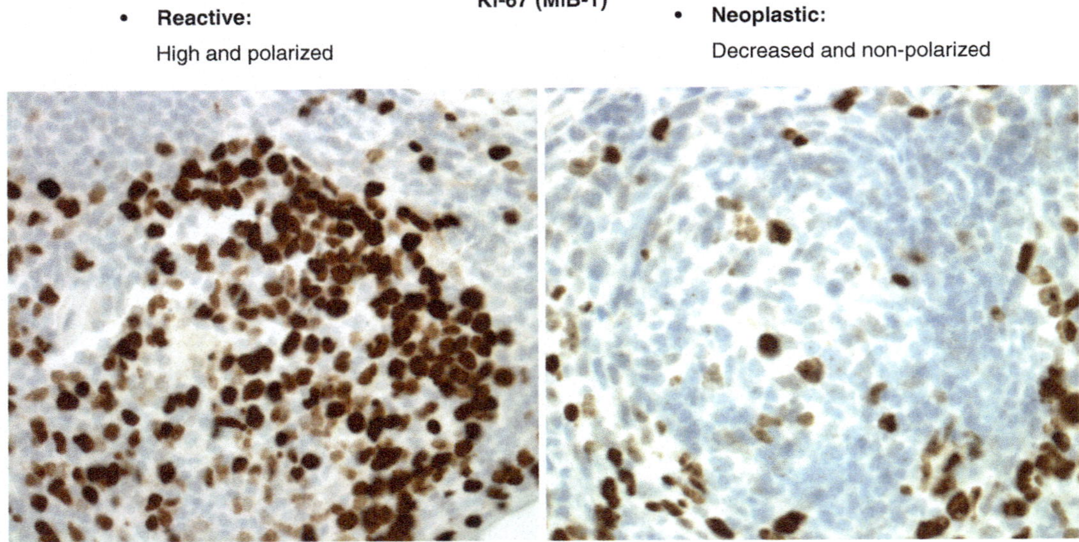

Fig. 40.9 Comparison of Ki-67 staining in reactive and neoplastic lymphoid follicles

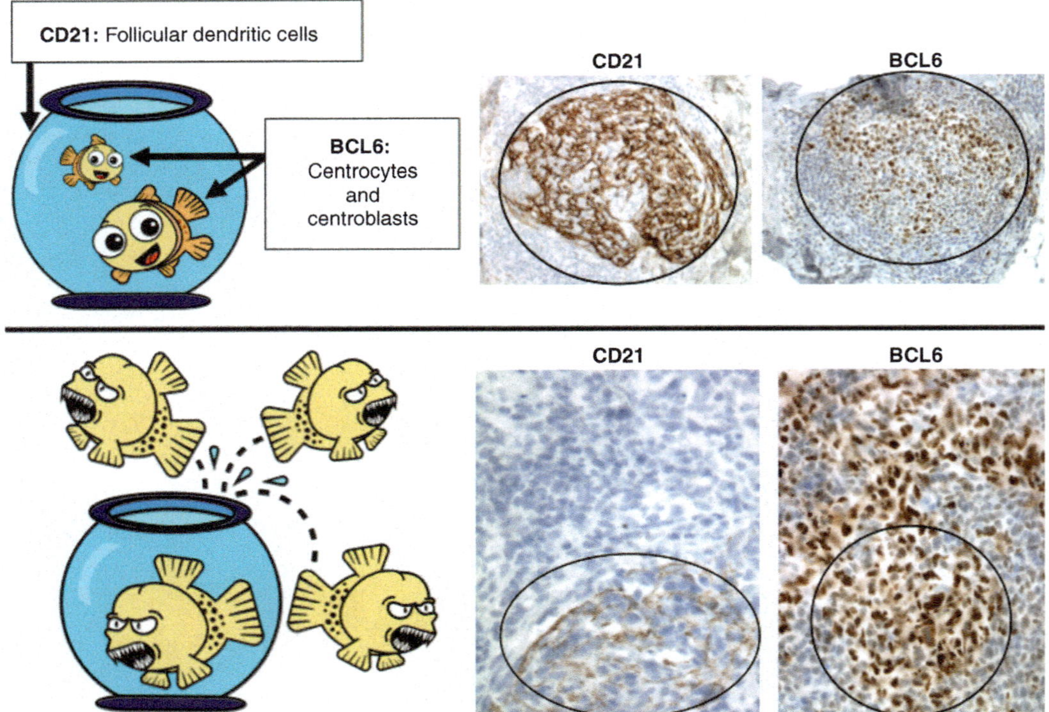

Fig. 40.10 Extrafollicular spread of neoplastic germinal center cells. BCL6 marks germinal center B cells (centrocytes and centroblasts), while CD21 highlights the lymphoid follicle by staining follicular dendritic cell meshworks. As an analogy, if centrocytes and centroblasts were fish, the follicular dendritic cell meshwork of the lymphoid follicle would be a fishbowl. In a benign process (reactive lymphoid hyperplasia, top panel), benign fish (goldfish) would stay inside the fishbowl (lymphoid follicle), and the foci of staining with both CD21 and BCL6 would match. In a malignant process (follicle center lymphoma, bottom panel), it would be common for malignant fish (piranhas) to jump out of the fishbowl (lymphoid follicle). This extrafollicular spread of germinal center B cells is highlighted by a mismatch between the staining pattern of BCL6 and CD21 (clusters of BCL6-positive cells are identified both within and outside the CD21-positive lymphoid follicle)

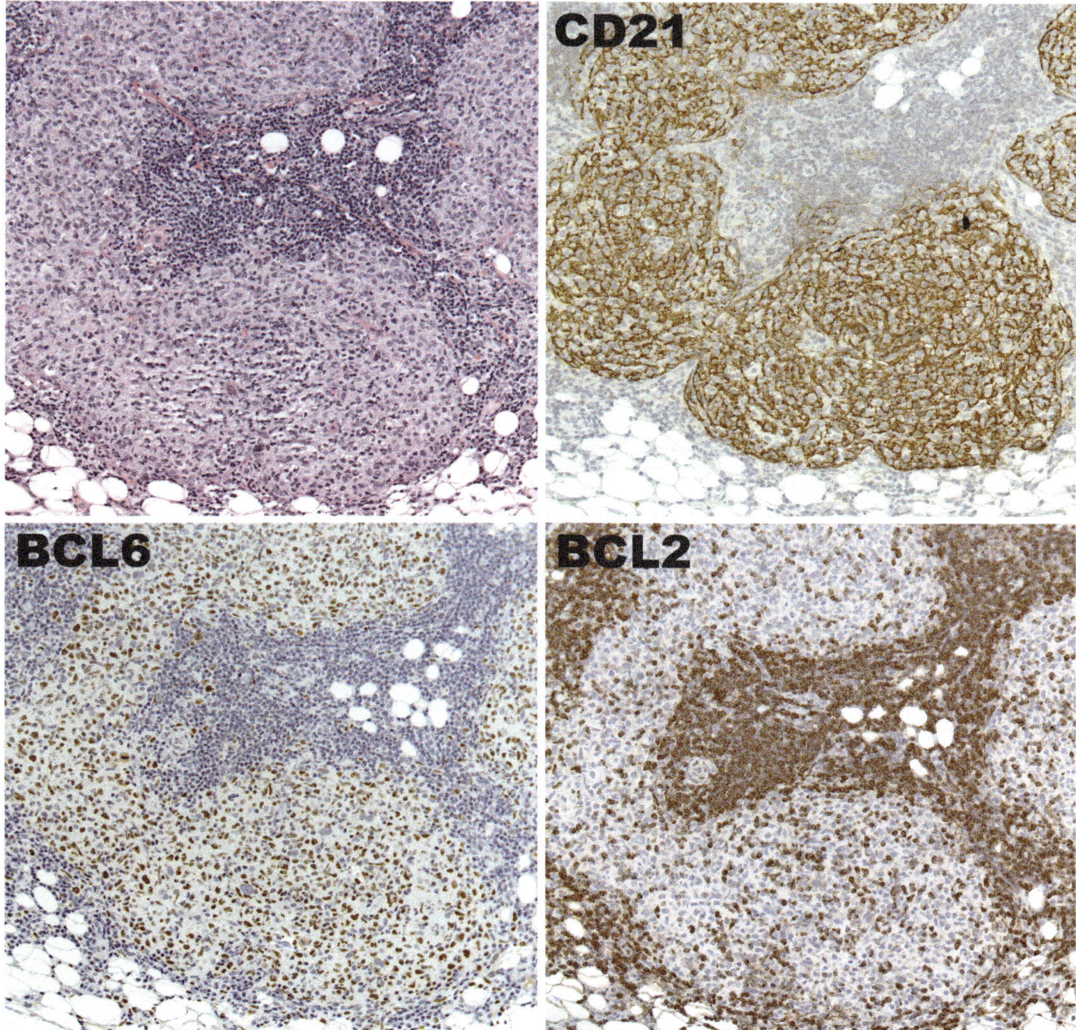

Fig. 40.11 BCL2-negative primary cutaneous follicle center lymphoma. The mantle zones are diminished to absent, and the germinal centers are crowded. CD21 stain highlights the irregular follicular dendritic cell meshworks of crowded follicles. Centrocytes and centroblasts are the main cellular component of the germinal centers and are highlighted by prominent BCL6 staining. BCL2 stain marks the mantle zone B cells and the follicular helper T cells in the germinal centers, while the neoplastic centrocytes and centroblasts are negative

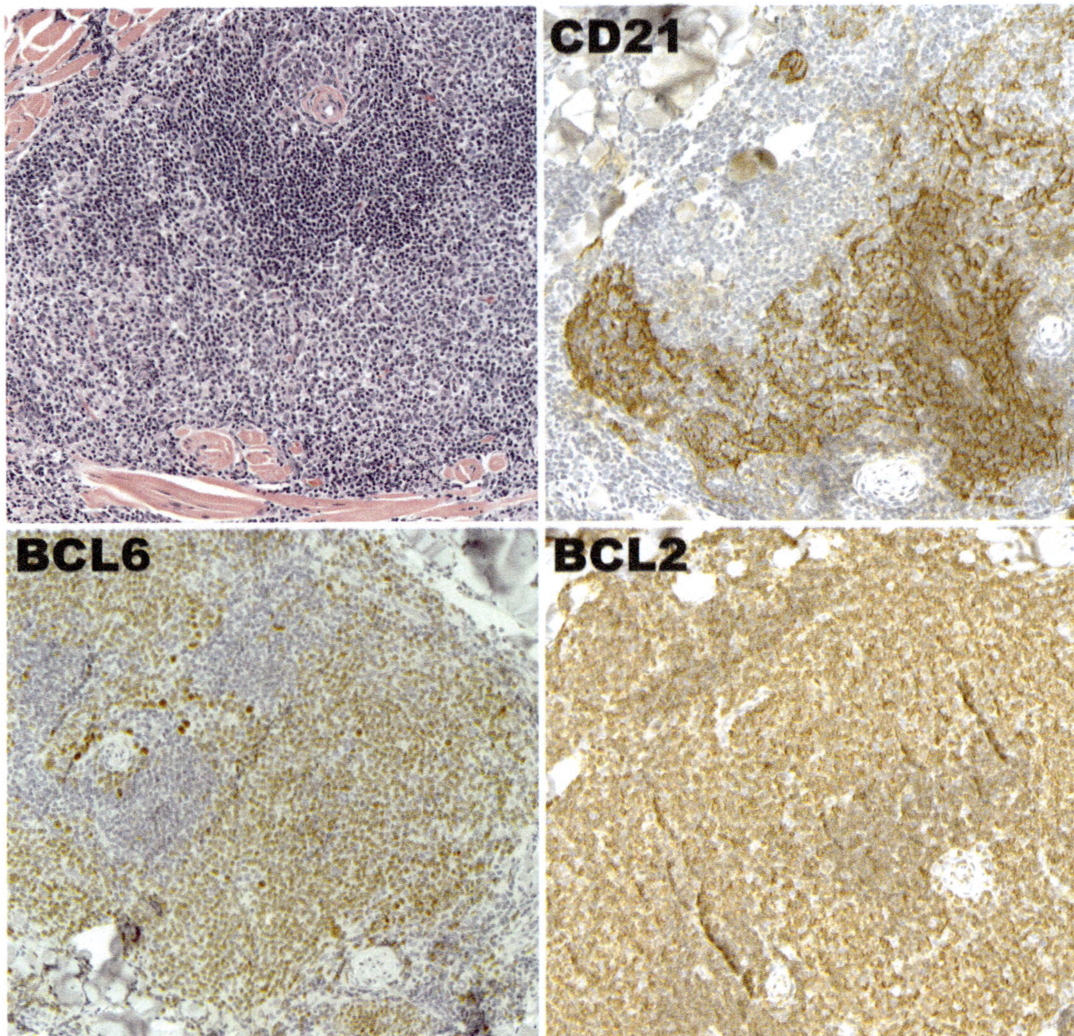

Fig. 40.12 BCL2-positive primary cutaneous follicle center lymphoma. The mantle zones are diminished to absent, and the germinal centers are crowded. CD21 stain highlights the irregular follicular dendritic cell meshworks of crowded follicles. Centrocytes and centroblasts are the main cellular component of the germinal centers and are highlighted by prominent BCL6 staining. BCL2 stain marks all cellular components, including the reactive mantle zone B cells and follicular helper T cells. The neoplastic centrocytes and centroblasts show aberrant expression of BCL2 protein

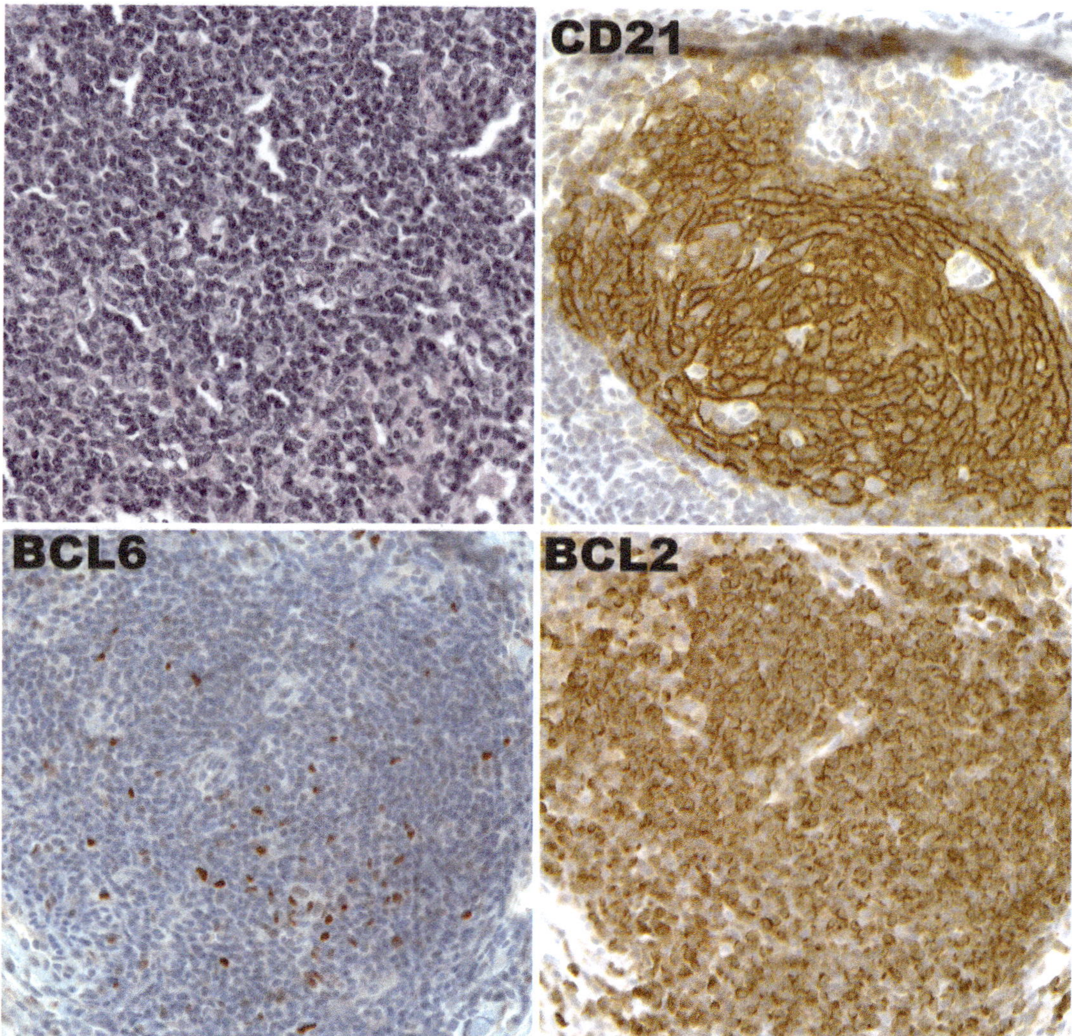

Fig. 40.13 BCL2-positive colonized lymphoid follicle in cutaneous marginal zone lymphoma (which can mimic BCL2-positive follicle center lymphoma). The majority of the infiltrate consists of small noncleaved lymphocytes. Follicles are difficult to visualize but are highlighted by CD21 staining of the follicular dendritic cell meshwork of the germinal center. Centrocytes and centroblasts are rare, and there is minimal to absent BCL6 staining. BCL2 stain marks the reactive mantle zone B cells and follicular helper T cells, as well as the small noncleaved marginal zone B cells colonizing the germinal center

Fig. 40.14 Comparison of cytomorphologic features of diffuse large B-cell lymphoma (admixture of immunoblasts and centroblasts) and cutaneous follicle center lymphoma (admixture of centroblasts and centrocytes)

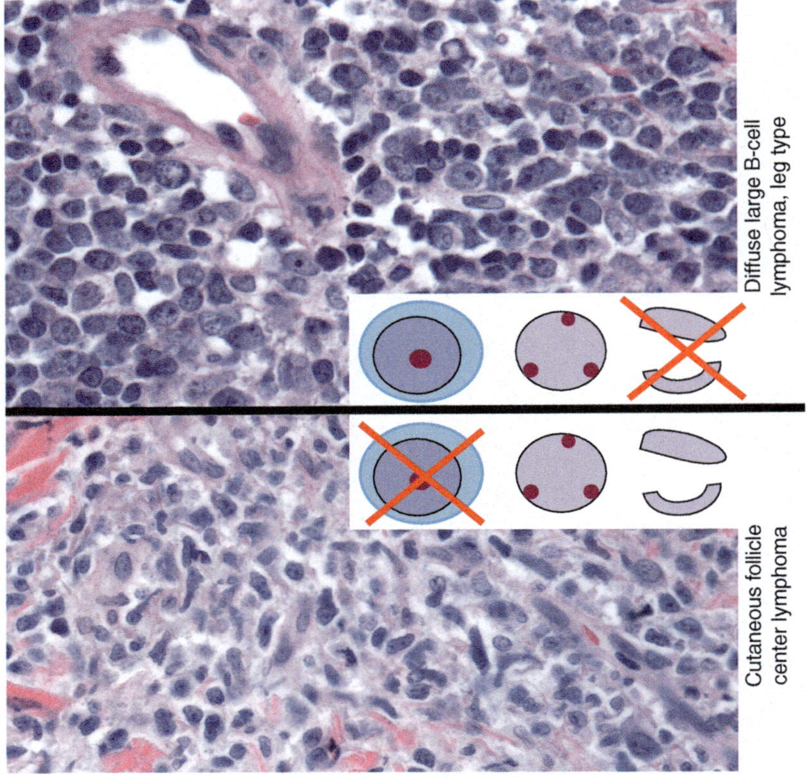

Disease Definition

– Primary cutaneous follicle center lymphoma is a tumor of neoplastic follicle center cells (centrocytes and a variable number of centro-blasts) with a follicular, follicular and diffuse, or diffuse growth pattern. It usually involves the head or trunk (Table 40.1).

Epidemiology

– Usually middle-aged adults
– Male predominance

Preferential Sites of Involvement

– The head (scalp, forehead) or trunk (Fig. 40.1).
– Solitary or localized skin lesions. Multifocal skin lesions or leg involvement are uncommon but may occur.

– Dissemination to extracutaneous sites is infrequent (10% of cases).

Clinical Features

– Papules, plaques, and/or nodules/tumors. Lesions are of variable size, firm, erythematous, violaceous, and infiltrated. Solitary or grouped lesions may be surrounded by erythematous patches or papules.
– *Less common presentations*: figurate plaques, ulceration, alopecia, anetoderma.

Histomorphology

– The cytomorphology of lymphocytes is part of the definition of several lymphomas (Tables 40.2 and 40.3). For example, the definition of follicle center lymphoma includes its composition of centrocytes and centroblasts (Fig. 40.2). In addition, it is important to recognize the architectural features of normal and abnormal lymphoid follicles (Figs. 40.3, 40.4, and 40.5).

- *Pattern*: Nodular (follicular) and/or diffuse interstitial growth pattern (Fig. 40.6). Dermal-based infiltrate with variable pannicular extension. Abnormal follicular architecture: crowding of germinal centers (back to back follicles), diminished to absent mantle zones, usually diminished proliferation rate with few mitotic figures, and usually scant tingible-body macrophages (Fig. 40.7). The epidermis is generally uninvolved.

- *Less common patterns*: Completely diffuse growth pattern (no nodularity but still composed of an admixture of centrocytes and centroblasts). Spindle cell lymphoma pattern composed predominantly of elongated centrocytes within myxoid stroma. Scattered large multilobated cells.

- *Neoplastic cells*: Germinal center B cells: centrocytes (small cleaved lymphocytes with scant cytoplasm) and centroblasts (large round/noncleaved lymphocytes with multiple peripheral nucleoli and scant cytoplasm).

- *Reactive cells*: small noncleaved reactive T cells, scattered histiocytes (some with features of tingible-body macrophages), and follicular dendritic cells (large round/noncleaved cells with prominent central nucleolus, often in overlapping small clusters). A significant component of plasma cells is generally not present.

Immunophenotype

- *Neoplastic cells*: CD20+, CD79a+, CD3−, BCL6+, MUM1−, CD5−, CD43−, and FOXP1− (Fig. 40.8). Ki-67 proliferation rate is generally less than 50%, though it may be higher in cases with a greater proportion of centroblasts (Fig. 40.9). Extrafollicular spread of centrocytes and centroblasts may be demonstrated in cases with at least partial diffuse growth pattern by comparing CD21 and BCL6 stains. CD21 highlights follicular dendritic cell meshworks, while BCL6 marks the germinal center B cells (centrocytes and centroblasts) (Fig. 40.10). CD10 expression is variable (more common in cases with nodular growth pattern). Most cases of primary cutaneous follicle center lymphoma (PCFCL) are BCL2-negative (Fig. 40.11). However, a significant subset of PCFCL and most (though not all) cases of systemic/nodal follicular lymphoma are positive with BCL2 immunohistochemistry (Fig. 40.12). Unlike marginal zone lymphoma, kappa and lambda immunostains are generally not helpful.

- *Reactive cells*: small T cells are positive with CD3, CD5, CD43, and BCL2 immunostains. Scattered CD68+ histiocytes.

Genetics

- Monoclonal rearrangement of immunoglobulin genes, but not always detectable due to somatic hypermutation.

Prognosis

- Indolent.
- 5-year survival: >95%.
- Adverse risk factors: presentation on the lower extremity and extracutaneous progression.
- Multifocal skin lesions, growth pattern, the presence of BCL2 expression or t(14;18) translocation, histologic grade, and number of centroblasts do not affect prognosis.
- Disease recurrence may occur in 30% of cases and tends to occur at the site of initial presentation. Cutaneous relapse is not associated with extracutaneous progression.

Differential Diagnosis

- Staging workup would demonstrate whether a follicular lymphoma in the skin is primary cutaneous or secondary cutaneous involvement by systemic/nodal follicular lymphoma. Staging should be performed after a lymphoma diagnosis at any organ.

- Numerous plasma cells would be unusual in cutaneous follicle center lymphoma. If frequent plasma cells are present in a dense dermal infiltrate with lymphoid follicles, consider the possibility of cutaneous marginal zone lymphoma with reactive follicles, and perform kappa and lambda light chain stains.
- Lymphoid follicles in marginal zone lymphoma (MZL) can be colonized by BCL2-positive neoplastic B cells and mimic BCL2-positive follicular lymphoma (ref. Chap. 20). In this differential, it is important to analyze the predominant cytomorphology (admixture of small cleaved/large noncleaved vs. predominantly small noncleaved) and the degree of BCL6 expression. Colonized follicles in MZL are often difficult to visualize but are highlighted by CD21 staining of the follicular dendritic cell meshwork of the germinal center. Centrocytes (small cleaved) and centroblasts (large noncleaved) are rare, and there is minimal to absent BCL6 staining. BCL2 stain marks the reactive mantle zone B cells and follicular helper T cells, as well as the small noncleaved marginal zone B cells colonizing the germinal center (Fig. 40.13).
- The cytomorphology of lymphocytes (as well as the growth pattern) is part of the definition of several lymphomas. For example, the definition of follicle center lymphoma includes centrocytes and centroblasts, while diffuse large B-cell lymphomas (DLBCL) are composed of immunoblasts and centroblasts. DLBCL lacks centrocytes (small cleaved cells) (Fig. 40.14). Therefore, being able to properly recognize different types of lymphocytes in a lymphoid infiltrate is critical for the correct diagnosis and classification of lymphomas. Strong expression of MUM1 and negative CD21 (due to absence of lymphoid follicles) by cutaneous DLBCL is also helpful in this differential. A lymphoma with a diffuse growth pattern (i.e., no nodular component due to lack of lymphoid follicles) and a monotonous proliferation of centroblasts and immunoblasts (i.e., without centrocytes) is classified as DLBCL (whether in the skin or elsewhere).

Table 40.2 Basic lymphoid cell morphologies

Lymphoid cell morphology	Dense chromatin	Nuclear shape	Prominent nucleolus	Cytoplasm
Small noncleaved	Yes (dark blue)	Round	No	Scant
Centrocyte (Small cleaved)	No	Elongated, spindle-like (cleaved)	No	Scant
Centroblast (Large noncleaved)	No	Round	Yes (multiple and peripheral)	Scant
Immunoblast	No	Round	Yes (single and central)	Moderate
Follicular dendritic cell	No	Round	Yes (single and central)	Scant

Table 40.3 Cellular components of lymphoid follicles

Cell type	Location in lymphoid follicle	Cytomorphologic features	Immunophenotype
Follicular dendritic cell (FDC)	Germinal center	Large round noncleaved nucleus with single central nucleolus	CD21+ (immunohistochemical stain highlights the dendritic processes)
Germinal center B cells (centrocytes and centroblasts)	Germinal center	Small cleaved and large noncleaved cells with scant cytoplasm	CD20+, BCL6+, BCL2−
(Tingible-body) Macrophages	Germinal center	Reniform, elongated nucleus and abundant cytoplasm with apoptotic debris	CD68+
Follicular helper T cells	Germinal center	Small noncleaved	CD3+, BCL2+
Mantle zone B cells	Mantle zone	Small noncleaved	CD20+, BCL6−, BCL2+

Table 40.4 Differential diagnosis of cutaneous lymphoid infiltrates with lymphoid follicle formation

Reactive/lymphoproliferative disorders	Lymphomas
Cutaneous reactive lymphoid hyperplasia (such as may occur due to vaccinations, arthropod bites, medications, and spirochetal infections)	Primary cutaneous follicle center lymphoma
Cutaneous Rosai-Dorfman disease	Secondary cutaneous involvement by systemic/nodal follicular lymphoma
Cutaneous IgG4-related disease	Cutaneous marginal zone lymphoma
Lupus panniculitis	Some cases of tumor-stage mycosis fungoides

Pearls and Pitfalls

1. Extrafollicular spread of germinal center B cells is a useful feature in the diagnosis of follicle center lymphoma; however, it is not always present. Cases of follicular lymphoma without a diffuse/interstitial component would lack this finding.

2. It is important to remember that there must be prominent clusters of BCL6-positive cells for an infiltrate to be considered BCL6-positive. Only a few scattered cells staining with BCL6 should be ignored.

3. BCL6 may be a technically difficult special stain, and it would be judicious to be careful with overstained or understained BCL6. Always confirm that the morphology of cells staining with BCL6 is that of centrocytes (cleaved) and centroblasts (large noncleaved cells with multiple peripheral nucleoli).

4. CD21 may be a technically difficult stain. If follicular dendritic cells (large noncleaved nucleus with single central nucleolus and scant cytoplasm, often in small clusters) are identified in a lymphoid infiltrate, there should be some staining with CD21. If follicular dendritic cells are visualized in the infiltrate (H&E stain) and CD21 stain looks completely negative, it likely represents a false negative, and the stain should be repeated.

5. In pseudolymphomas and in marginal zone lymphoma, lymphoid follicles are reactive, while in follicle center (follicular) lymphoma, lymphoid follicles are neoplastic.

6. Cutaneous marginal zone B-cell lymphoma often exhibits multifocal skin lesions (on trunk and extremities), while cutaneous follicle center lymphoma tends to be more localized/grouped (on the scalp or back).

7. B-cell lymphomas are associated with light chain restriction. While this is easily identifiable with flow cytometry, the demonstration of light chain restriction via tissue immunohistochemistry (of formalin-fixed, paraffin-embedded tissue) would generally require significant cytoplasmic immunoglobulin (i.e., plasmacytic differentiation in a substantial subset of the neoplastic B cells). Since follicle center lymphoma generally lacks plasmacytic differentiation (unlike marginal zone lymphoma), kappa and lambda immunohistochemistry is usually not helpful in the diagnosis of follicle center lymphoma. As reviewed in this chapter, the diagnosis of follicle center lymphoma is based on a combination of architectural, cytomorphologic, and immunophenotypic features. Flow cytometry would require fresh tissue and is not commonly used in skin lesions.

8. Because the diagnosis of follicle center lymphoma is based on a combination of architectural, cytomorphologic,

and immunophenotypic features, small or superficial biopsies will generally be nondiagnostic.

9. The presence of a nodular pattern in a dermal lymphoid infiltrate would suggest the presence of lymphoid follicles (Table 40.4).

10. Reticulohistiocytoma of the dorsum (Crosti lymphoma) is the historic term for primary cutaneous follicle center lymphoma involving the back.

11. The gold standard for determining primary cutaneous follicle center lymphoma versus cutaneous presentation of systemic/nodal follicular lymphoma is the staging workup (not whether BCL2 and/or CD10 are present). The standard of care is that a staging workup is performed after a diagnosis of lymphoma (at any organ).

12. Unlike nodal follicular lymphoma, histologic grading (based on the number of centroblasts per high-power microscopic field) is not reported in primary cutaneous follicle center lymphoma and does not affect prognosis. Routinely reporting histologic grade in cutaneous follicle center lymphomas prior to staging workup may lead to overtreatment of grade 3 cases.

13. Rarely, systemic follicular lymphomas may present with secondary skin involvement. These cases are diagnosed by the demonstration of extracutaneous disease via staging workup after the initial skin biopsy. In this uncommon situation, a histologic grade for the cutaneous infiltrate can be reported in an addendum after the positive staging workup.

Suggested Reading

Leinweber B, Colli C, Chott A, Kerl H, Cerroni L. Differential diagnosis of cutaneous infiltrates of B lymphocytes with follicular growth pattern. Am J Dermatopathol. 2004;26(1):4–13.

Orazi A, Weiss LM, Foucar K, Knowles DM. Knowles' neoplastic hematopathology. 3rd ed. Philadelphia: Lippincott Williams & Wilkins; 2014.

Swerdlow SH, et al., editors. WHO classification of tumors of hematopoietic and lymphoid tissues. Lyon: IARC; 2008.

Swerdlow SH, Campo E, Pileri SA, et al. The 2016 revision of the WHO classification of lymphoid neoplasms. Blood. 2016;127(20):2375–90.

Swerdlow SH, et al., editors. WHO classification of tumors of hematopoietic and lymphoid tissues (revised 4th edition). Lyon: IARC; 2017.

Willemze R, Jaffe ES, Burg G, et al. WHO-EORTC classification for cutaneous lymphomas. Blood. 2005;105(10):3768–85.

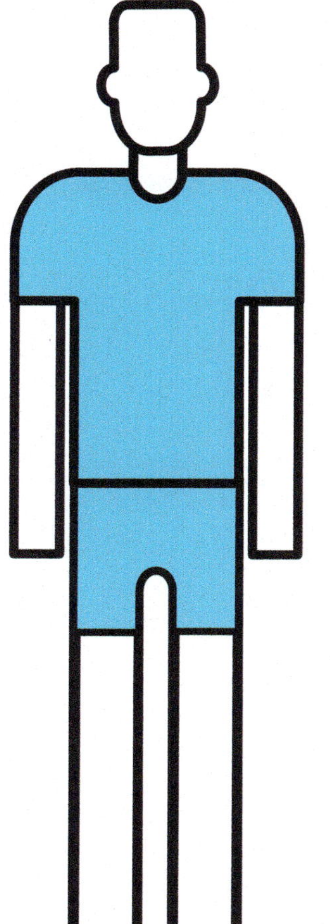

Fig. 41.1 Cutaneous marginal zone B-cell lymphoma is an indolent process with preferential involvement of trunk and/or proximal extremities

Table 41.1 Key facts

Definition

Primary cutaneous marginal zone B-cell lymphoma (PCMZL) is an indolent skin lymphoma composed of morphologically heterogeneous small B cells, including marginal zone (centrocyte-like) cells, lymphoplasmacytoid cells, and plasma cells, admixed with small numbers of scattered centroblast- or immunoblast-like cells. A variable component of reactive T cells and reactive lymphoid follicles is frequently present

Prototypic clinical presentation

Multifocal papules and/or nodules on trunk and/or proximal extremities

Histopathologic findings

Superficial and deep dermal, nodular, interstitial, and/ or perifollicular, heterogeneous infiltrate composed of a variable admixture of predominantly small lymphocytes, lymphoplasmacytoid, and plasma cells. Common vertical orientation adjacent to a hair follicle ("blue column in the dermis"), though epithelial infiltration (epitheliotropism) is uncommon. Reactive lymphoid follicles are common and may be colonized. Most common immunophenotype: marginal zone B cells (CD20+, CD79a+, CD5−, CD10−, BCL6−, BCL2+, low Ki-67) and lymphoplasmacytoid and/or plasma cells (CD20-, CD79a+, monotypic lambda or kappa). CD43 expression may be seen

Prognosis

Excellent

© Springer Nature Switzerland AG 2019
A. Subtil, *Diagnosis of Cutaneous Lymphoid Infiltrates*,
https://doi.org/10.1007/978-3-030-11654-5_41

Fig. 41.2 Cutaneous marginal zone B-cell lymphoma. A vaguely nodular, superficial, and deep dermal lymphoid infiltrate with perifollicular accentuation is present

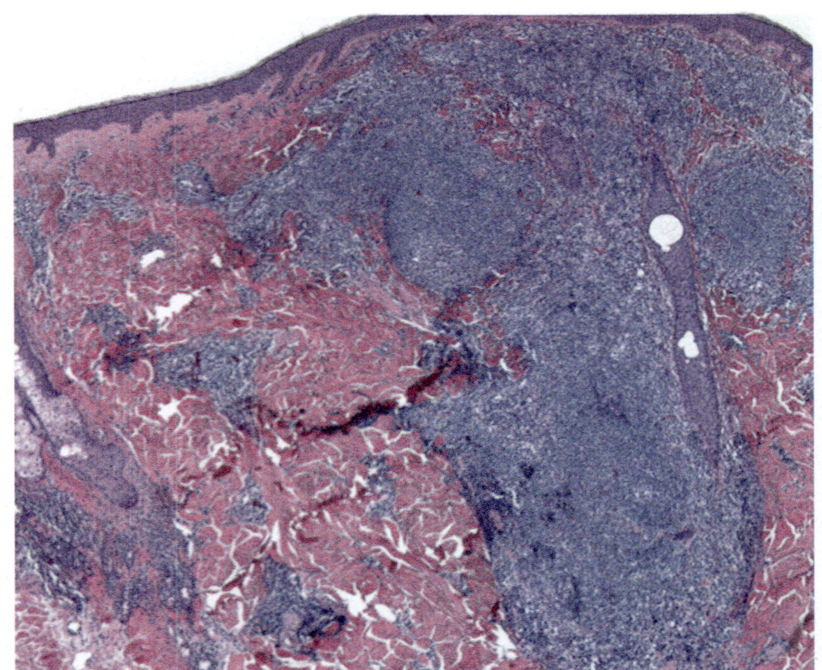

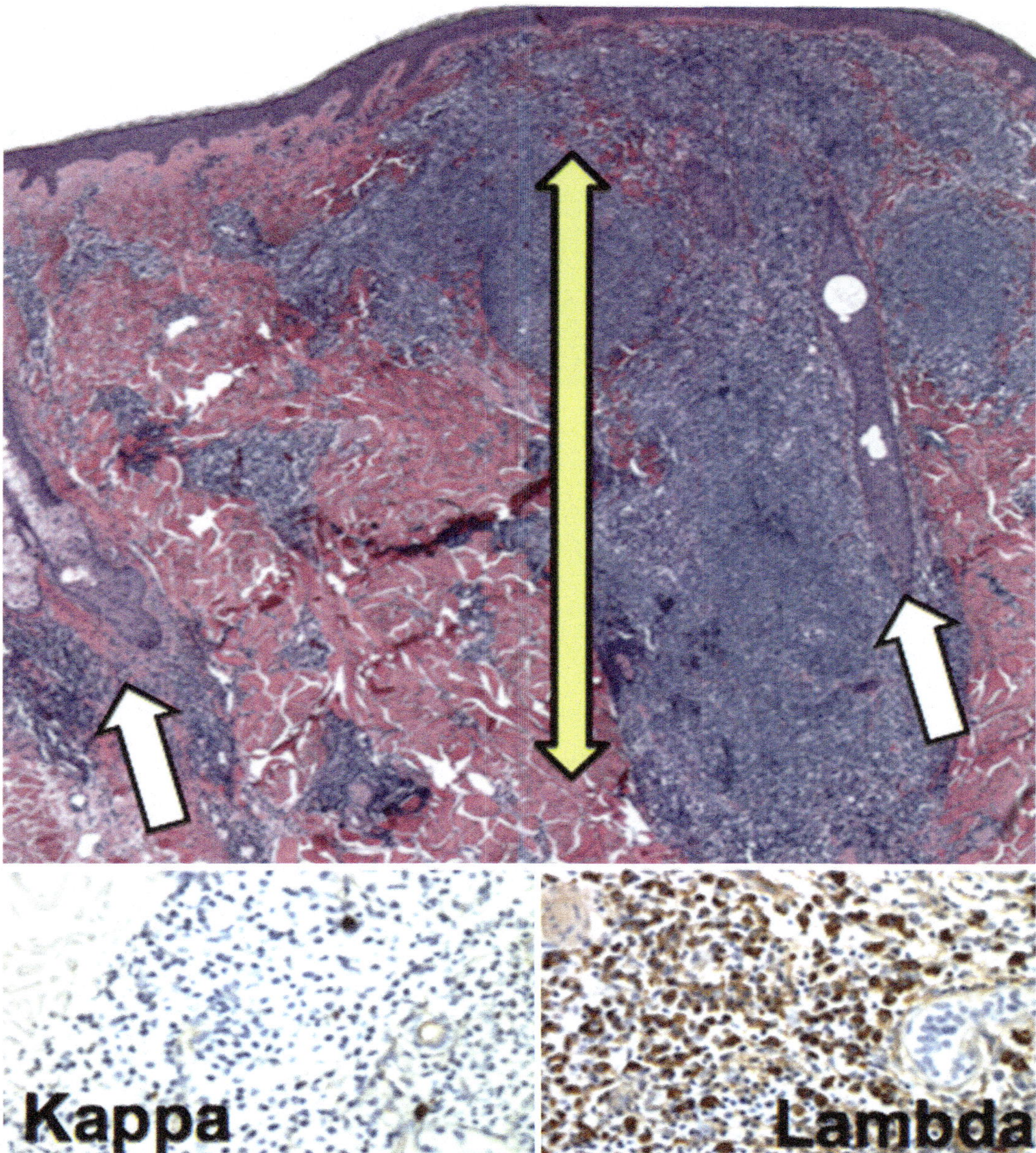

Fig. 41.3 Cutaneous marginal zone B-cell lymphoma showing perifollicular accentuation. A vertical orientation (yellow arrow) of the infiltrate resembling a column adjacent to a hair follicle (white arrow) is a common pattern. Immunoglobulin light chain stains demonstrate a marked predominance of lambda compared to that seen with kappa, consistent with a monotypic pattern

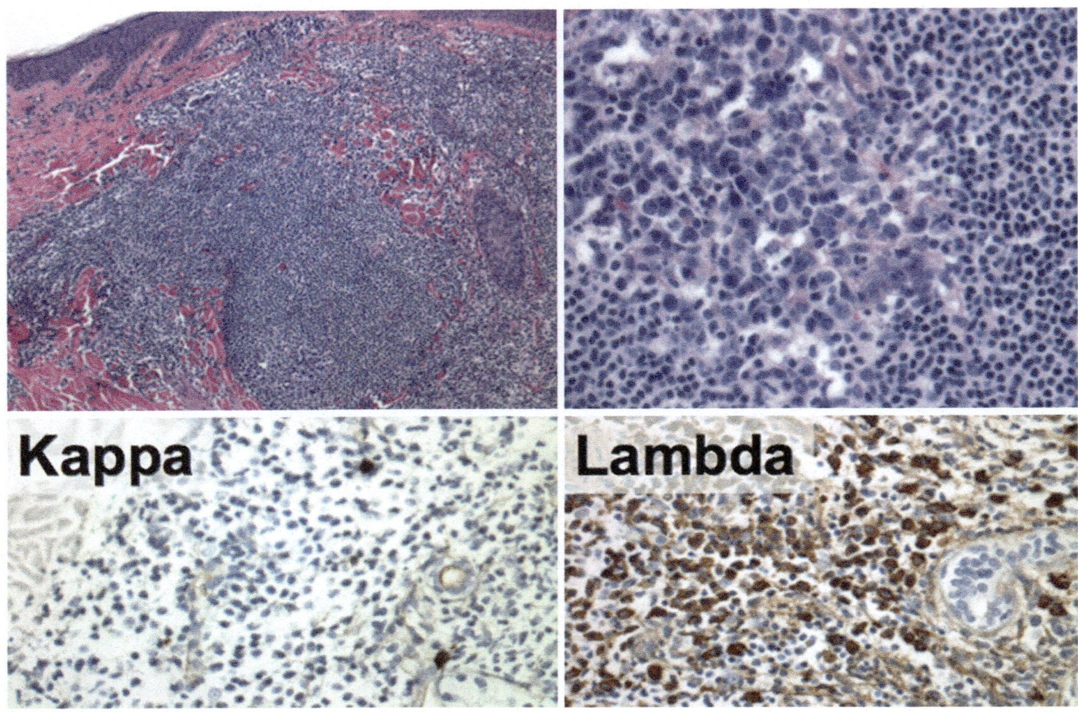

Fig. 41.4 Reactive lymphoid follicles are frequently present in cutaneous marginal zone B-cell lymphoma. The lymphoid follicles are well spaced and show preserved mantle zones and reactive germinal centers. However, unlike reactive lymphoid hyperplasia, the plasma cells show light chain restriction

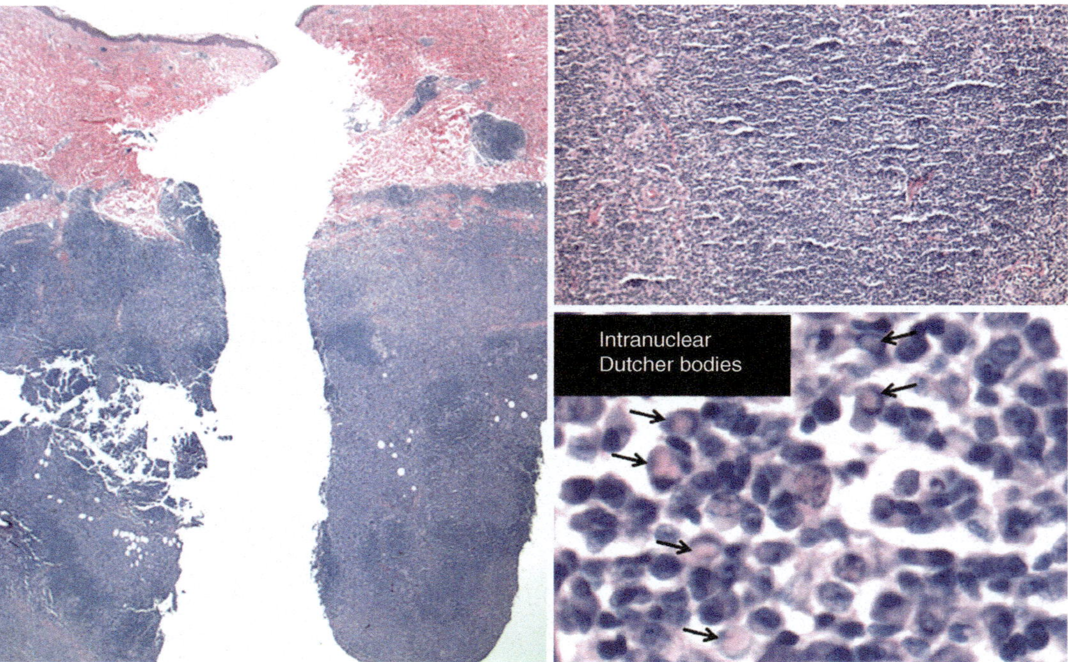

Fig. 41.5 Cutaneous marginal zone B-cell lymphoma with intranuclear Dutcher bodies (arrows) ("lymphoplasmacytic variant," "cutaneous immunocytoma")

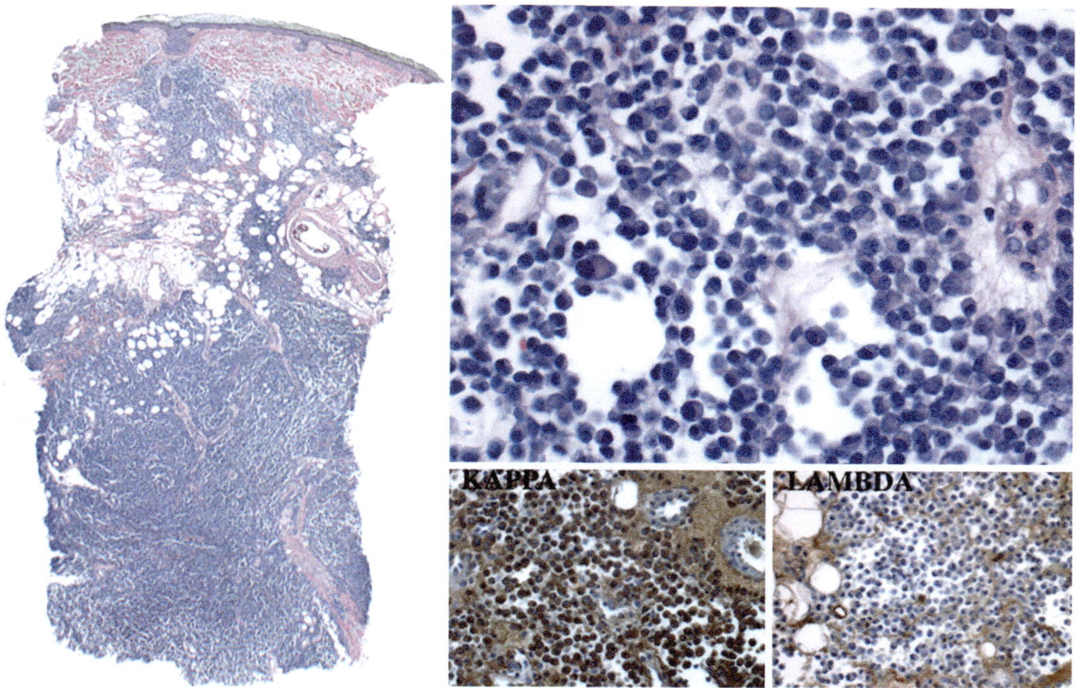

Fig. 41.6 Cutaneous marginal zone B-cell lymphoma composed exclusively of monotypic plasma cells ("plasmacytic variant of PCMZL," "primary cutaneous plasmacytoma without underlying plasma cell myeloma")

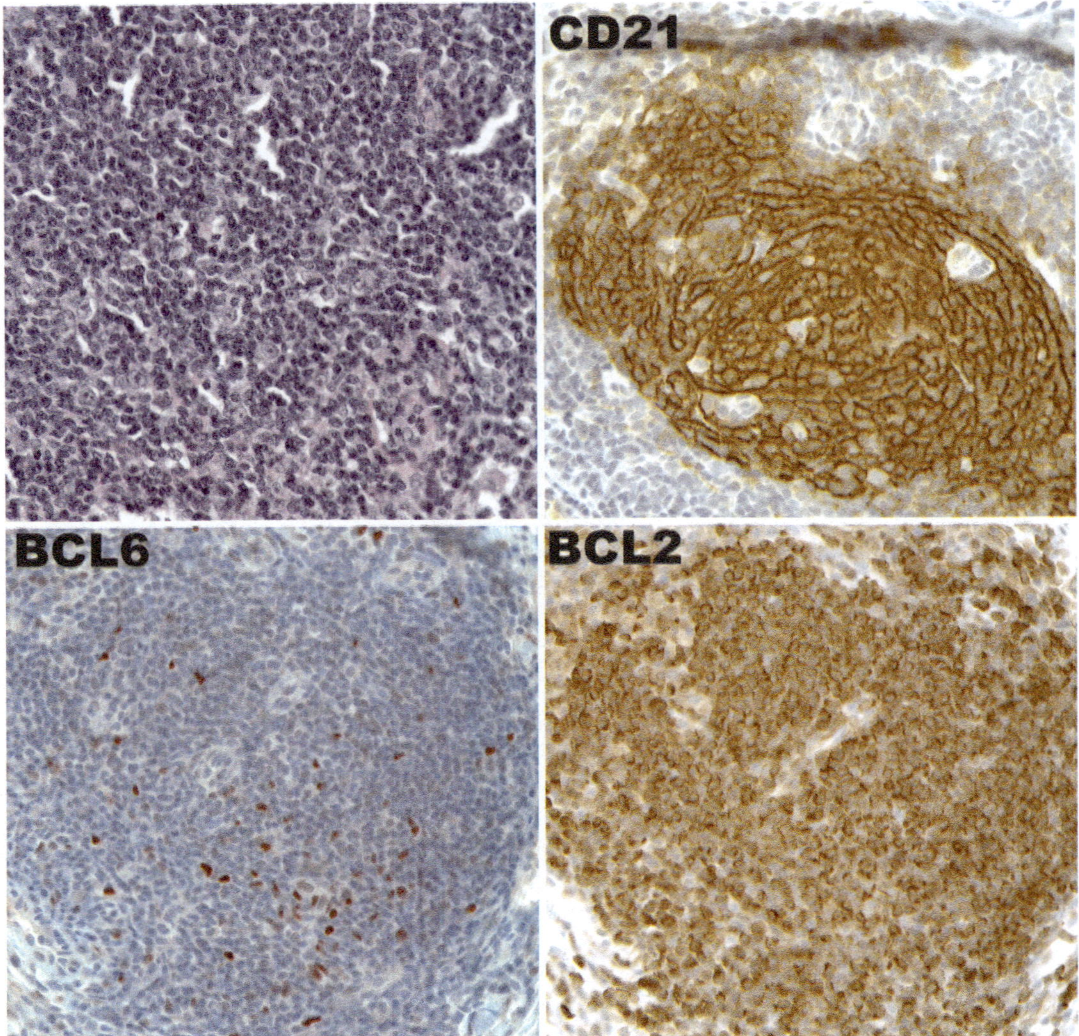

Fig. 41.7 BCL2-positive, colonized lymphoid follicle in cutaneous marginal zone lymphoma. Follicles are difficult to visualize but are highlighted by CD21 staining of the follicular dendritic cell meshwork of the germinal center. Centrocytes and centroblasts are rare, and there is mini-mal BCL6 staining. BCL2 stain marks the reactive mantle zone B cells and follicular helper T cells, as well as the small noncleaved marginal zone B cells colonizing the germinal center

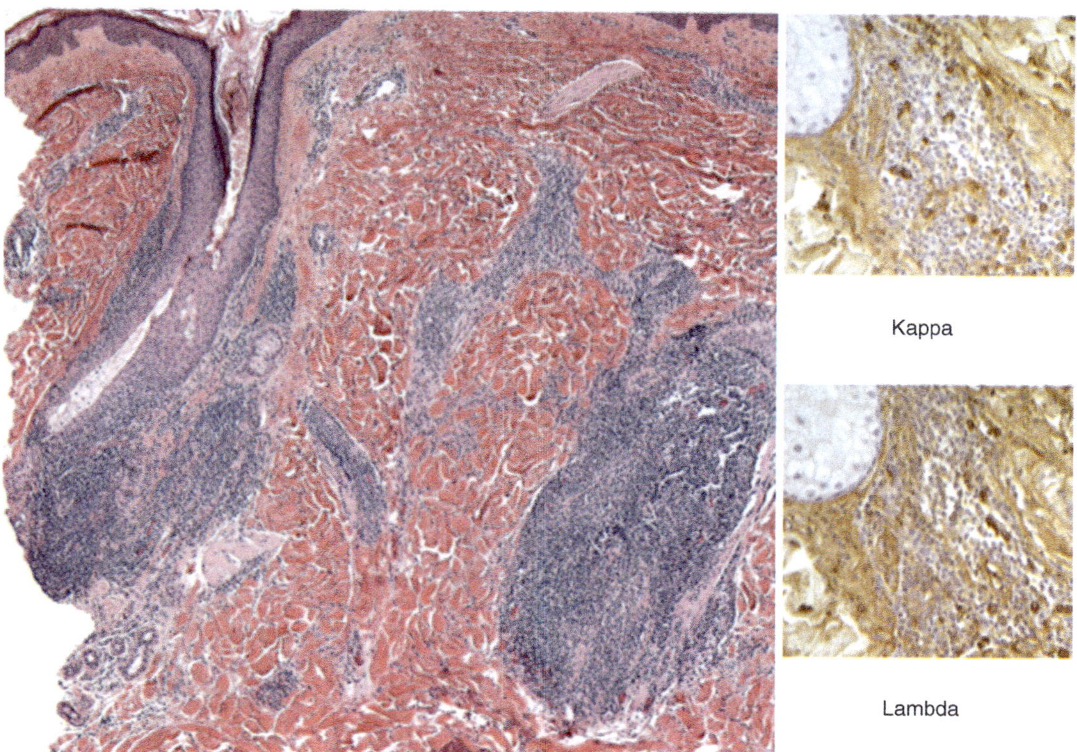

Fig. 41.8 Lymphomatoid drug eruption due to carbamazepine showing vertical orientation of the infiltrate adjacent to a hair follicle. Kappa and lambda immunoglobulin light chain stains demonstrate a polytypic pattern in scattered plasma cells

Disease Definition

- Primary cutaneous marginal zone B-cell lymphoma (PCMZL) is an indolent skin lymphoma composed of morphologically heterogeneous small B cells, including marginal zone (centrocyte-like) cells, lymphoplasmacytoid cells, and plasma cells, admixed with small numbers of scattered centroblast- or immunoblast-like cells. A variable component of reactive T cells and reactive lymphoid follicles is frequently observed (Table 41.1).
- PCMZL may show a variety of histopathologic patterns and includes cases previously designated as cutaneous follicular lymphoid hyperplasia with monotypic plasma cells, primary cutaneous immunocytoma, and primary cutaneous plasmacytoma without underlying plasma cell myeloma ("extramedullary plasmacytoma of the skin"). Some patients with PCMZL may show different histopathologic patterns in different lesions.
- PCMZL is considered part of the broad group of extranodal marginal zone lymphomas commonly involving mucosal sites, called MALT (mucosa-associated lymphoid tissue) lymphomas.

Epidemiology

- Usually adults but may occur in children and young adults

Preferential Sites of Involvement

- Trunk and extremities (especially upper extremities) (Fig. 41.1)

Clinical Features

- Multiple or solitary, erythematous to violaceous, non-ulcerated papules and/or nodules. Often multifocal skin lesions. Lesions may be clustered.
- *Less common presentations*: Large dome-shaped tumor on lower extremity. Spontaneous resolution and anetoderma.

Histomorphology

- *Pattern*: variably dense, superficial, and deep dermal, nodular, interstitial, and/or perifollicular lymphoid infiltrate. The infiltrate is generally heterogeneous and is composed of a variable admixture of predominantly small lymphocytes, lymphoplasmacytoid, and plasma cells (Fig. 41.2). Common vertical orientation of the lymphoplasmacytic dermal infiltrate adjacent to a hair follicle ("blue column in the dermis," Fig. 41.3 and Table 41.2), though epithelial infiltration (epitheliotropism) is uncommon. Small numbers of scattered centroblast- or immunoblast-like cells may be seen. Reactive lymphoid follicles are common and may be surrounded by cells with abundant cytoplasm (Fig. 41.4). Focal superficial pannicular extension may occur.
- *Less common patterns*: dense heterogeneous infiltrates with intranuclear Dutcher bodies ("cutaneous immunocytoma," "lymphoplasmacytic variant of PCMZL") (Fig. 41.5). Primary cutaneous plasmacytoma without underlying plasma cell myeloma ("extramedullary plasmacytoma of the skin"): skin-only infiltrates composed almost exclusively of monotypic plasma cells ("plasmacytic variant of PCMZL") (Fig. 41.6). Rare cases of PCMZL lack significant plasmacytic differentiation and may be difficult to diagnose due to noncontributory kappa and lambda stains.
- *Neoplastic cells*: marginal zone B cells (small lymphocytes with dense chromatin and variable cytoplasm), lymphoplasmacytoid, and plasma cells.
- *Reactive cells*: Small T cells (which may predominate). Reactive lymphoid follicles are common.

Immunophenotype

- PCMZL is usually composed of a heterogeneous infiltrate with a variable proportion of neoplastic and reactive cells. Depending on the composition and proportion of these different subsets, variations in the predominant immunophenotype will occur. Therefore, it is important to correlate the cytomorphologic features with the immunohistochemical stains.
- *Neoplastic cells*: small marginal zone B cells (CD20+, CD79a+, CD5−, CD10−, BCL6−, BCL2+, low Ki-67), lymphoplasmacytoid, and/or plasma cells (CD20−, CD79a+, CD138+, monotypic lambda or kappa via immunohistochemistry, or in situ hybridization). CD43 expression may be seen.
- *Reactive cells*: small T cells (CD3+, CD20−) and lymphoid follicles with reactive germinal centers (CD20+, CD79a+, CD21+, BCL6+, BCL2−, high Ki-67).

Genetics

- Monoclonal rearrangement of immunoglobulin genes in majority of cases.
- While the same clone is usually identified in different lesions, some patients may have different clones at different sites.

Prognosis

- Excellent. Cutaneous recurrence is common, but extracutaneous dissemination is rare.
- 5-year survival: 99–100%.
- Adverse risk factors: transformation to diffuse large B-cell lymphoma (rare).

Differential Diagnosis

- Numerous plasma cells would be unusual in cutaneous follicle center lymphoma. If frequent plasma cells are present in a dense dermal infiltrate with lymphoid follicles, consider the possibility of cutaneous marginal zone lymphoma with reactive follicles, and perform kappa and lambda light chain stains.

– Lymphoid follicles in marginal zone lymphoma (MZL) can be colonized by BCL2-positive neoplastic B cells and mimic BCL2-positive follicular lymphoma (ref. Chap. 20). In this differential, it is important to analyze the predominant cytomorphology (admixture of small cleaved/large noncleaved vs. predominantly small noncleaved) and the degree of BCL6 expression. Colonized follicles in MZL are often difficult to visualize but are highlighted by CD21 staining of the follicular dendritic cell meshwork of the germinal center. Centrocytes (small cleaved) and centroblasts (large noncleaved) are rare, and there is minimal to absent BCL6 staining. BCL2 stain marks the reactive mantle zone B cells and follicular helper T cells, as well as the small noncleaved marginal zone B cells colonizing the germinal center (Fig. 41.7).

– Cutaneous marginal zone lymphomas generally exhibit polymorphic infiltrates and may resemble reactive lymphoid hyperplasia (pseudolymphoma). Kappa and lambda immunoglobulin light chain stains are usually helpful in this differential (Fig. 41.8 and Table 41.3).

Table 41.2 Differential diagnosis of cutaneous lymphocytic infiltrates with perifollicular accentuation

Lymphomas/lymphoproliferative disorders	Benign dermatoses
Cutaneous marginal zone B-cell lymphoma	Lymphomatoid drug eruption
Folliculotropic mycosis fungoides	Pseudolymphomatous folliculitis
Follicular lymphomatoid papulosis	Primary follicular mucinosis
Primary cutaneous aggressive epidermotropic CD8-positive cytotoxic T-cell lymphoma	Arthropod bite reaction (including persistent nodular scabies)
	Herpes folliculitis
	Lichen striatus
	Lupus erythematosus
	Lichen planopilaris
	Alopecia areata
	Graft-versus-host disease
	Infundibulofolliculitis

Table 41.3 Differential diagnosis of cutaneous lymphoid infiltrates with lymphoid follicle formation

Reactive/lymphoproliferative disorders	Lymphomas
Cutaneous reactive lymphoid hyperplasia (may occur due to vaccinations, arthropod bites, medications, and spirochetal infections)	Primary cutaneous follicle center lymphoma
Cutaneous Rosai-Dorfman disease	Secondary cutaneous involvement by systemic/nodal follicular lymphoma
Cutaneous IgG4-related disease	Cutaneous marginal zone lymphoma
Lupus panniculitis	Some cases of tumor-stage mycosis fungoides

Pearls and Pitfalls

1. In pseudolymphomas and in marginal zone lymphoma, lymphoid follicles are reactive, while in follicle center (follicular) lymphoma, lymphoid follicles are neoplastic.

2. In cutaneous marginal zone B-cell lymphoma, monotypic plasma cells are often located at the periphery of nodular infiltrates (semicircular arrangement) and in clusters near the papillary dermis.

3. Cutaneous marginal zone B-cell lymphoma often exhibits multifocal skin lesions (on trunk and extremities), while

cutaneous follicle center lymphoma tends to be more localized (on the scalp or back).

4. B-cell lymphomas are associated with light chain restriction. While this is easily identifiable with flow cytometry, demonstration of light chain restriction via tissue immunohistochemistry (of formalin-fixed, paraffin-embedded tissue) would generally require significant cytoplasmic immunoglobulin (i.e., plasmacytic differentiation in a substantial subset of the neoplastic B cells). Flow cytometry would require fresh tissue and is not commonly used in skin lesions. However, flow cytometry may be considered in the occasional cases of cutaneous marginal zone B-cell lymphoma without significant plasmacytic differentiation.

Suggested Reading

Leinweber B, Colli C, Chott A, Kerl H, Cerroni L. Differential diagnosis of cutaneous infiltrates of B lymphocytes with follicular growth pattern. Am J Dermatopathol. 2004;26(1):4–13.

Swerdlow SH, et al., editors. WHO classification of tumors of hematopoietic and lymphoid tissues. Lyon: IARC; 2008.

Swerdlow SH, Campo E, Pileri SA, et al. The 2016 revision of the WHO classification of lymphoid neoplasms. Blood. 2016;127(20):2375–90.

Willemze R, Jaffe ES, Burg G, et al. WHO-EORTC classification for cutaneous lymphomas. Blood. 2005;105(10):3768–85.

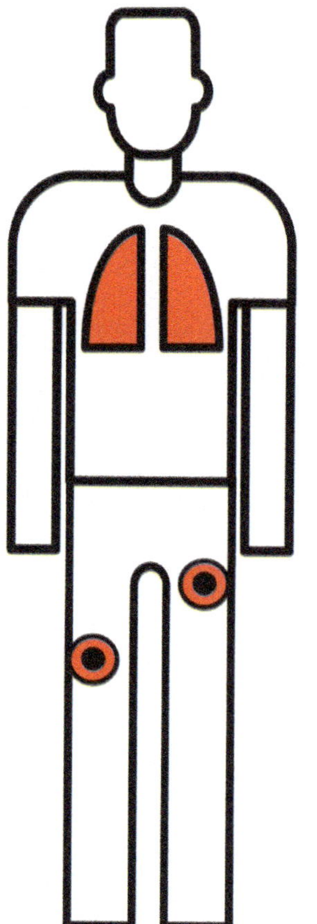

Table 42.1 Key facts

Definition	
Lymphomatoid granulomatosis (LYG) is an angiocentric and angiodestructive lymphoproliferative disease involving extranodal sites composed of EBV-positive B cells admixed with reactive T cells	
Prototypic clinical presentation	
Lesions in the skin and lung. Ulceration is common. Trunk and extremities	
Histopathologic findings	
Angiocentric and angiodestructive polymorphous infiltrate in the dermis and/or panniculus. Necrosis and granulomatous inflammation are common. Most common immunophenotype (large atypical cells): CD20+, CD15−, variable CD30, variable LMP1, and EBV+	
Prognosis	
Variable	

Fig. 42.1 Lymphomatoid granulomatosis (LYG) is an angiocentric and angiodestructive lymphoproliferative disease involving extranodal sites (particularly the lung and skin)

© Springer Nature Switzerland AG 2019
A. Subtil, *Diagnosis of Cutaneous Lymphoid Infiltrates*,
https://doi.org/10.1007/978-3-030-11654-5_42

Fig. 42.2
Lymphomatoid
granulomatosis. This
skin biopsy shows an
atypical dermal and
pannicular lymphoid
infiltrate with
angiocentrism. There is
prominent necrosis

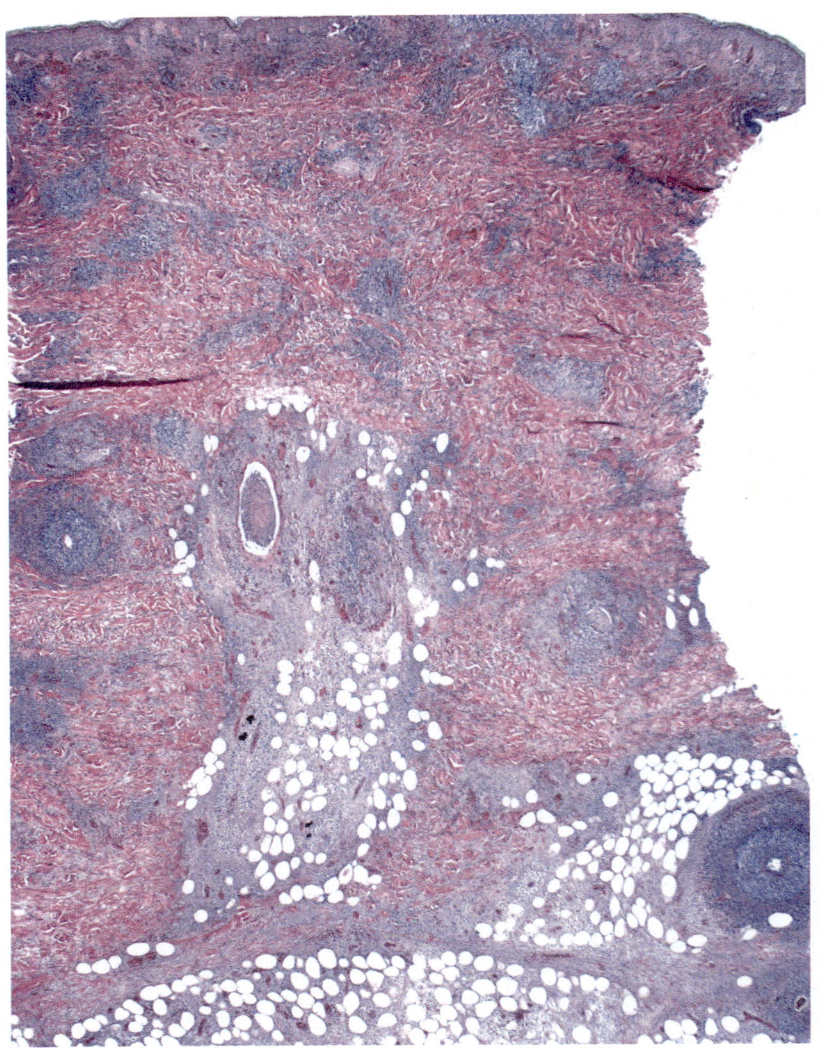

Fig. 42.3
Lymphomatoid granulomatosis. This atypical cutaneous lymphoid infiltrate shows angiocentrism and necrosis. Two affected vessels are highlighted. One of the vessels is completely necrotic (arrowhead)

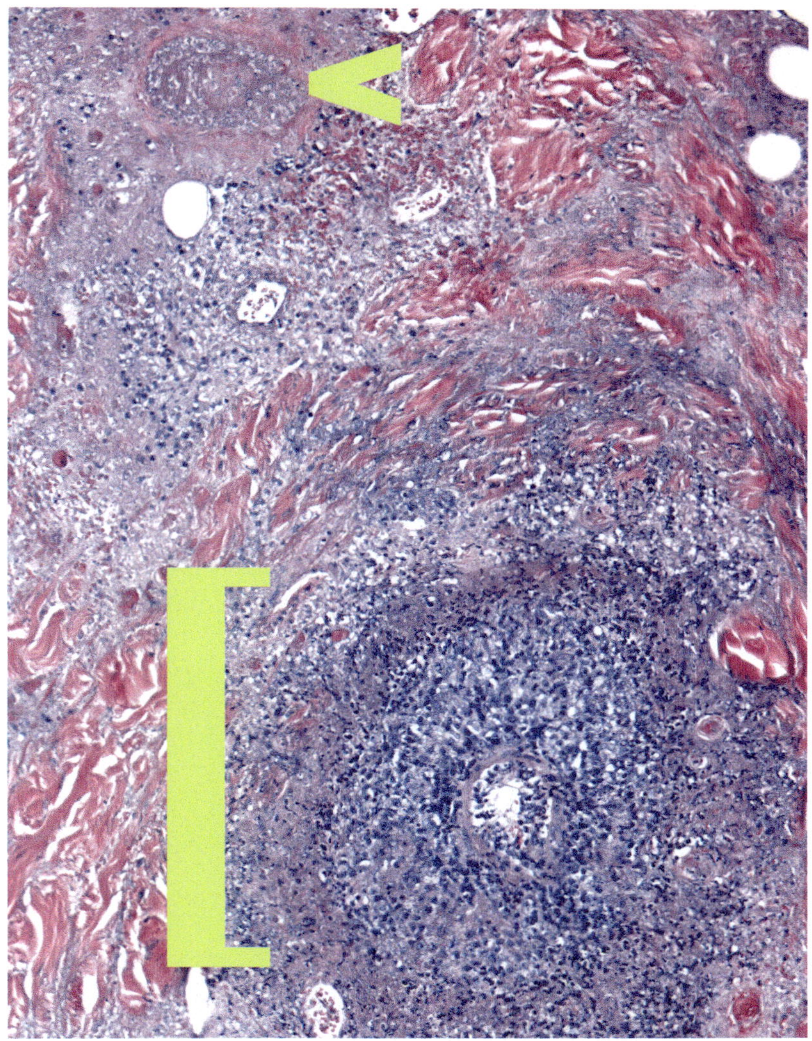

Fig. 42.4
Lymphomatoid
granulomatosis. The
overlying epidermis and
dermis exhibit marked
necrosis due to
angiodestruction

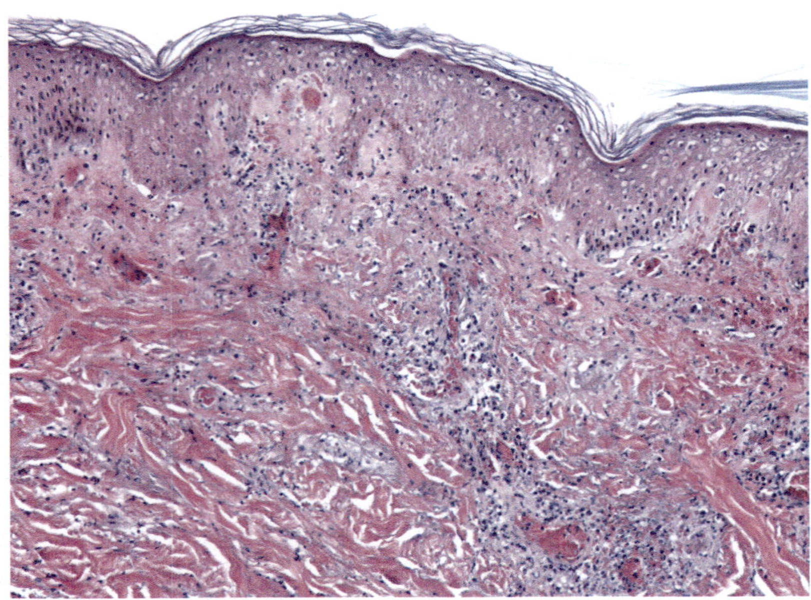

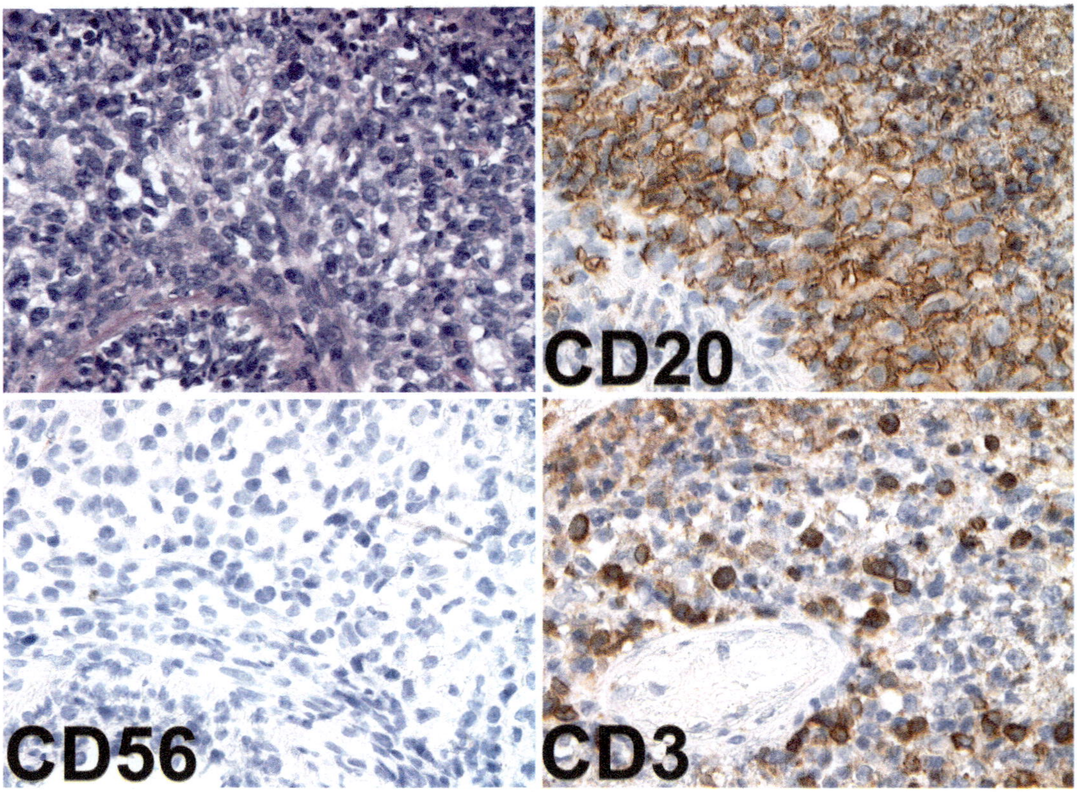

Fig. 42.5 Lymphomatoid granulomatosis. The large atypical lymphocytes infiltrating the blood vessel walls are predominantly CD20-positive B cells. There is a smaller subset of reactive CD3-positive T cells. CD56 is negative

Fig. 42.6
Lymphomatoid
granulomatosis. EBV in
situ hybridization is
positive in the
angiocentric lymphoid
infiltrate

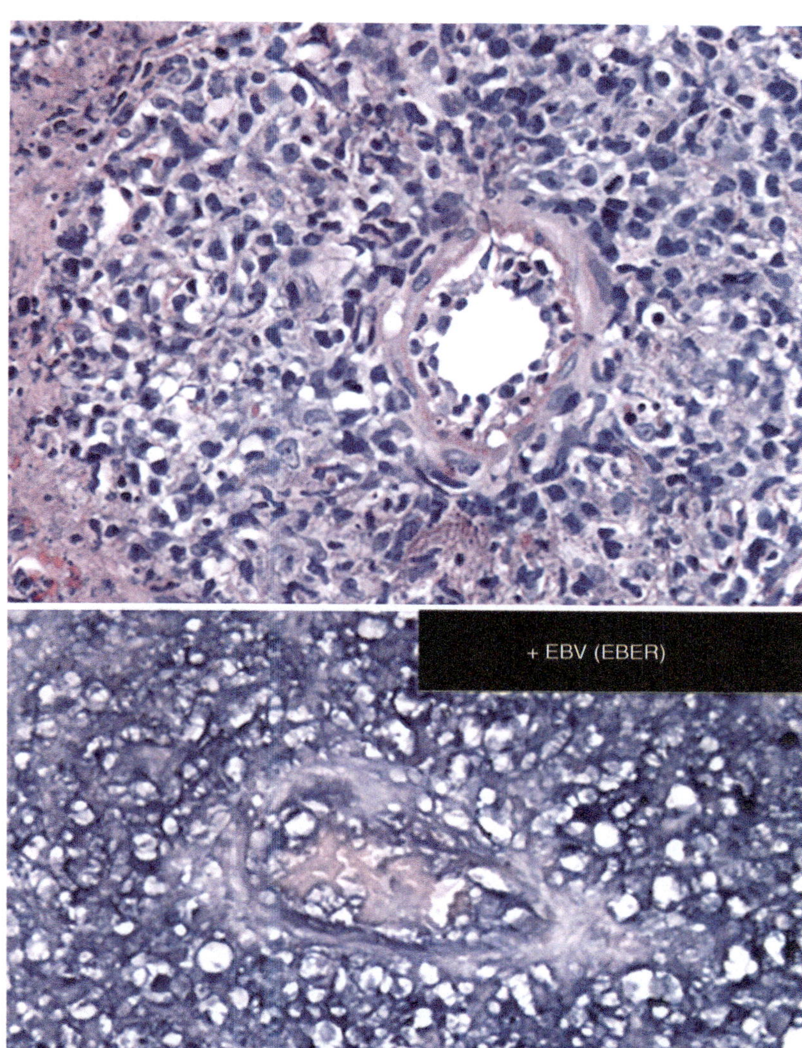

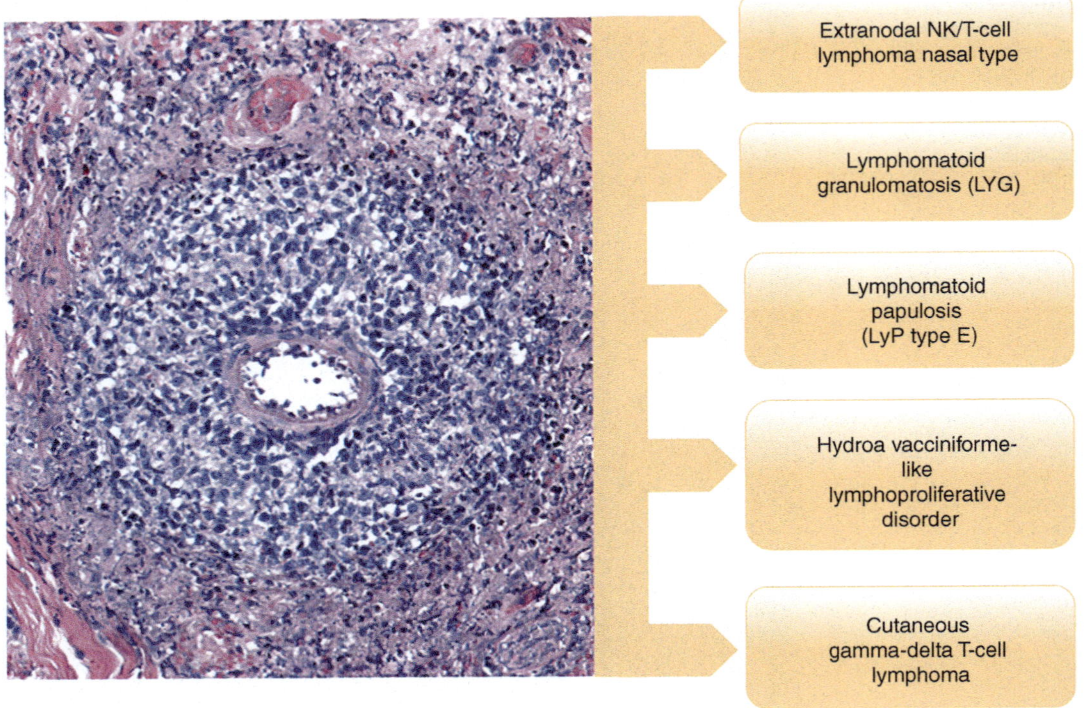

Fig. 42.7 Differential diagnosis of atypical lymphoid infiltrate with angiocentrism

Disease Definition

- Lymphomatoid granulomatosis (LYG) is an angiocentric and angiodestructive lymphoproliferative disease involving extranodal sites (particularly the lung and skin) composed of Epstein-Barr virus (EBV)-positive B cells admixed with reactive T cells (Table 42.1).
- LYG shows a spectrum of histopathologic grades and clinical behavior related to the proportion of large B cells.

Epidemiology

- Rare
- Usually adults and male predominance
- Children with immunodeficiency

Preferential Sites of Involvement

- The lung (>90% of cases, predilection for lower lobes) and skin (up to 50%) are the most common sites of involvement (Fig. 42.1).
- Less common: the central nervous system, kidney, liver, upper respiratory tract, and gastrointestinal tract. Lymph node, bone marrow, or spleen involvement is very rare.

Clinical Features

- Variable depending on involved organs. Respiratory (cough, dyspnea) and constitutional (fever, weight loss) symptoms are common. EBV viral load is usually normal or minimally elevated.
- Skin lesions are diverse: maculopapular rash, multiple erythematous papules, plaques,

tumors, or subcutaneous nodules. Usually on trunk and extremities. Ulceration is common.
- *Less common presentations*: asymptomatic disease.

Histomorphology

- *Pattern*: Angiocentric (infiltration of vascular walls) polymorphous infiltrate in the dermis and/or panniculus (Figs. 42.2 and 42.3). Infarct-like and fibrinoid necrosis from angiodestruction is frequent (Fig. 42.4). Granulomatous inflammation is common in the skin.
- *Less common patterns*: Pleomorphic neoplastic cells resembling Hodgkin cells. Nonspecific perivascular and periadnexal lymphohistiocytic infiltrate of small- and intermediate-sized cells. Subcutaneous pannicular infiltrates with non-necrotizing granulomas.
- *Neoplastic cells*: Variable number of large atypical EBV-positive neoplastic B cells resembling immunoblasts (large noncleaved nuclei with prominent central nucleoli).
- *Reactive cells*: Plasma cells, reactive lymphocytes, and histiocytes. Neutrophils and eosinophils are usually rare. Reactive T cells and inflammatory background are often more prominent than neoplastic B cells.
- Grading is based on proportion of EBV-positive B cells relative to reactive inflammatory background (Table 42.2).

Immunophenotype

- *Neoplastic cells*: CD20+, CD15−, variable CD30, variable LMP1, EBV+ (EBER in situ hybridization), and frequent MUM1 expression; light chain restriction may occasionally be identified with kappa and lambda stains (Figs. 42.5 and 42.6).
- *Reactive cells*: CD3+ T cells (CD4+ cells more frequent than CD8+).

Genetics

- Monoclonal rearrangement of immunoglobulin genes in majority of grade 2 and grade 3 cases (variable results in grade 1). Rarely, monoclonal rearrangement of T-cell receptor gene may occur.

Prognosis

- Variable but usually aggressive
- Adverse risk factors: histological grade, underlying immunodeficiency disorder, extent of extracutaneous disease

Differential Diagnosis

- Angioinvasion may be a feature of aggressive lymphomas, such as extranodal NK/T-cell lymphoma nasal type and gamma-delta T-cell lymphoma. However, it may also occur in an indolent process, such as angioinvasive lymphomatoid papulosis (LyP type E). The differential diagnosis for angiodestruction would also include hydroa vacciniforme-like lymphoproliferative disorder, an EBV-positive condition with NK- or T-cell phenotype that affects children and usually presents with ulcerated necrotic lesions on sun-exposed skin. Considering the disparate prognoses of the entities with an angiocentric pattern, it is critical to obtain comprehensive immunophenotyping, EBV in situ hybridization, and careful clinical correlation for accurate classification (Tables 42.3 and 42.4; Fig. 42.7). Lymphomatoid granulomatosis (LYG) is an angiocentric lymphoproliferative disease of EBV-positive B cells, while other processes in the differential diagnosis are of T- or NK-cell origin.

Table 42.2 Histological grading of lymphomatoid granulomatosis

	Grade 1	Grade 2	Grade 3
Atypical large lymphoid cells in polymorphous inflammatory background	Absent or rare	Occasional (small clusters with CD20 stain)	Easily identified (larger aggregates with CD20), may see pleomorphic and Hodgkin-like cells
Necrosis	Absent or focal	Common	Usually extensive
EBV+ cells (EBER in situ hybridization)	Infrequent (<5 per high-power field), may be absent	Easily identified (variable but usually 5–20 per high-power field)	Numerous (usually >50 per high-power field), may form small confluent sheets

Table 42.3 Differential diagnosis of an atypical angiocentric lymphoid infiltrate in relation to Epstein-Barr virus (EBV) and immunophenotype

EBV	Angiocentric process	Immunophenotype
Positive (+)	Extranodal NK/T-cell lymphoma nasal type	T cell or NK cell
	Hydroa vacciniforme-like lymphoproliferative disorder	T cell or NK cell
	Lymphomatoid granulomatosis (LYG)	B cell
Negative (−)	Cutaneous gamma-delta T-cell lymphoma	Gamma-delta T cell
	Lymphomatoid papulosis (LyP type E)	CD30-positive T cell

Table 42.4 Lymphoproliferative diseases with frequent EBV expression

Extranodal NK/T-cell lymphoma, nasal type
EBV+ diffuse large B-cell lymphoma
Systemic EBV+ T-cell lymphoma of childhood
Hydroa vacciniforme-like lymphoproliferative disorder
Lymphomatoid granulomatosis (LYG)
EBV+ mucocutaneous ulcer
Aggressive NK-cell leukemia
Posttransplant lymphoproliferative disorders
Plasmablastic lymphoma
Primary effusion lymphoma
Diffuse large B-cell lymphoma associated with chronic inflammation
Angioimmunoblastic T-cell lymphoma
Classical Hodgkin lymphoma
Burkitt lymphoma

Pearls and Pitfalls

1. Angiocentrism (infiltration of vascular walls) is not always present in a biopsy of an angioinvasive lymphoid process. Clues for the diagnosis would include infarct-like necrosis and cytotoxic immunophenotype. EBV in situ hybridization and careful clinical pathologic correlation would be essential for proper classification.

2. Infiltration and destruction of blood vessel walls is generally not a feature of intravascular lymphomas (atypical lymphocytes within vessel lumens).

3. While several lymphomas may express EBV, the identification of EBV may or may not be part of the minimum diagnostic criteria for a particular lymphoma. For example, Burkitt lymphoma is frequently EBV-positive; however, if a case of Burkitt lymphoma were EBV-negative, this would not change the diagnosis. In contrast, a nasal T-cell lymphoma that is CD3-positive and CD56-negative but negative for EBV would not be classified as extranodal NK/T-cell lymphoma nasal type.

4. In situ hybridization for Epstein-Barr-encoded RNA (EBER) is the most reliable method to demonstrate the presence of EBV. Immunohistochemical stains for EBV often yield variable and inconsistent results. However, angiocentric processes are frequently associated with necrosis, which may cause technical difficulties due to poor RNA preservation. EBNA2 PCR may be considered in technically suboptimal cases.

Suggested Reading

Song JY, Pittaluga S, Dunleavy K, et al. Lymphomatoid granulomatosis. A single institution experience: pathologic findings and clinical correlations. Am J Surg Pathol. 2015;39(2):141–56.

Swerdlow SH, et al., editors. WHO classification of tumors of hematopoietic and lymphoid tissues. Lyon: IARC; 2008.

Swerdlow SH, Campo E, Pileri SA, et al. The 2016 revision of the WHO classification of lymphoid neoplasms. Blood. 2016;127(20):2375–90.

Willemze R, Jaffe ES, Burg G, et al. WHO-EORTC classification for cutaneous lymphomas. Blood. 2005;105(10):3768–85.

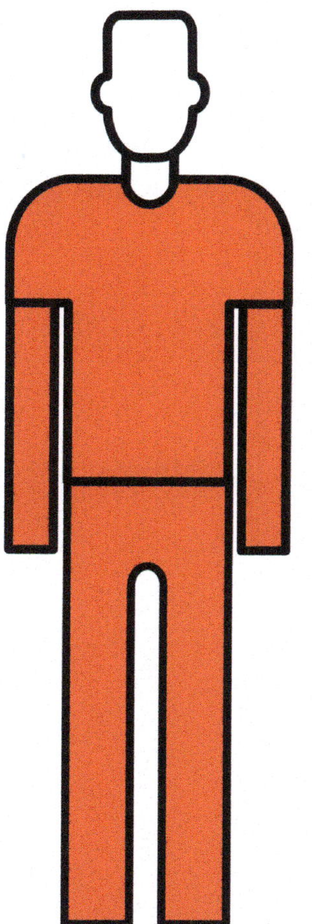

Fig. 43.1 Blastic plasmacytoid dendritic cell neoplasm. Patients usually present with multiple nodules and plaques. Bruise-like patches and disseminated disease are common

Table 43.1 Key facts

Definition
Blastic plasmacytoid dendritic cell neoplasm (BPDCN) is a clinically aggressive hematopoietic neoplasm of precursors of plasmacytoid dendritic cells with a high frequency of skin and bone marrow involvement and leukemic dissemination
Prototypic clinical presentation
Multiple nodules, plaques, and/or bruise-like patches. Bone marrow involvement at presentation is common
Histopathologic findings
Interstitial, perivascular, periadnexal, and/or diffuse dermal infiltrate of variable density and without epidermotropism. Cytomorphology is usually blastic, but some cases show cleaved nuclei
Most common immunophenotype: CD3−, CD20−, CD79a−, CD4+, CD56+, TIA1−, CD43+, MPO−, EBV−, with expression of plasmacytoid dendritic cell-associated antigens (CD123, TCL1, or CD303)
Prognosis
Poor

A. Subtil, *Diagnosis of Cutaneous Lymphoid Infiltrates*,
https://doi.org/10.1007/978-3-030-11654-5_43

Fig. 43.2 Blastic plasmacytoid dendritic cell neoplasm. The pattern of dermal infiltration resembles that of myeloid leukemia cutis: triple combination of perivascular, interstitial, and periadnexal distribution

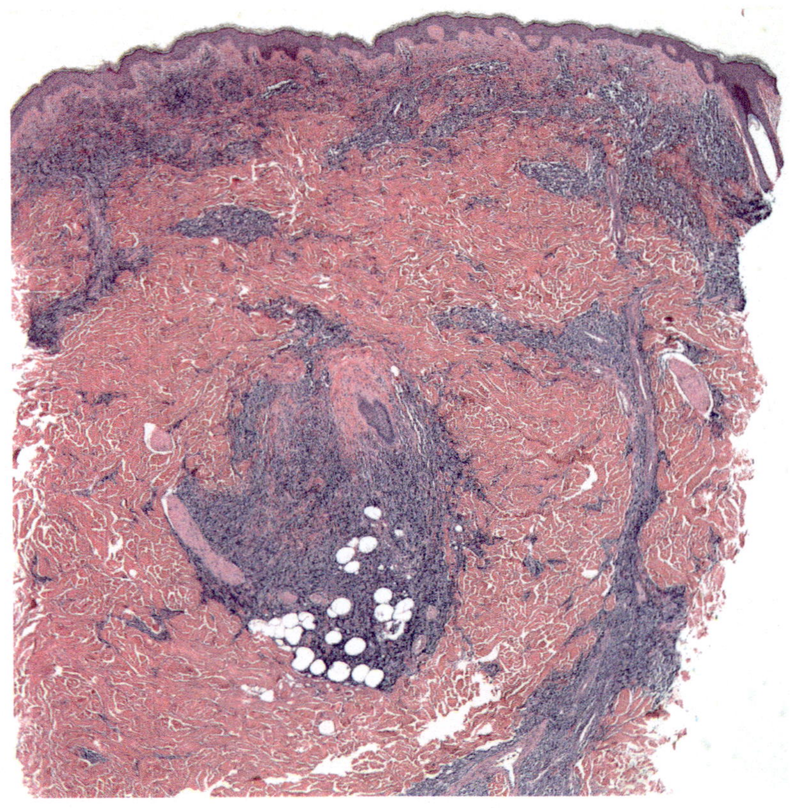

Fig. 43.3 Blastic plasmacytoid dendritic cell neoplasm. Non-epidermotropic dermal infiltrate with perivascular and interstitial pattern

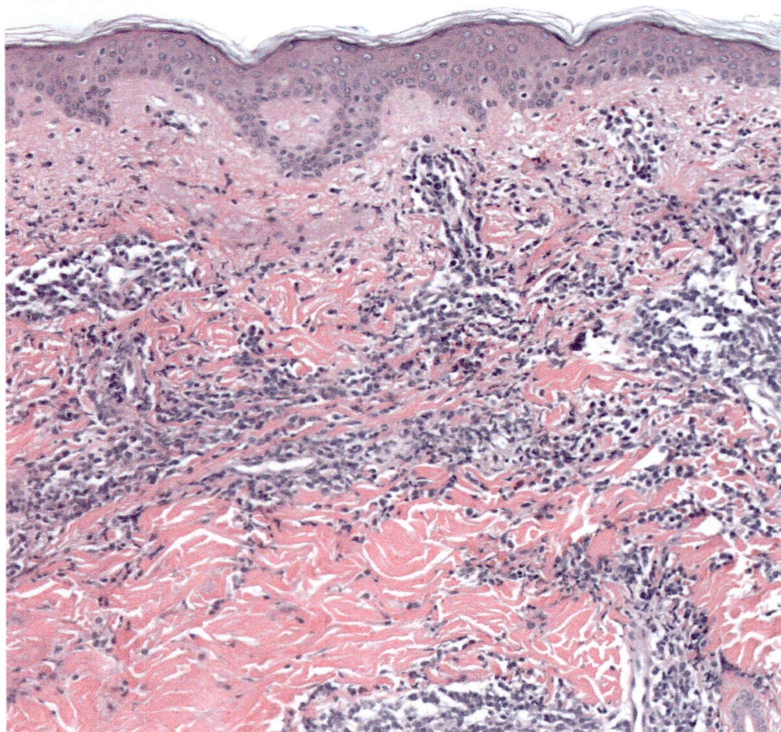

Fig. 43.4 Blastic plasmacytoid dendritic cell neoplasm. Dermal infiltrate with perivascular and periadnexal pattern

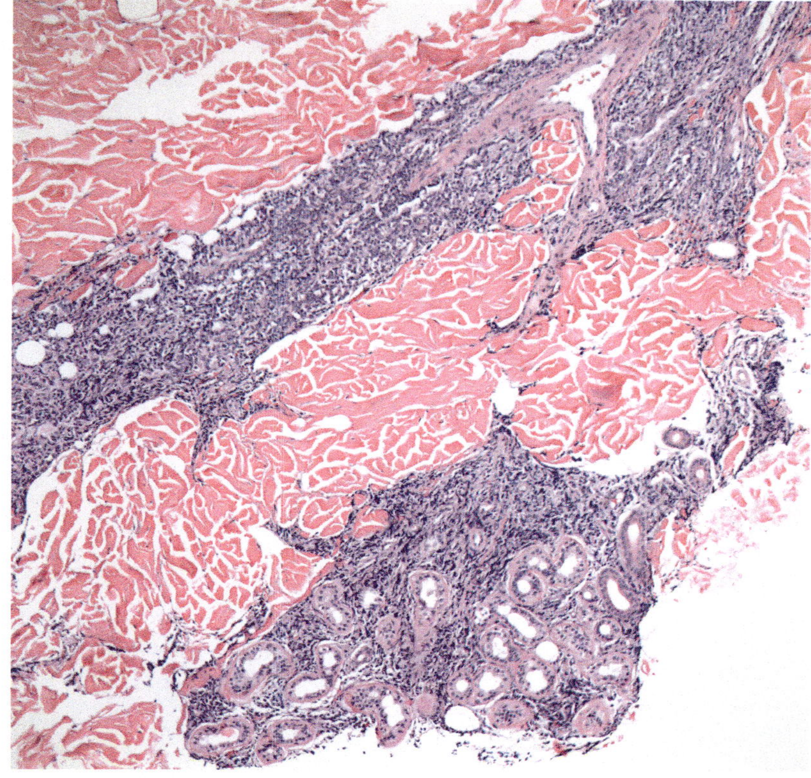

Fig. 43.5 Blastic plasmacytoid dendritic cell neoplasm. Atypical lymphoid-appearing cells with blastic features

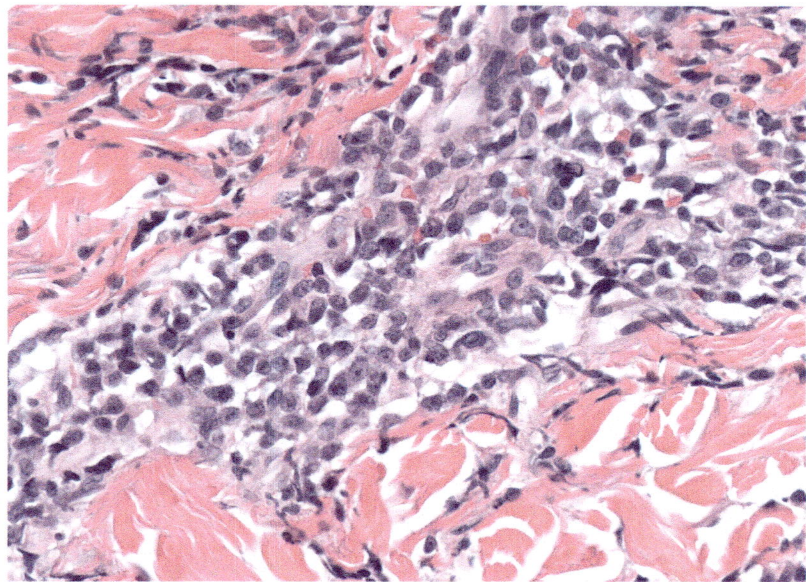

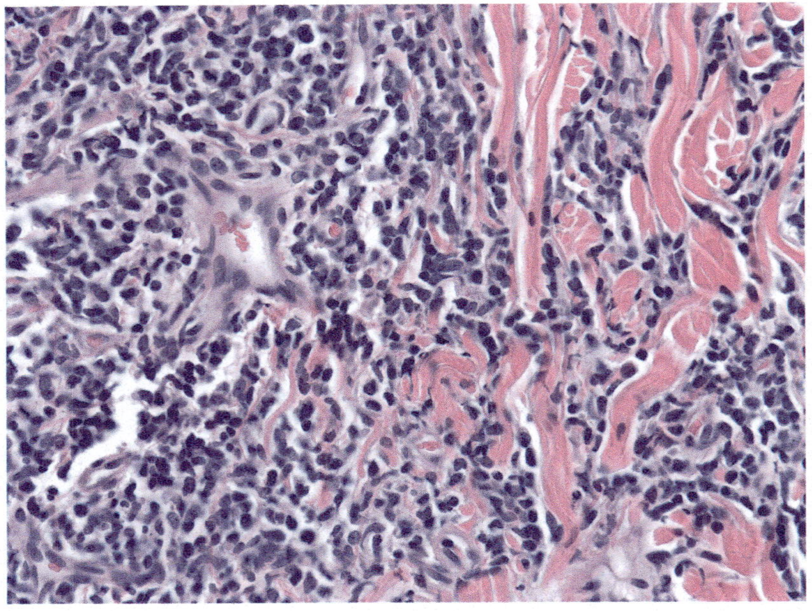

Fig. 43.6 Blastic plasmacytoid dendritic cell neoplasm. Cytologic variant mimicking centrocytes of follicle center lymphoma

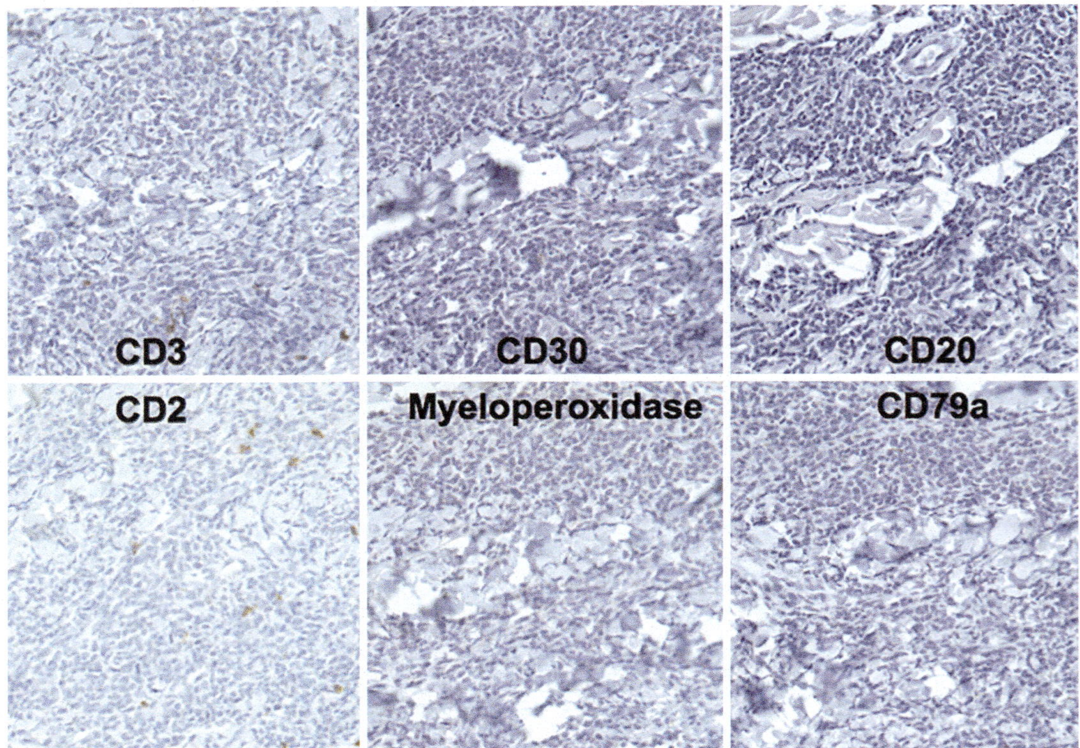

Fig. 43.7 Multiple negative markers (T cell, B cell, and myeloid) in a lymphoid-appearing infiltrate are a clue to the diagnosis of blastic plasmacytoid dendritic cell neoplasm

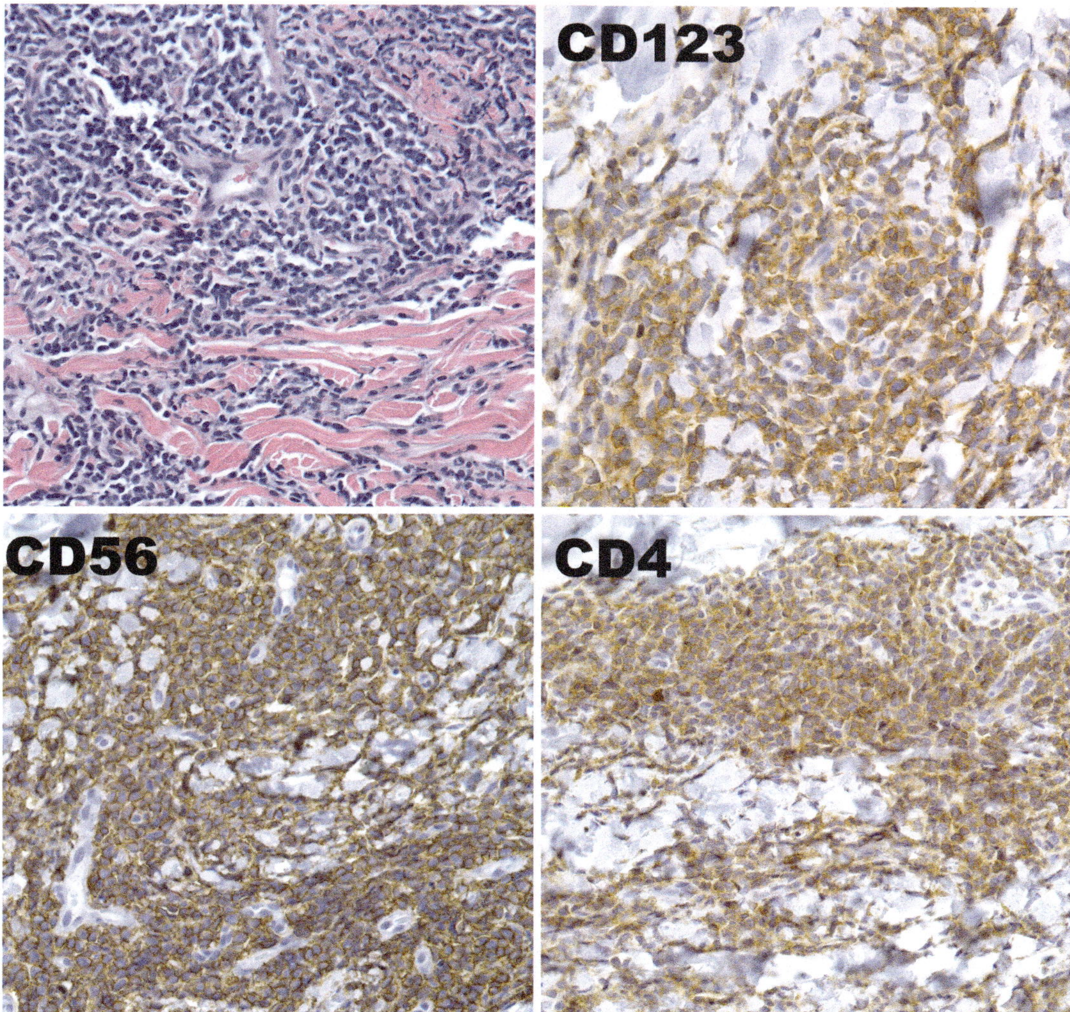

Fig. 43.8 Blastic plasmacytoid dendritic cell neoplasm. This aggressive hematopoietic neoplasm was previously known as "CD4+/CD56+ hematodermic neoplasm." In addition to the classic expression of both CD4 and CD56, plasmacytoid dendritic cell markers (such as CD123) are present

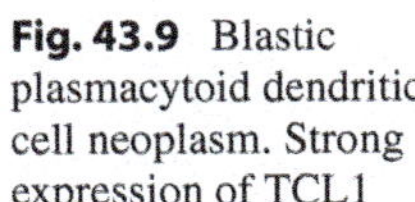

Fig. 43.9 Blastic plasmacytoid dendritic cell neoplasm. Strong expression of TCL1

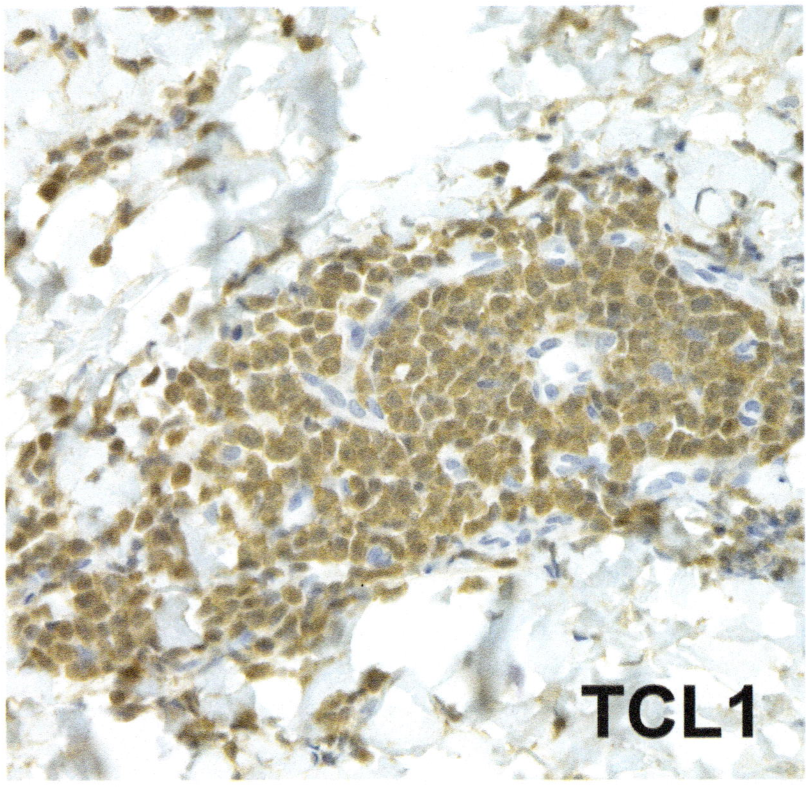

Disease Definition

- Blastic plasmacytoid dendritic cell neoplasm (BPDCN) is a clinically aggressive hematopoietic neoplasm of precursors of plasmacytoid dendritic cells with a high frequency of skin and bone marrow involvement and leukemic dissemination (Table 43.1).
- Before the cell of origin was elucidated, BPDCN was previously termed "agranular CD4+ natural killer (NK) cell leukemia," "blastic NK-cell lymphoma," "CD4+/CD56+ hematodermic neoplasm," and "blastic natural killer leukemia/lymphoma."
- The blastic cytomorphology and CD56 expression had initially suggested an NK-cell precursor origin. Since 2008, BPDCN has been classified by the WHO as part of the group of acute myeloid leukemias and related precursor neoplasms.

Epidemiology

- Male predominance.
- Most patients are adults, but children may also be affected.

Preferential Sites of Involvement

- High frequency of cutaneous, peripheral blood, and bone marrow involvement at presentation.
- Lymphadenopathy may be identified in 20% of cases at presentation.
- While multiple sites are often involved (Fig. 43.1), some cases may present with disease localized to the skin.

Clinical Features

- Patients usually present with multiple nodules and plaques. Bruise-like patches and mucosal involvement may also occur.
- *Less common presentations*: solitary skin lesion.

Histomorphology

- *Pattern*: Interstitial, perivascular, periadnexal, and/or diffuse dermal infiltrate of variable density and without epidermotropism (Figs. 43.2, 43.3, and 43.4).
- *Less common patterns*: Pannicular involvement may be seen.
- *Neoplastic cells*: Monomorphous, medium-sized blastoid cells exhibit fine chromatin, one to several small nucleoli, and generally scant cytoplasm (Fig. 43.5). A morphologic variant of BPDCN with cleaved nuclei may morphologically resemble the centrocytes of cutaneous follicle center lymphoma; however, the infiltrate is negative with B-cell markers (Fig. 43.6).
- *Reactive cells*: Usually scant (scattered lymphocytes). Vast majority of cells in the infiltrate are neoplastic.

Immunophenotype

- *Neoplastic cells*: A clue to the diagnosis of BPDCN is the presence of multiple negative markers (T cell, B cell, and myeloperoxidase) (Fig. 43.7). In addition to CD4 and CD56, plasmacytoid dendritic cell-associated antigens (such as CD123, TCL1, and CD303) are typically expressed (Figs. 43.8 and 43.9). Rare cases may lack CD4 or CD56.
- An extensive immunohistochemical panel is often necessary to exclude other hematolymphoid neoplasms and to document plasmacytoid dendritic cell origin (Table 43.2).
- Almost always positive: CD4, CD56, CD43, CD45RA, CD123, and TCL1.

- Regularly negative markers: CD3, CD5, CD13, CD16, CD19, CD20, CD79a, CD34, CD117, TIA1, lysozyme, myeloperoxidase (MPO), and EBV (Epstein-Barr virus) in situ hybridization (EBER).
- Variable expression: CD68 (50% of cases, cytoplasmic dot pattern), TdT (33% of cases), CD2, CD7, CD33, and CD38.
- *Reactive cells*: Usually scant CD3-positive T cells. Reactive plasmacytoid dendritic cells lack CD56 and TdT.

Genetics

- Negative for clonal B- or T-cell gene rearrangement in the majority of cases, though rare cases may demonstrate T-cell clonality.

Prognosis

- Poor.
- Median survival is 12–14 months.
- Adverse risk factors: Young age, CD303 expression, and high proliferative index (Ki-67) have been reported to be associated with longer survival.

Differential Diagnosis

- A comprehensive immunohistochemical panel is necessary to differentiate BPDCN from myeloid leukemia cutis, which may occasionally express CD56. CD33 may be expressed by BPDCN, which may cause further diagnostic confusion with myeloperoxidase-negative myeloid leukemia cutis. MNDA (myeloid cell nuclear differentiation antigen) may be helpful in this differential given its absence in BPDCN.
- Cutaneous gamma-delta T-cell lymphoma (GDTCL) is an important differential diagnosis in an atypical CD56-positive lymphoid infiltrate. GDTCL is an aggressive cytotoxic cutaneous lymphoma of gamma-delta T cells (betaF1−, CD3+, CD5−,

CD4−, CD8−/+, CD56+, TIA1+) that may involve any or all layers of the skin (epidermis, dermis, and/or panniculus). Ulceration and angiocentrism may also occur. CD3 is negative in BPDCN.

– Extranodal NK/T-cell lymphoma, nasal type, most commonly involves the upper aerodigestive tract but frequently presents in the skin. This aggressive EBV-positive angiodestructive malignant process is designated "NK/T" because the immunophenotype can be NK cell or cytotoxic T cell. CD56 expression is generally present. In the setting of angiocentrism and cytotoxic phenotype, EBV in situ hybridization (EBER) should be obtained. EBV is negative in BPDCN.

Table 43.2 Immunophenotype of blastic plasmacytoid dendritic cell neoplasm

Frequency	Markers
Almost always positive (+)	CD4, CD56, CD43, CD45RA, CD123, TCL1
Regularly negative (−)	CD3, CD5, CD13, CD16, CD19, CD20, CD79a, CD34, CD117, TIA1, lysozyme, myeloperoxidase, EBV (EBER)
Variable expression	CD68 (50% of cases; cytoplasmic dot pattern), TdT (33% of cases), CD2, CD7, CD33, CD38

Table 43.3 Differential diagnosis of CD56 expression in the skin

Lymphoid/hematopoietic	Non-lymphoid
Rare cases of mycosis fungoides	Merkel cell carcinoma
Rare cases of CD30-positive lymphoproliferative disorders	Schwannoma
Cutaneous gamma-delta T-cell lymphoma	Neuroblastoma
Extranodal NK/T-cell lymphoma, nasal type	Cellular neurothekeoma
Blastic plasmacytoid dendritic cell neoplasm	Plexiform fibrohistiocytic tumor
Some cases of myeloid leukemia cutis	Metastatic renal cell carcinoma
Most cases of plasma cell myeloma	Damaged muscle fibers

Pearls and Pitfalls
1. The identification of CD56 expression in a cutaneous lymphoid infiltrate is not enough to make a diagnosis (Table 43.3). Additional immunophenotyping and clinical correlation are necessary for proper classification.
2. Merkel cell carcinoma (MCC) is immunoreactive with CD56. While most cases would not resemble a lymphoma, some cases of MCC may be discohesive, poorly fixed, and/or partially obscured by inflammation and may resemble a CD56-positive lymphoma or leukemia.
3. Plasmacytoid dendritic cells are also known as professional type 1 interferon-producing cells and plasmacytoid monocytes.

Suggested Reading

Cota C, Vale E, Viana I, et al. Cutaneous manifestations of blastic plasmacytoid dendritic cell neoplasm-morphologic and phenotypic variability in a series of 33 patients. Am J Surg Pathol. 2010;34(1):75–87.

Julia F, Petrella T, Beylot-Barry M, et al. Blastic plasmacytoid dendritic cell neoplasm: clinical features in 90 patients. Br J Dermatol. 2013;169(3):579–86.

Julia F, Dalle S, Duru G, et al. Blastic plasmacytoid dendritic cell neoplasms: clinico-immunohistochemical correlations in a series of 91 patients. Am J Surg Pathol. 2014;38(5):673–80.

Petrella T, Comeau MR, Maynadié M, et al. Agranular CD4+ CD56+ hematodermic neoplasm (blastic NK-cell lymphoma) originates from a population of CD56+ precursor cells related to plasmacytoid monocytes. Am J Surg Pathol. 2002;26(7):852–62.

Swerdlow SH, et al., editors. WHO classification of tumors of hematopoietic and lymphoid tissues. Lyon: IARC; 2008.

Swerdlow SH, Campo E, Pileri SA, et al. The 2016 revision of the WHO classification of lymphoid neoplasms. Blood. 2016;127(20):2375–90.

Willemze R, Jaffe ES, Burg G, et al. WHO-EORTC classification for cutaneous lymphomas. Blood. 2005;105(10):3768–85.

Appendix 1 Main Immunohistochemical Stains Used in the Diagnosis of Lymphoproliferative Disorders

Antibody	Predominant cells labeled
CD1a	Langerhans cells, precursor T cells
CD2	T cells
CD3	T cells
CD4	T-helper cells, blastic plasmacytoid dendritic cell neoplasm
CD5	T cells, chronic lymphocytic leukemia/small lymphocytic lymphoma, mantle cell lymphoma
CD7	T cells
CD8	T-cytotoxic cells
CD10	(CALLA, common acute lymphoblastic leukemia antigen); germinal center B cells, follicular lymphoma, B-ALL (acute lymphoblastic leukemia/lymphoma), Burkitt lymphoma
CD15	Neutrophils, Reed-Sternberg cells of classic Hodgkin lymphoma
CD20	B cells
CD21	Follicular dendritic cells
CD23	Follicular dendritic cells, B-cell subsets, chronic lymphocytic leukemia/small lymphocytic lymphoma
CD30	Activated lymphocytes, anaplastic large cell lymphoma, lymphomatoid papulosis, Reed-Sternberg cells of classic Hodgkin lymphoma
CD34	Endothelial cells, precursor cells
CD43	T cells, myeloid cells, mast cells, T-cell lymphomas, some B-cell lymphomas (chronic lymphocytic leukemia/small lymphocytic lymphoma, mantle cell lymphoma)
CD45	(LCA, leukocyte common antigen); hematolymphoid cells, most B- and T-cell lymphomas
PAX-5	B cells (nuclear staining pattern)

Antibody	Predominant cells labeled
CD56	(NCAM, neural cell adhesion molecule); NK cells, NK-cell lymphomas, some T-cell lymphomas, most gamma-delta T-cell lymphomas, neuroendocrine tumors, blastic plasmacytoid dendritic cell neoplasm
CD68	Histiocytes/macrophages, mast cells
CD79a	Immature and mature B cells, plasma cells. Useful stain in B-cell lymphoma patients being treated with rituximab
CD117	(c-Kit) mast cells
CD138	Plasma cells, plasmacytic differentiation
TIA-1	Cytotoxic cells, cytotoxic T-/NK-cell lymphomas (cytoplasmic granular staining pattern)
Granzyme B	Cytotoxic cells, cytotoxic T-/NK-cell lymphomas (cytoplasmic granular staining pattern)
Perforin	Cytotoxic cells, cytotoxic T-/NK-cell lymphomas (cytoplasmic granular staining pattern)
BCL-2 protein	T cells, non-germinal center B cells, most follicular lymphomas (cytoplasmic staining pattern)
BCL-6	Germinal center B cells, lymphomas of germinal center origin, cutaneous follicle center lymphoma (nuclear staining pattern)
ALK1	ALK+ anaplastic large cell lymphoma, ALK+ diffuse large B-cell lymphoma
TdT	Precursor cells, B- and T-ALL (acute lymphoblastic leukemia/lymphoma)
Kappa	Plasma cells, plasmacytic differentiation
Lambda	Plasma cells, plasmacytic differentiation

© Springer Nature Switzerland AG 2019
A. Subtil, *Diagnosis of Cutaneous Lymphoid Infiltrates*,
https://doi.org/10.1007/978-3-030-11654-5

A significant amount of genetic data has been obtained over the years from several research studies and has improved our understanding of disease mechanisms and histogenesis. However, their clinical use has been limited by lack of clinical validation or test availability, small sample size, and/or low frequency of certain genetic abnormalities. The gold standard for the diagnosis of cutaneous lymphomas continues to be the correlation of clinical and histopathologic findings. Only genetic features of current clinical use are included in the lymphoma chapters. This appendix lists genetic abnormalities that are currently of research interest.

Chapter 22. Classic Mycosis Fungoides

- Complex karyotypes, particularly in advanced disease
- Chromosomal loss at 10q
- Abnormalities in p15, p16, and p53 tumor suppressor genes
- Activating JAK3 mutations
- Constitutive activation of STAT3
- Inactivation of CDKN2A and PTEN
- Point mutations and genomic gains in TNFRSF1B
- Alterations in TOX and PDCD1

Chapter 25. Granulomatous Slack Skin

- t(3;9)(q12;p24) translocation in one case

Chapter 26. Sézary Syndrome

- Common complex numerical and structural alterations
- Loss of 1p, 6q, 10q
- Gain of 8q
- Isochromosome 17q
- Overexpression of PLS3, DNM3, TWIST1, EPHA4
- Underexpression of STAT4
- Constitutive activation of STAT3
- Loss-of-function mutations in POT1, ARID1A, and ATM
- Gain-of-function mutations in CARD11, CD28, PLCG1, and TNFRSF1B
- Inactivating mutations of TP53

Chapter 27. Primary Cutaneous CD30+ Lymphoproliferative Disorders: Cutaneous Anaplastic Large Cell Lymphoma

- DUSP22-IRF4 rearrangement in a minority of cases (20–25%). Epidermotropism is often marked in these cases.
- Most cases do not have ALK translocations.
- Gain of 7q31 and losses at 6q16-21 and 13q34 are common.
- NPM1-TYK2 gene fusion resulting in constitutive STAT signaling.
- High expression of skin-homing chemokine receptor genes CCR8 and CCR10.

Chapter 28. Primary Cutaneous CD30+ Lymphoproliferative Disorders, Lymphomatoid Papulosis

- DUSP22-IRF4 rearrangement at 6p25.3 in <5% of cases.
- t(2;5)(p23;q35) involving ALK is not identified.

Chapter 30. Subcutaneous Panniculitis-Like T-Cell Lymphoma (Alpha-Beta)

- Gains in chromosomes 2q and 4q.
- Losses in chromosomes 16, 19, 20, and 22.
- Allelic NAV3 aberrations.
- Expression of CCL5 ligand may explain preferential pannicular involvement due to adipocyte expression of CCR5 receptor.

Chapter 31. Cutaneous Gamma-Delta T-Cell Lymphoma

- Monoclonal rearrangement of T-cell receptor gamma genes in majority of cases. T-cell receptor beta genes may be clonally rearranged or deleted but are not expressed.
- Epstein-Barr virus (EBV) is negative.
- Cases with predominant subcutaneous involvement usually express Vδ2.
- Overexpression of NK-cell-associated genes (KIR3DL1, KIR2DL4, KIR2DL2, KLRC4, KLRD1, KLRC2).
- Chromosomal aberrations may involve WWOX-TCL and BCL11B.

Chapter 32. Primary Cutaneous CD8-Positive Aggressive Epidermotropic Cytotoxic T-Cell Lymphoma

- Monoclonal rearrangement of T-cell receptor genes in most (but not all) cases.
- EBV (EBER) is negative.

- Gains (predominantly in chromosomes 3, 7, 8, 11, 17, 18, and 22) are more common than losses (particularly 9p21).

Chapter 33. Extranodal NK/T-Cell Lymphoma, Nasal Type

- As the name indicates, extranodal NK-/T-cell lymphoma, nasal type may be of NK-cell origin or T-cell origin. Depending on the cell of origin, PCR results will be different. NK-cell origin (most common type) will be associated with negative T-cell clonality (germline configuration). Monoclonal rearrangement of T-cell receptor genes occurs in a minority of cases (cytotoxic T-cell origin).
- EBV in situ hybridization (EBER) is positive.
- EBV is present in clonal episomal form with type II latency pattern (EBNA1+, EBNA2−, LMP1+).
- A 30-base pair deletion in latent membrane protein-1 gene is common.
- EBV is usually of subtype A.
- Del(6)(q21q25) and i(6)(p10) are common cytogenetic abnormalities.
- Aberrant methylation of promoter CpG regions of multiple genes, including p73.
- Other chromosomal aberrations include gain of 2q and loss of 1p36.23-p36.33, 6q16.1−q27, 4q12, 5q34−q35.3, 7q21.3−q22.1, 11q22.3−q23.3, and 15q11.2−q14.
- Loss of 6q may affect transcription factors PRDM1and FOXO3 and result in cellular proliferation.
- Partial deletion of FAS gene and/or loss or mutation in TP53, beta-catenin, K-RAS, c-Kit, or CDKN2A genes in a subset of cases.

Chapter 38. Primary Cutaneous Diffuse Large B-Cell Lymphoma, Leg Type

- Monoclonal rearrangement of immunoglobulin genes in majority of cases.
- Gene expression profile of activated B-cell-like diffuse large B-cell lymphoma.

- Frequent translocations involving c-MYC, BCL6, and IGH genes.
- Mutations in MYD88 gene and 9p21 deletions are common.
- Frequent DNA amplifications of 18q21.31–q21.33, including MALT1 and BCL2 genes (may explain strong BCL2 expression since t(14;18) not found).

Chapter 40. Primary Cutaneous Follicle Center Lymphoma

- BCL2 rearrangements are less common than in nodal follicular lymphoma but occur in a significant subset of primary cutaneous cases (10–40%).
- REL amplification is common.
- 14q32.33 deletion has been identified.
- Inactivation of CDKN2A and CDKN2B in 9p21.3 by deletion or promoter hypermethylation is rare.

Chapter 41. Primary Cutaneous Marginal Zone B-Cell Lymphoma

- Monoclonal rearrangement of immunoglobulin genes in majority of cases
- Low frequency of several chromosomal abnormalities: t(11;18) API2-MALT1 (0–8% of cases), t(14;18) IGH-MALT1 (0–14%), t(3;14) FOXP1-IGH (0–10%), +3 (20%), and +18 (4%)

Suggested Reading

Choi J, Goh G, Walradt T, Hong BS, Bunick CG, Chen K, Bjornson RD, Maman Y, Wang T, Tordoff J, Carlson K, Overton JD, Liu KJ, Lewis JM, Devine L, Barbarotta L, Foss FM, Subtil A, Vonderheid EC, Edelson RL, Schatz DG, Boggon TJ, Girardi M, Lifton RP. Genomic landscape of cutaneous T cell lymphoma. Nat Genet. 2015;47(9):1011–9.

Elder DE, Massi D, Scolyer RA, Willemze R, editors. WHO classification of skin tumors. 4th ed. Lyon: IARC; 2018.

Swerdlow SH, Campo E, Pileri SA, et al. The 2016 revision of the WHO classification of lymphoid neoplasms. Blood. 2016;127(20):2375–90.

Willemze R, Jaffe ES, Burg G, et al. WHO-EORTC classification for cutaneous lymphomas. Blood. 2005;105(10):3768–85.

Appendix 3 Basic Features of Cutaneous Pseudolymphomas

The gold standard for the diagnosis of cutaneous lymphomas and pseudolymphomas is the correlation of clinical and histopathologic findings. Several benign entities may mimic different types of skin lymphoma due to the density of the inflammatory infiltrate, presence of immunoblasts in the infiltrate ("atypia"), and/or epithelial exocytosis. Below are clinical and/or histopathologic clues for the diagnosis of cutaneous pseudolymphomas.

Lymphoma	Mimic	Clinical clues	Histopath clues
Mycosis fungoides (MF)	Lymphomatoid lichenoid keratosis	Small solitary lesion	Interface change, mixed infiltrate
	Pigmented purpuric dermatosis	Small lesions below waist	Edema, lack of significant cytologic atypia
	Inflammatory stage of vitiligo	Symmetric/periorificial distribution of eventually depigmented lesions with well-demarcated borders	Complete destruction of melanocytes
	CD8+ cutaneous infiltrates in acquired immunodeficiency syndrome (AIDS)	Clinical history of advanced AIDS, regression with anti-retroviral treatment	CD8+ infiltrate, negative PCR
	Lymphomatoid drug reaction	Medication history, resolution after discontinuation of culprit medication	Mixed infiltrate, lack of significant cytologic atypia
	Lymphomatoid tattoo reaction	Clinical appearance of lesions restricted to tattoo (often in areas with red pigment)	Presence of tattoo pigment in dermis
	Pityriasis lichenoides	Small lesions	Lack of significant cytologic atypia
Sézary syndrome (SS)	Benign erythrodermas (spongiotic/eczematous dermatitis, psoriasis, drug eruption, etc.)	Significant clinical overlap	Histopathology of benign and malignant erythrodermas often nonspecific, but negative blood flow and lack of matching T-cell clones in blood and skin

© Springer Nature Switzerland AG 2019
A. Subtil, *Diagnosis of Cutaneous Lymphoid Infiltrates*,
https://doi.org/10.1007/978-3-030-11654-5

Lymphoma	Mimic	Clinical clues	Histopath clues
CD30+ lymphoproliferative disorders	Viral infection (herpes folliculitis, inflamed molluscum)	Clinical presentation and distribution of lesions	Necrotic sebaceous glands (herpes folliculitis), identification of viral cytopathic effect, large cells are relatively infrequent and are immunoblasts
	Arthropod bite reaction, including scabies	Clinical history	Lack of marked cytologic atypia, large cells are relatively infrequent and are immunoblasts, prominent eosinophils
	Lymphomatoid drug reaction	Medication history, resolution after discontinuation of culprit medication	Mixed infiltrate, lack of marked cytologic atypia
Subcutaneous panniculitis-like T-cell lymphoma (SPTCL)	Lupus panniculitis	Significant clinical overlap, some patients may have both lupus panniculitis and lymphoma	Prominent component of CD20+ B cells, CD21+ lymphoid follicles, frequent plasma cells and CD123+ plasmacytoid dendritic cells, hyaline fat necrosis, lack of prominent lymphocytic atypia, limited to absent adipocyte rimming, low proliferation rate
Cutaneous B-cell lymphomas	Pseudolymphoma after vaccination	Clinical history, localized lesion developing after vaccine administration	Mixed infiltrate, lymphoid follicles with reactive germinal centers
	Lymphomatoid drug reaction	Medication history, resolution after discontinuation of culprit medication	Mixed infiltrate with polytypic plasma cells
	Cutaneous plasmacytosis and plasma cell-rich reactive infiltrates	Variable but clinical overlap may occur	Polytypic plasma cells
	Rosai-Dorfman disease	Significant clinical overlap	Emperipolesis, polytypic plasma cells, lymphoid follicles with reactive germinal centers, S100+ histiocytes

Index

© Springer Nature Switzerland AG 2019
A. Subtil, *Diagnosis of Cutaneous Lymphoid Infiltrates*,
https://doi.org/10.1007/978-3-030-11654-5

The manufacturer's authorised representative in the EU is Springer
Nature Customer Service Centre GmbH, Europaplatz 3, 69115 Heidelberg,
Germany. If you have any concerns regarding our products, please
contact ProductSafety@springernature.com

Printed and bound by CPI Group (UK) Ltd, Croydon, CR0 4YY
05/06/2026
02128933-0002